AF412380

Atlas of **Vitrified Blastocysts** in **Human Assisted Reproduction**

Atlas of Vitrified Blastocysts in Human Assisted Reproduction

THOMAS EBNER
Department of Gynecological Endocrinology and Kinderwunsch Zentrum,
Landes–Frauen–und Kinderklinik Linz, and Faculty of Medicine, Johannes Kepler
University of Linz, Linz, Austria

PIERRE VANDERZWALMEN
The IVF Centres of Professor Zech in Bregenz, Austria; the IVF unit at the Centre
Hospitalier Inter-régional Edith Cavell (CHIREC) in Braine l'alleud-Brussels,
Belgium

BARBARA WIRLEITNER
The IVF Centres of Professor Zech in Bregenz, Austria

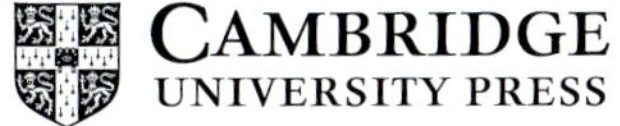

CAMBRIDGE
UNIVERSITY PRESS

CAMBRIDGE
UNIVERSITY PRESS

University Printing House, Cambridge CB2 8BS, United Kingdom

Cambridge University Press is part of the University of Cambridge.

It furthers the University's mission by disseminating knowledge in the pursuit of
education, learning and research at the highest international levels of excellence.

www.cambridge.org
Information on this title: www.cambridge.org/9781107074095

© Thomas Ebner, Pierre Vanderzwalmen and Barbara Wirleitner 2015

First published 2015

Printed in the United Kingdom by Bell and Bain Ltd

A catalog record for this publication is available from the British Library

Library of Congress Cataloging in Publication data
Ebner, Thomas, author.
Atlas of vitrified blastocysts in human assisted reproduction / Thomas Ebner,
Pierre Vanderzwalmen,
Barbara Wirleitner.
    p. ; cm.
Includes bibliographical references and index.
ISBN 978-1-107-07409-5 (hardback)
I. Vanderzwalmen, Pierre, author.   II. Wirleitner, Barbara, author.   III. Title.
[DNLM: 1. Blastocyst – Atlases.   2. Blastocyst – Case Reports.   3. Vitrification –
Atlases.   4. Vitrification – Case Reports.   5. Reproductive Techniques, Assisted –
Atlases.   6. Reproductive Techniques, Assisted – Case Reports. QS 17]
QP252
612.6–dc23

                                                                2014042963

ISBN 978-1-107-07409-5 Hardback

CONTENTS

Part B   Closed Vitrification Method   155

PREFACE

In Assisted Reproduction Technologies we live in times when pictures have already started moving. Time-lapse imaging has taken over control of non-invasive embryo selection. However, the quality and the success of the previous *Atlas on Oocytes, Zygotes and Embryos in Reproductive Medicine* (edited by M. Van den Bergh, T. Ebner and K. Elder) emphasize the value of static images in the field of IVF.

It is especially in cryopreservation that it is almost impossible to create proper video sequences since during the cooling and warming steps several cryopreservation media have to be used, thus requiring numerous transfers of the embryos from one drop to another. In addition to this technical limitation, the different concentrations of cryoprotectants used change media viscosity which will lead to floating of the embryos not allowing for proper focusing. As a matter of fact, in these cases serial images may provide for a better view of morphological changes during cryopreservation and subsequent embryo viability.

Since slow freezing has virtually been replaced by vitrification this Atlas is exclusively focused on the latter technique representing the state of the art in cryopreservation. Embryologists performing vitrification may be divided into two groups: those who allow direct contact between the embryos and liquid nitrogen, thus optimizing cooling and warming rates, and advocates of the closed system, who hermetically seal the embryos before vitrifying them, which avoids theoretical contamination due to impure nitrogen.

The book in hand is the first to cope with both vitrification strategies – the open and the closed one. This dichotomy is also reflected by the contents of the Atlas. The open system is covered by the Kinderwunsch Zentrum Linz, Austria, and the cases of the closed system stem from the team of the IVF Centers Prof. Zech in Bregenz, Austria. Regardless of the mode of vitrification chosen it was decided to include at least three images per case, one before vitrification, one immediately after warming, and one prior to transfer. This not only illustrates morphological changes of the embryos but also documents their survival.

Treatment outcome up to birth in combination with the clinical data provided makes this Atlas unique. It should provide valuable insight into daily practical procedures such as controlled ovarian hyperstimulation, embryo culture and selection, and vitrification as performed by two experienced and successful IVF teams.

We are confident that this collection will provide a helpful learning and reference tool, not only for students and trainees but also for experienced clinical embryologists and clinicians.

ABBREVIATIONS

AMH	anti-Müllerian hormone	IVF	in vitro fertilization
AW	after warming	LH	luteinizing hormone
BMI	body mass index	MH	menstrual history
BT	blastocyst transfer	NAD	no abnormality detected
BV	before vitrification	OHSS	ovarian hyperstimulation syndrome
COC	cumulus–oocyte complex	PCO	polycystic ovaries/polycystic ovarian syndrome
ET	embryo transfer		
FSH	follicle stimulating hormone	PVS	perivitelline space
HMG	human menopausal gonadotropin	TE	trophectoderm
ICM	inner cell mass	TESE	testicular sperm extraction
ICSI	intracytoplasmic sperm injection	ZP	zona pellucida
IUI	intrauterine insemination		

Introduction

Vitrification of blastocysts: the evolving "state of the art" freezing technique

The proportion of births following transfer of cryopreserved blastocysts has increased dramatically during the last 10 years due to a remarkable improvement in the efficiency of vitrification techniques as alternatives to the classical slow freezing procedure (Vanderzwalmen *et al.*, 2002, 2003, 2010; Mukaida *et al.*, 2003a; Stehlik *et al.*, 2005; Liebermann and Tucker, 2006; Stachecki *et al.*, 2008; Van Landuyt *et al.*, 2011; Panagiotidis *et al.*, 2013). With the policy of single blastocyst transfer an increasing proportion of supernumerary blastocysts is vitrified either on day 5 or 6 (Liebermann and Tucker, 2006). Also, there is an increasing tendency to shift from fresh blastocyst transfer to vitrified blastocyst transfer to circumvent an inadequate uterine environment due to risk of ovarian hyperstimulation syndrome, inappropriate endometrium build up, endometrial polyps or uterine myomas. Moreover, vitrification of blastocysts is a valuable option when they originate from in vitro maturation cycles (Vanderzwalmen *et al.*, 2010; Ortega-Hrepich *et al.*, 2013).

Furthermore, several studies have reported that the safety of vitrified blastocysts in terms of obstetric outcome did not differ either from those of fresh blastocysts or blastocysts cryopreserved by slow-freeze methods (Takahashi *et al.*, 2005; Liebermann, 2009; Wikland *et al.*, 2010).

Principle and description of the different phases of a vitrification procedure

It is entirely the skill of being able to prevent ice crystals forming inside the cell (which can happen during the cooling as well as during the warming process) that will determine the viability of the embryos (Quinn, 2010). When the temperature decreases, liquid water can be converted either to a solid crystal or to a solid amorphous glass when the supercooled water is dropped instantaneously below the glass transition temperature. The physical process by which a viscous solution supercools to very low temperatures and finally solidifies into a meta-stable glass, without undergoing crystallization at a practical cooling rate, is called vitrification (Rall and Fahy, 1985). According to this definition, with the application of vitrification, formation of ice crystals is not theoretically possible in the intra-cellular or extra-cellular spaces.

The fundamental issue in all vitrification methods is to achieve and maintain conditions within the cells which guarantee an amorphous state throughout the cooling as well as during the warming process. Independent of the carrier device that determines the cooling and/or the warming rate, the key of success in order to achieve a "glass-like" state depends on an optimal balance between the speed of cooling/rewarming (time and temperature) and the optimal cell dehydration and penetration of cryoprotectant (CP) when cells are exposed to concentrated hypertonic solutions (Leibo and Pool, 2011).

Vitrification and warming of blastocysts consists of several steps irrespective of whether an open or a closed system is used:

(i)   selection of blastocysts before vitrification;
(ii) exposure of blastocysts to the CP solutions;
(iii) loading on the carrier device and plunging into liquid nitrogen (LN_2);
(iv) storage in LN_2 containers;
(v)   the warming process;
(vi) dilution of the CP;
(vii) selection of warmed blastocysts before embryo transfer (ET).

Step one: selection of blastocysts before vitrification

It should be obligatory to cryopreserve supernumerary blastocysts of moderate to good quality in order to increase cumulative pregnancy rates. With regard to this, it is very important to achieve a reproducible outcome, especially in terms of survival after warming independently of the quality, to allow high success rates after vitrified/warmed blastocyst transfer.

Grading of blastocyst morphology incorporates assessment of degree of expansion of the blastocyst and the quality of the inner cell mass and the trophectoderm (Alpha Scientists in Reproductive Medicine and ESHRE Special Interest Group of Embryology, 2011; Ebner *et al.*, 2011). Several studies have shown that trophectoderm was statistically significantly related to the rate of ongoing pregnancy and miscarriage. By contrast, neither inner cell mass nor blastocyst expansion was statistically significantly related (Ahlström *et al.*, 2011; Honnma *et al.*, 2012). In a more recent article, Ahlström *et al.* (2013) analysed which pre-freeze morphological parameters can be used to predict live birth outcomes after vitrified/warmed blastocyst transfer cycles. They stated that blastocoel expansion and trophectoderm grade were identified as the most significant pre-freeze morphological predictors of live birth.

Acceptable results were also obtained after vitrification of blastocysts that originated from embryos that were not selected either for fresh ET or cryopreservation on day 3 because of their poor quality. Fifty blastocyst warming cycles resulted in a 76% survival rate, 44% clinical pregnancy rate, and 39% implantation rate (Shaw-Jackson *et al.*, 2013).

With respect to blastocyst quality and survival, the question arises whether artificial shrinkage or collapsing is mandatory.

Since the size of the blastocoel corresponds to the amount of water in this cavity, larger blastocysts might show reduced cryopreservation potential due to ice crystal formation during the cooling step and devitrification during the warming step.

In order to reduce the likelihood of ice crystal formation artificial shrinkage or collapsing of expanded blastocysts has been suggested, using either micropipettes (Vanderzwalmen *et al.*, 2002) or laser pulses (Mukaida *et al.*, 2006).

However, with the use of a vitrification solution containing a higher sucrose concentration of 0.75 M instead of 0.5 M, we observe that artificial shrinkage of the blastocoelic cavity is not necessary for preventing injury from intracellular ice because there is sufficient dehydration during the exposure to the vitrification solution.

In addition, Zech *et al.* (2005) showed the benefit of opening the zona pellucida some hours before the vitrification process. They observed that blastocysts with a larger blastocoelic cavity survived vitrification better when they partially or completely hatched even with short exposure to cryoprotectant solutions.

Step two: exposure of blastocysts to the CP solutions

Before the blastocysts are immersed in LN_2, they are exposed to a CP solution in order to increase the intra- and extracellular viscosity to a level that the liquid water molecules will solidify so quickly that they will not have time to rearrange themselves into a crystalline structure. To achieve this objective, in nearly all vitrification methods the blastocysts are exposed to a minimum of two steps of gradually increasing concentrations of non-vitrifying solution (nVS) and vitrifying solution (VS) (Vanderzwalmen *et al.*, 2013a).

In a single or sequential steps the blastocysts are first exposed to nVS. During this step, a certain amount of CP enters the cells. It may take 3–15 minutes according to the type of CP and the cooling rate which in turn depends on the carrier device. The length of time of exposure to the nVS at a defined temperature (T°) is of utmost importance and determines the amount of intracellular CP. The duration of exposure to the permeable CPs is determined by several biophysical factors such as the membrane properties (cellular permeability to water and CP), the type and concentration of CP, the surface/volume ratio of the cells, and the rate of cooling and warming (Leibo, 1980; Kasai and Edashige, 2010; Vanderzwalmen *et al.*, 2013a). The nVS is exclusively composed of permeable CP (e.g., DMSO, ethylene glycol, 1,2-propanediol, glycerol).

In the final step, the biological material is exposed for a shorter time to the VS (30–90 seconds). An intracellular vitrifying state is obtained due to the dehydration of the inner cell mass and trophectoderm cells in contact with the VS that concentrates the intracellular solutions of salts, proteins, and CP that have penetrated the cell in the course of exposure to nVS. This strategy will generate an intracellular environment that is compatible with a vitreous state when cells are directly plunged into LN_2. The extracellular vitrifying state is obtained by the high concentration of CP in the VS that encapsulates the embryo in a vitrifying sheath. Additionally, non-permeable CPs with low (sucrose, trehalose) or high molecular weight (Ficoll) are present in the VS.

Although the solutions used to vitrify blastocysts contain high concentrations of permeable cryoprotectants as compared with the conventional slow freezing procedure, it has been observed that, contrary to common belief, the intracellular concentration of cryoprotectant is almost one-third of the concentration of the VS and even lower than after a slow freezing procedure (Vanderzwalmen *et al.*, 2013b). We may therefore state that although slow freezing has been the standard cryopreservation method for more than 25 years, few were aware that cell survival is the consequence of the presence of an intracellular vitrified state. This vitrified state is a result of a long-term effect of solution during cooling and is a reflection of a very high concentration of CP. We may therefore suggest that a drop in survival after slow freezing is probably more related to osmotic shock after warming than to mechanical injuries due to the formation of intracellular ice crystals. Moreover, in order to avoid the use of highly concentrated CP solution, it is not justified to continue with slow freezing procedures.

To conclude we may advise that slow freezing is ultimately another way to do vitrification.

Step three: loading on a carrier device and plunging in LN_2

Open system

It was postulated that ultra-rapid cooling and warming rates (as high as 20,000–30,000°C/minute) are mandatory during the vitrification process to reduce the risk of intracellular crystal formation and the concomitant damage to the cell structures (Lane *et al.*, 1999). To achieve ultra-rapid cooling rates, a very small volume of VS of less than 1 µl is deposited on an open carrier device (e.g., Cryotop, Vitriplug, Cryoloop, copper electron microscopical grids), which is directly plunged into LN_2 (Vanderzwalmen *et al.*, 2002; Mukaida *et al.*, 2003a, 2003b; Kuwayama, 2007).

The advantage of such an approach is that blastocysts are exposed in two steps to increasing concentrations of CP. However, this exposure is only for a short period of time – long enough to permit the extraction of the intracellular water while limiting the amount of CP permeating into cells, thus reducing osmotic stress.

One drawback of the "open" carrier devices is that the blastocysts are directly exposed to LN_2 during the cooling process as well as during the whole storage time. Although the theoretical risk of cross-contamination by bacteria, viruses, or fungi during cooling or storage in LN_2 has been widely debated (AbdelHafez *et al.*, 2011), the potential for contamination with reactive chemical compounds raises safety concerns (Bielanski, 2009).

Various methods for sterilizing LN_2 have been proposed or are under development, including ceramic filters (Cobo *et al.*, 2011) or ultraviolet light with subsequent hermetic cryostorage (Parmegiani *et al.*, 2010, 2011), or using LN_2 vapor for storage (Grout and Morris, 2009). Although the probability of an impairment of cellular structures by contact with LN_2 is still being discussed, this risk is important and the ongoing discussion indicates that the storage system, especially in the long term, should be revised. Even the standard storage conditions and refilling of the tanks pose a hazard when oxygen from surrounding air condenses and mixes with LN_2 during the regular opening of the nitrogen tank for routine refilling or whenever straws are added or withdrawn. Although it is generally assumed that thermally driven reactions do not occur in cells at −196° C, it has been reported that in the case of radiation of an LN_2/oxygen mixture a synthesis of oxygen radicals resulting from ozone formation and decomposition cannot be excluded and is even enhanced by the catalytic effect of nitrogen. Mouse oocytes show impaired survival, fertilization rates, and embryonic development after prolonged contact with LN_2 (Yan *et al.*, 2011).

Closed system

The European Directives (2004/23/EC) as well as the FDA directives on tissue and cell storage dictate the adherence to certain safety regulations, ensuring that gametes and embryos are protected from any possible contamination with pathogens and to prevent them from any harmful physical conditions during storage. To achieve the EU directive, a valuable option consists of switching from an open vitrification carrier device to a protocol that entails complete isolation of the biological samples from LN_2 during both the cooling process as well as storage by hermetically isolating the embryos from LN_2 in the tanks.

A huge difference exists in the cooling rate is the subject of an ongoing debate as the cooling rate is widely believed to be an important factor for success of the vitrification protocols. Several studies have shown that vitrification of oocytes (Papatheodorou *et al.*, 2013), zygotes (Vanderzwalmen *et al.*, 2012), and blastocysts in closed carriers achieves good results in clinical studies (Kuwayama *et al.*, 2005; Liebermann and Tucker, 2006; Stachecki *et al.*, 2008; Vanderzwalmen *et al.*, 2010; Panagiotidis *et al.*, 2013).

In a recent study, Chatzimeletiou *et al.* (2012) investigated the effects of aseptic vitrification on the cytoskeleton and development of human blastocysts, by analyzing survival rates and spindle and chromosome configurations by fluorescence and confocal laser scanning microscopy. Although there was a significantly higher incidence of abnormal spindles in the vitrified group compared with the fresh group, the high survival rate following warming and the large proportion of normal spindle/chromosome configurations suggest that aseptic vitrification at the blastocyst stage on day 5 does not adversely affect the development of human embryos and the ability of spindles to form and continue normal cell divisions.

Step four: storage in LN₂ containers

Little is known about the risks of prolonged storage of cryopreserved cells as vitrification is the solidification of a fluid without formation of crystalline structures – a physically disorganized unstable system. This raises the question as to whether this state changes over time, thus impairing survival and implantation potential of vitrified gametes and embryos. Subsequently, any potential impact on the health of the newborn is unknown. Results after vitrification of blastocysts in a closed system show no alterations with respect to survival and live birth rates irrespective whether storage lasted for 1, 2, 3, 4, 5, or 6 years. A mean pregnancy rate (PR) of 43.6%; an ongoing PR of 35.8%, and a live birth rate of 29.0% were observed. More interestingly, no malformations were reported (Wirleitner *et al.*, 2013). From these observations covering a storage period of 6 years it may be concluded that vitrification of blastocysts is a safe technique.

Step five: the warming process

Since the rate of cooling engendered a hot debate, it is surprising that little emphasis is put on the warming procedure. However, it has become obvious that the warming rate might play a more essential role in modulating survival after vitrification than the cooling rate.

A fast warming rate prevents the vitreous water from re-crystallizing during the warming phase (Seki and Mazur, 2008, 2009). In fact, during the process of warming, cells first devitrify when they are warmed above the glass transition temperature. If the warming rate is not fast enough the supercooled liquid is transformed with high speed into small ice crystals. If the appropriate timing is not used or if warming rates are too slow, small ice crystals are subjected to the phenomenon referred to as re-crystallization, which may have lethal consequences.

It is well known that for any given concentration of CP the critical warming rate is much higher than the critical cooling rate (Fahy *et al.*, 1987). Consequently, the minimum concentration of CP to prevent crystallization during warming must be higher than during cooling. This means that it might be easier to maintain a vitrified state during the cooling than during the warming process for the same concentration of CP. If the warming rate is reduced by using devices isolating the drop containing the embryos, higher intracellular concentrations of CP are needed in order to reduce the likelihood of re-crystallization. However, these higher concentrations of CP might be toxic to the cells. Hence, in order not to increase the concentration of CP above the toxic level the biological material has to be warmed extremely rapidly.

Step six: dilution of the CP

During warming water re-enters the cells and the CP is washed out. This has to be performed in a controlled way in order to avoid cellular damage. A too rapid influx of water is circumvented by a stepwise exposure to solutions containing reducing sucrose concentrations.

Step seven: selection of warmed blastocysts before ET

ALPHA Scientists in Reproductive Medicine and ESHRE Special Interest Group Embryology (2011) published key performance indicators for all steps of cryopreservation procedures including minimum performance and aspirational benchmark values. Morphological parameters, however, were not in the scope of this workshop.

Though some post-thaw morphological predictors have been investigated in slow freezing of blastocysts, e.g., immediate re-expansion (Van den Abbeel *et al.*, 2005; Shu *et al.*, 2008) or 24-hour survival, no such data have yet been published for vitrified blastocysts. It has been suggested that as the result of the presence and size of the blastocoelic cavity, vitrified/warmed blastocysts experience several morphologic changes and become collapsed during cryopreservation. Thus, it is more difficult to score a vitrified blastocyst after warming than a fresh one (Shu *et al.*, 2008).

Several factors (unrelated to vitrification method) are known to directly influence the fate of a cryopreserved blastocyst after thawing/warming and transfer. It is important to realize that survival rates in the literature are hardly comparable due to the fact that some embryologists focus on immediate survival while others suggest an additional waiting period of 24 hours to facilitate control of growth (Vanderzwalmen *et al.*, 2003). Differences in implantation rates may also be attributed to the fact that not all working groups apply assisted hatching to the thawed blastocysts (whilst shrunk), though this was found to improve outcome (Vanderzwalmen *et al.*, 2003).

In detail, re-expansion of the blastocoel (and consequently the blastocyst) after thawing is expected within 24 hours after thawing (Vanderzwalmen *et al.*, 2003; Van den Abbeel *et al.*, 2005). However, immediate re-expansion, e.g., within the first 2 hours after warming, has not been used for prognostic purposes in vitrified blastocysts. Since in slow freezing approximately half of the frozen blastocysts turned out to re-expand immediately after 2–4 hours in culture (Shu *et al.*, 2008), it is indicated that using vitrification a higher rate of re-expansion might be observed (Ebner *et al.*, 2009).

Even if it can be assumed that all viable blastocysts will re-expand after several more hours, any delay in this process could be the manifestation of altered osmotic and/or metabolic conditions (comparable to the situation found during blastocoel development when water enters the blastocoelic cavity via tight junctions, either diffusing passively or being pumped actively).

A recent publication (Ebner *et al.*, 2009) introduced a grading system based on re-expansion, hatching (out of the artificial gap in the ZP), cytoplasmic granulation, and presence of necrotic foci.

Vitrification in an open system (Linz, cases 1–70)
Vitrification
Routine in vitro culture for cases 1–70 was either performed in sequential media (EmbryoAssist and BlastAssist, Origio, Denmark) or global media (GM501 Cult, Gynemed, Lensahn, Germany). Irrespective of the type of medium, culture was performed in 30 µl drops under sterile mineral oil (GM501 Mineral Oil, Gynemed). Both approaches had the medium changed on day 3. All embryos that were not transferred in a fresh cycle were cultured up to day 5, the day vitrification was performed routinely. It should be noted that some patients needed special media to get blastocysts at all. In detail, those patients (cases 43, 65, 67) who suffered from azoospermia had their testicular tissue treated with collagenase (GM501 Collagenase) in order to facilitate collection of testicular spermatozoa. In these cases TESE sperm were further treated with theophylline (GM501 SpermMobil) to improve/restore motility. Others (cases 12, 27, 47, 53) had their oocytes cultured in an ionophore (GM508 Cult-Active) bath immediately after ICSI in order to overcome low fertilization (Ebner and Montag, 2014) or severe male factor infertility (Ebner *et al.*, 2012).

Prior to vitrification all blastocysts were scored according to the guidelines of Gardner and Schoolcraft (1999) focusing on expansion, inner cell mass, and trophectoderm. Only morulae and early blastocysts without fragments or blastocysts with both adequate ICM and trophectoderm were considered for cryostorage (Figure 1). According to in-house definitions, an adequate quality was reached if early blastocysts had only minor fragmentation and full to expanded blastocysts showed either a perfect ICM and/or TE (with none of these cell types allowed to be of worst quality according to the Gardner score).

In all cases, vitrification was done utilizing a commercially available kit (GM501 VitriStore Freeze, Gynemed) at room temperature (RT). All morulae/blastocysts were pre-incubated in a medium containing PBS and HSA for 1 minute (Figure 2). This step was followed by two media, a nVS and a classical VS with different composition. The time blastocysts were kept in the nVS (PBS, HSA, ethylene glycol, and DMSO) depended on the individual degree of expansion. In detail, morulae and early blastocysts were incubated for 1 minute, full blastocysts for 2 minutes and expanded or hatching blastocysts for 3 minutes (Figure 3). Partial shrinkage of the blastocysts was controlled under a microscope. Since in the VS (PBS, HSA, ethylene glycol, DMSO, and sucrose) CPs were at a higher concentration, as far as possible the exposure time was kept to a minimum (30 seconds) (Figure 4).

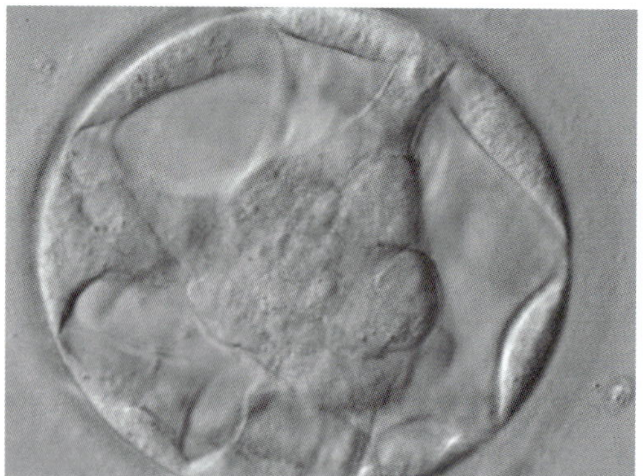

1

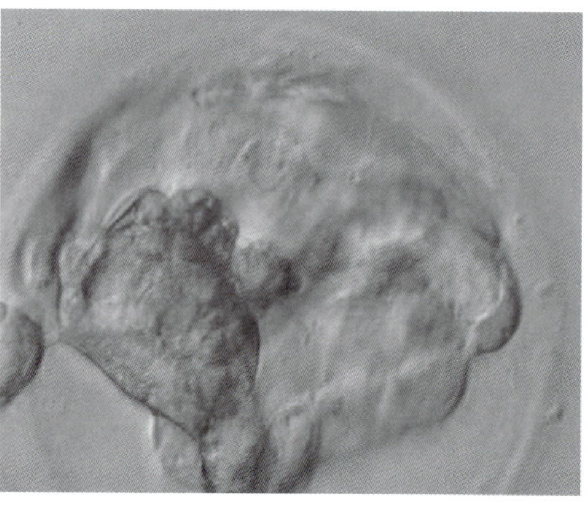

2

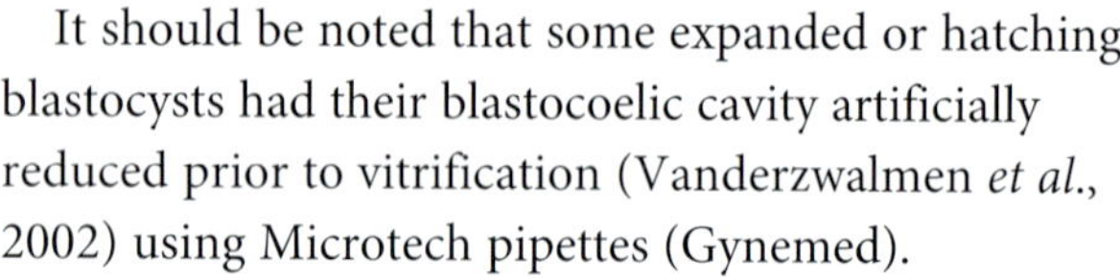

3

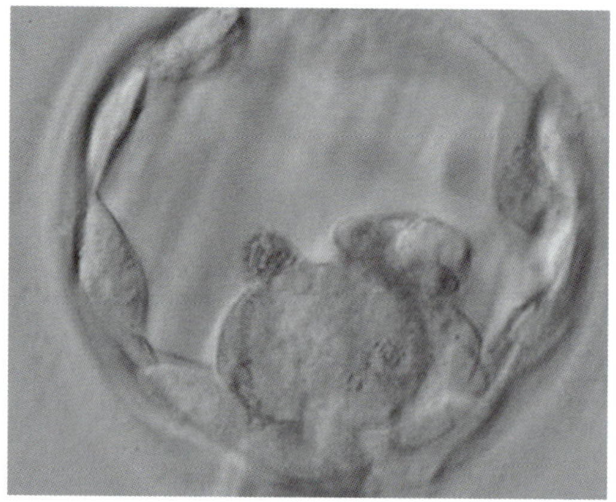

4

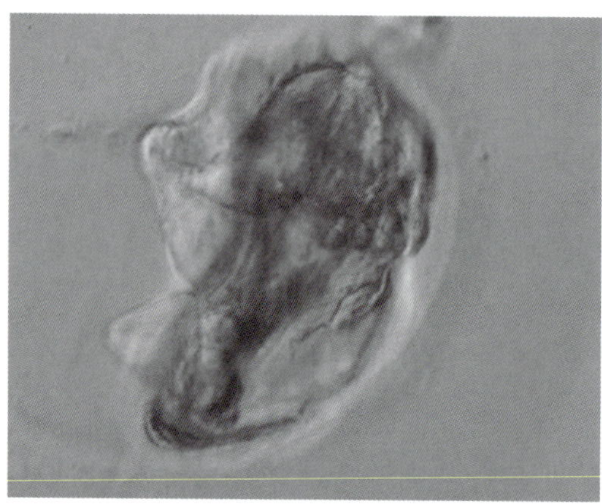

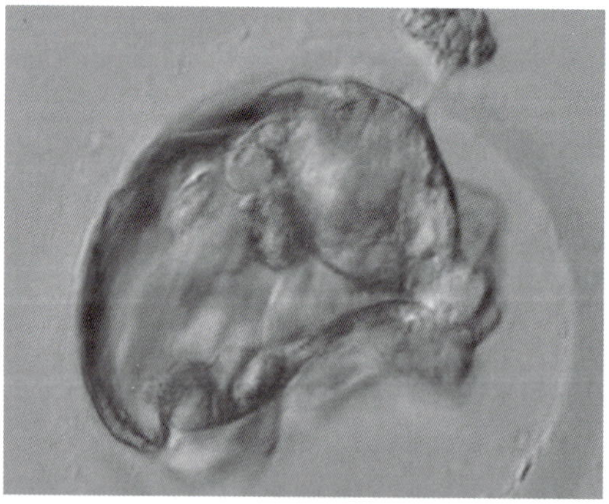

5

It should be noted that some expanded or hatching blastocysts had their blastocoelic cavity artificially reduced prior to vitrification (Vanderzwalmen *et al.*, 2002) using Microtech pipettes (Gynemed).

Within this last crucial period a maximum of two shrunk morulae/blastocysts were placed on the tip of a Hemi-straw (VitroPlug, Astro Med Tec, Salzburg, Austria) in a very small volume of vitrification medium 2 (<0.5 µl) followed by direct plunging into LN_2. Before storage in a special container (Arpege 170, Air Liquid, Vienna, Austria) all semi-straws were sealed with high security straws (Cryo Bio System, L´Aigle, France).

Warming
Special care was taken to ensure very fast warming rates which required rapid separation of the semi- and the protective high security straw followed by immediate plunging into the first warming solution at 37°C (Figure 5).

The other three media of the GM501 VitriStore Thaw kit (Gynemed) were kept at RT (Figures 6–8). All four warming media were based on PBS and HSA but had descending concentrations of sucrose (0.5 M,

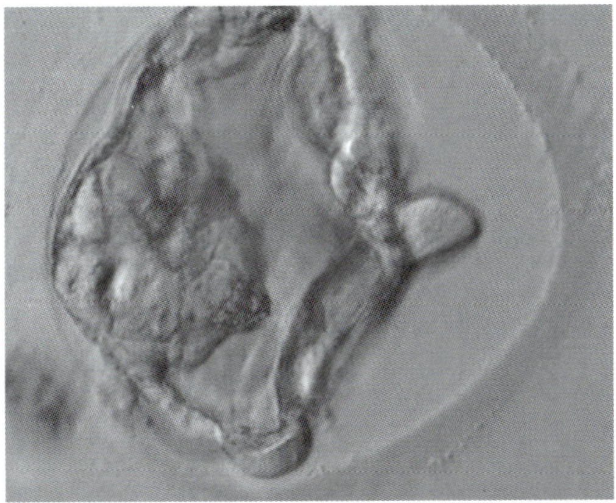

6

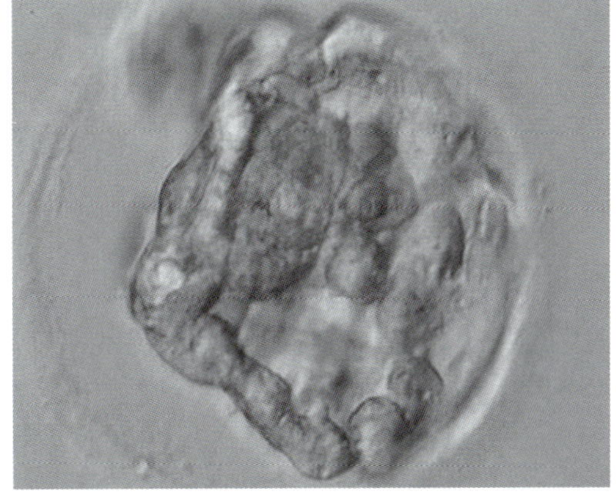

7

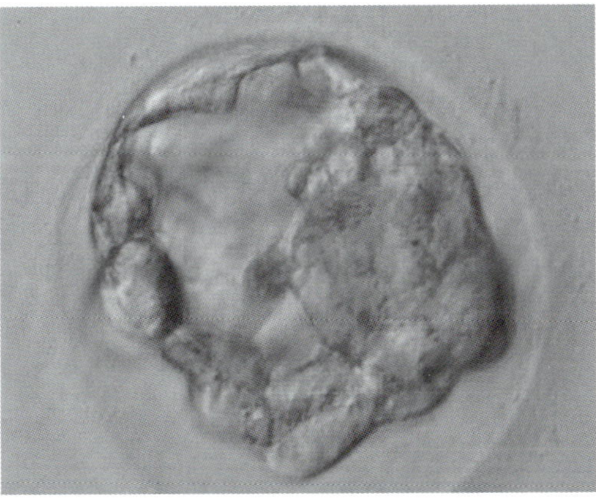

8

0.25 M, 0.125 M, 0 M). After this warming process direct transfer into a pre-warmed culture medium, either GM501 (Gynemed) or BlastAssist (Origio, Måløv, Denmark), was performed.

All warmed blastocysts (except those that had started to leave the zona before vitrification) were hatched by means of a laser in order to minimize any theoretical impact of cryopreservation on ZP constitution (Vanderzwalmen *et al.*, 2003; Liebermann and Tucker, 2006).

All blastocysts considered to be viable after warming were scored according to a previously published grading system based on re-expansion, hatching out of the artificial gap in the ZP, cytoplasmic granulation, and presence of necrotic foci (Ebner *et al.*, 2009). Routinely warmed blastocysts were kept in culture for at least 2 hours prior to scoring and transfer.

Vitrification in a closed system (Bregenz, cases 71–100)

Exposure to the cryoprotectant

All the procedures occurred at RT utilizing a commercially available kit (VitriFreeze ES: Fertipro, Bernem, Belgium). The blastocysts were exposed to two nVS. The nVS1 was composed of 5% EG and 5% DMSO in PBS–HSA, whereas the nVS2 had double concentration. The VS was composed of 20% EG (v/v), 20% DMSO (v/v), 25 µmol/l (10 mg/mL) Ficoll (70,000 MW), and 0.75 mol/l sucrose.

Drops of 50 µl of nVS1 and nVS2 were deposited in a Petri dish and covered with oil. A maximum of two blastocysts were exposed for 5 and 4 minutes in nVS1 and nVS2 respectively. Except for expanded blastocysts the time in the nVS1 solution may be prolonged up to 7 min (Figure 9a).

The blastocysts were placed in the nVS2 drop and three elongated drops of VS (50 µl, 50 µl, 100 µl) were deposited in a Petri dish without oil overlay (Figure 9b). To avoid an osmotic shock, blastocysts were then transferred to the first VS drop with a small volume of nVS2 and left for 10 s before placing them in the second drop for 10 s more. Before transfer of the blastocysts in the second and third VS drops, the pipette was washed with pure VS solution. Finally the blastocysts were placed in the third drop and by gentle washing and rotating for almost 10 to 15 s encapsulation of the blastocyst in the VS was guaranteed. The VS induces a pronounced collapsing of the blastocysts, strong enough to permit an acceptable survival rate without previous artificial shrinkage of the blastocoel cavity.

Loading on the closed carrier device "VitriSafe" and plunging in LN$_2$

After incubating the biological material in the VS, a maximum of two blastocysts was deposited in the gutter of the Vitrisafe (Figure 10b, c) (IVF Distribution, Bregenz, Austria). When expanded blastocysts and blastocysts exhibited an inner cell mass and trophectoderm of quality A or B, vitrification of only one at a time was done.

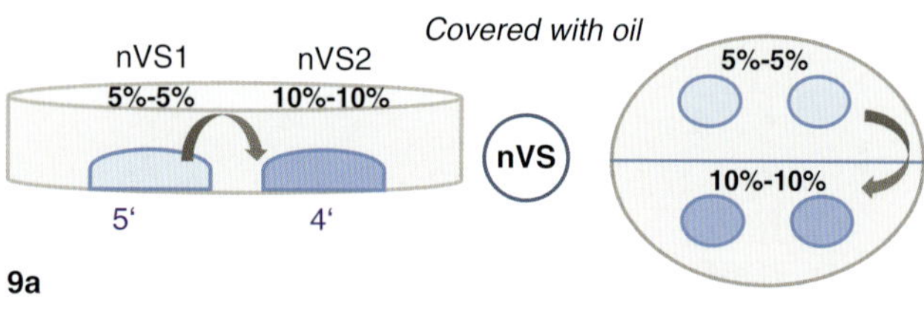

9a

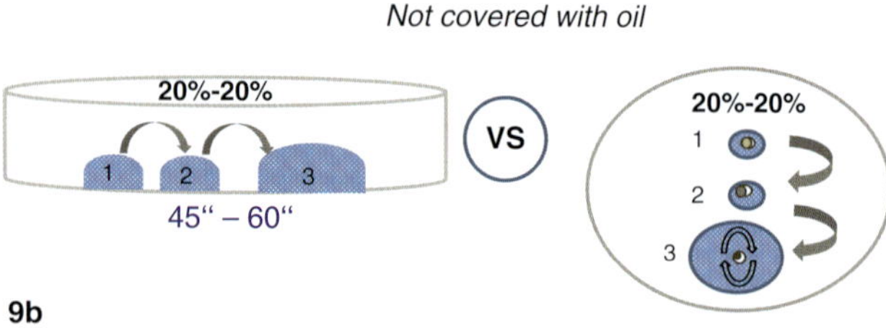

9b

9 General procedure for vitrification of blastocysts

The Vitrisafe consists of a large gutter (Figure 10a) that is inserted into a protective outer straw of 0.3 mL (CBS, Cryo Bio System, France) (Figure 10d). The edges of the protective 0.5 mL straw are welded (Figure 10e) ensuring a complete isolation of the biological sample from LN$_2$. The hermetically closed straw is then directly plunged into LN$_2$ (Figure 10f). A cooling rate of 1300°C/min is achieved. The total time necessary to place and mix the blastocysts into the VS, load them on the carrier device and finally plunge them into LN$_2$ after welding the protective straw is 50 to 70 s. Afterwards the cooled straws were placed in a long-term LN2 tank (Figure 10g).

Warming steps and dilution of the CP

The solutions for warming were made of 1, 0.5, 0.25, and 0.125 M sucrose with 20% HSA (VitriThaw ES: Fertipro, Bernem, Belgium). An extra 0.75 M sucrose solution was made by mixing 1 M and 0.5 M sucrose V/V.

The Vitrisafe is designed to guarantee high warming rates of >25,000°C/min. The Dewar vessel with LN$_2$ containing the straw was placed close to the stereomicroscope. Avoiding contact with LN$_2$, the outer straw was cut with scissors and an extractor (a small straw with a conical end that entraps the Vitrisafe plug (Figure 11a)) was inserted to fix the Vitrisafe plug (Figure 11b). The plug was pulled out of the protective

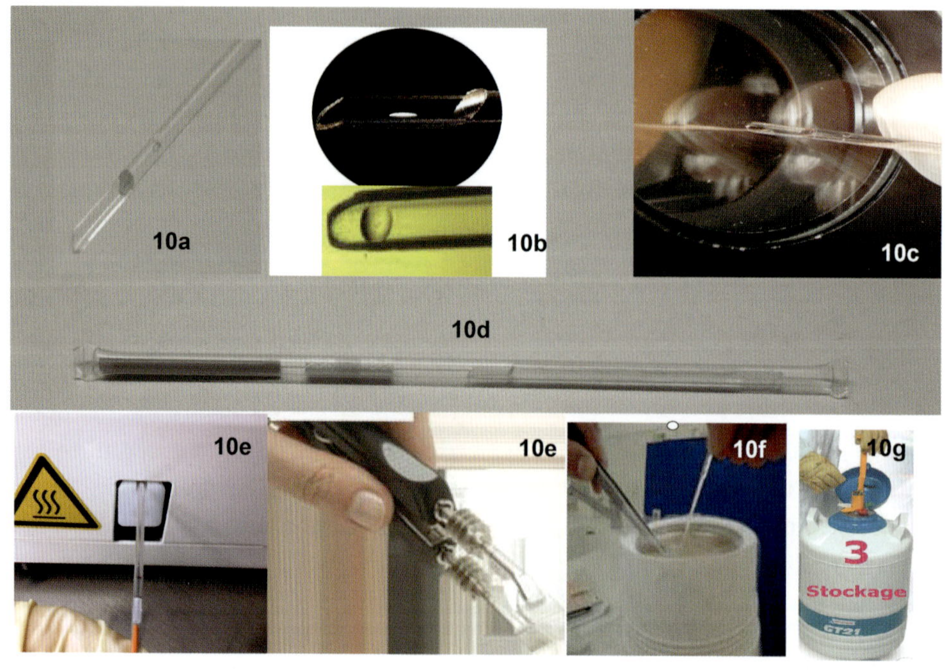

10 Loading on the closed carrier device VitriSafe and plunging in LN$_2$

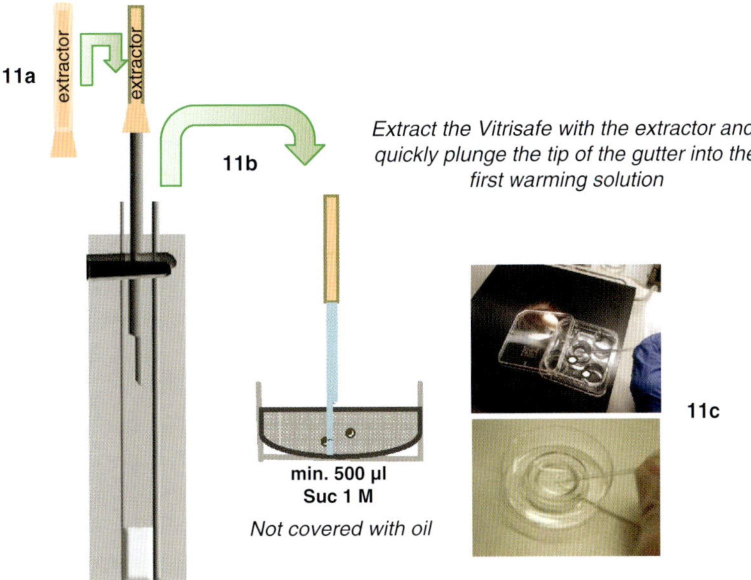

11 Loading on the closed carrier device VitriSafe and plunging in LN_2

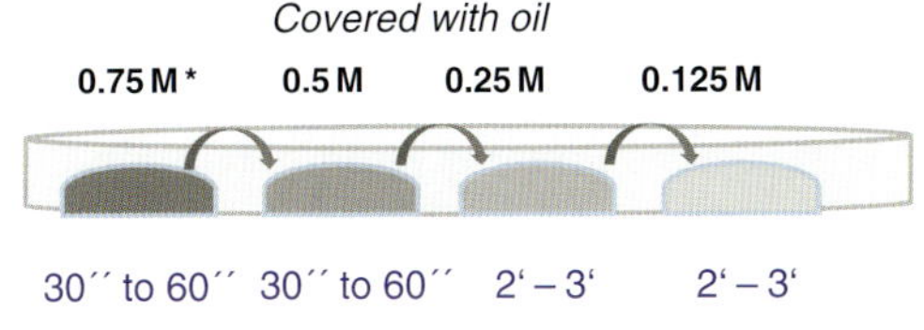

* Suc 1 M + Suc 0.5 M : 1/1 (V/V)

12 General procedure of warming of blastocysts

larger straw and the tip of the gutter holding the blastocysts immediately immersed in a 4-well or a 1-well dish containing a minimum of 500 µl of 1 M sucrose (Figure 11 c). After 1 minute the blastocysts were transferred to a Petri dish containing drops of 50 µl of 0.75 M, then 0.5 M sucrose, for 30–60 s. Subsequently they were transferred for 2–3 min in 0.25 M, then 0.125 M sucrose (Figure 12). All procedures were performed at room temperature. The embryos were then washed several times in the culture medium. Transfer of a maximum of two blastocysts was scheduled after an additional culture period of 4–24 hours. All blastocysts considered to be viable after warming were scored according to a previously published grading system based on re-expansion, hatching out of the artificial gap in the ZP, cytoplasmic granulation, and presence of necrotic foci (Ebner *et al.*, 2009).

REFERENCES

AbdelHafez F, Xu J, Goldberg J, *et al.* Vitrification in open and closed carriers at different cell stages: assessment of embryo survival, development, DNA integrity and stability during vapor phase storage for transport. *BMC Biotechnology* 2011; 11: 29.

Ahlström A, Westin C, Reismer E *et al.* Trophectoderm morphology: an important parameter for predicting live birth after single blastocyst transfer. *Human Reproduction* 2011; 26: 3289–3296.

Ahlström A, Westin C, Wikland M *et al.* Prediction of live birth in frozen–thawed single blastocyst transfer cycles by pre-freeze and post-thaw morphology. *Human Reproduction* 2013; 28: 1199–1209.

ALPHA Scientists in Reproductive Medicine, ESHRE Special Interest Group Embryology. Istanbul consensus workshop on embryo assessment: proceedings of an expert meeting. *Reproductive BioMedicine Online* 2011; 22: 632–646.

Bielanski A. A review of the risk of contamination of semen and embryos during cryopreservation and measures to limit cross-contamination during banking to prevent disease transmission in ET practices. *Theriogenology* 2009; 77: 467–482.

Chatzimeletiou K, Morrison EE, Panagiotidis Y *et al.* Cytoskeletal analysis of human blastocysts by confocal laser scanning microscopy following vitrification. *Human Reproduction* 2012; 27: 106–113.

Cobo A, Castello D, Weiss B *et al.* Highest liquid nitrogen quality for vitrification process: micro bacteriological filtration of LN2. 16th World Congress on In Vitro Fertilization, 2011; Abstract P052: 289.

Ebner T, Vanderzwalmen P, Shebl O *et al.* Morphology of vitrified/warmed day-5 embryos predicts rates of implantation, pregnancy and live birth. *Reproductive Biomedicine Online* 2009; 19: 72–78.

Ebner T, Vanderzwalmen P, Shebl O *et al.* Morphological aspects of human blastocysts and the impact of vitrification. *Journal für Reproduktionsmedizin und Endokrinologie* 2011; 8: 13–20.

Ebner T, Köster M, Shebl O *et al.* Application of a ready-to-use calcium ionophore increases rates of fertilization and pregnancy in severe male factor infertility. *Fertility and Sterility* 2012; 98: 1432–1437.

Ebner T, Montag M, Oocyte Activation Study Group. Live birth after artificial oocyte activation using a ready-to-use ionophore: a prospective multicentre study. *Reproductive Biomedicine Online* 2014.

European Parliament Directive (EU Tissues and Cells Directive 2004/23/EC). http://eurlex.europa.eu/LexUriServ/site/fr/oj/2004/l_102/l_10220040407fr00480058.pdf.

Fahy GM, Levy DI, Ali SE. Some emerging principles underlying the physical properties, biological actions, and utility of vitrification solutions. *Cryobiology* 1987; 24: 196–213.

Gardner DK, Schoolcraft WB. In vitro culture of human blastocysts. In Jansen R, Mortimer D (eds) *Towards Reproductive Certainty: Infertility and Genetics Beyond 1999.* Parthenon Press, Carnforth, 1999, pp. 378–388.

Grout BW, Morris GJ. Contaminated liquid nitrogen vapour as a risk factor in pathogen transfer. *Theriogenology* 2009; 71: 1079–1082.

Honnma H, Baba T, Sasaki M *et al.* Trophectoderm morphology significantly affects the rates of ongoing pregnancy and miscarriage in frozen-thawed single-blastocyst transfer cycle in vitro fertilization. *Fertility and Sterility* 2012; 98: 361–367.

Kasai M, Edashige K. Movement of water and cryoprotectants in mouse oocytes and embryos at different stages: relevance to cryopreservation. In Ri-Cheng C, Quinn P (eds) *Fertility Cryopreservation.* Cambridge University Press, Cambridge, 2010, pp. 16–23.

Kuwayama M, Vajta G, Leda S *et al.* Comparison of open and closed methods for vitrification of human embryos and the elimination of potential contamination. *Reproductive BioMedicine Online* 2005; 11: 608–614.

Kuwayama M. Highly efficient vitrification for cryopreservation of human oocytes and embryos: the CryoTop method. *Theriogenology* 2007; 67: 73–80.

Lane M, Schoolcraft WB, Gardner DK. Vitrification of mouse and human blastocysts using a novel cryoloop container-less technique. *Fertility and Sterility* 1999, 72: 1073–1078.

Leibo S. Water permeability and its activation energy of fertilized and unfertilized mouse ova. *Journal of Membrane Biology* 1980; 53: 179–188.

Leibo SP, Pool TB. The principal variables of cryopreservation: solutions, temperatures, and rate changes. *Fertility and Sterility* 2011; 96: 269–276.

Liebermann J, Tucker MJ. Comparison of vitrification and conventional cryopreservation of day 5 and day 6 blastocysts during clinical application. *Fertility and Sterility* 2006; 86: 20–26.

Liebermann J. Vitrification of human blastocysts: an update. *Reproductive BioMedicine Online* 2009; 19 (Suppl 4): 4328.

Mukaida T, Nakamura S, Tomiyama T *et al.* Vitrification of human blastocysts using cryoloops: clinical outcome of 223 cycles. *Human Reproduction* 2003a; 18: 384–391.

Mukaida T, Takahashi K, Kasai M. Blastocyst cryopreservation: ultrarapid vitrification using cryoloop technique. *Reproductive BioMedicine Online* 2003b; 6: 221–225.

Mukaida T, Oka C, Goto T *et al.* Artificial shrinkage of blastocoeles using either a micro-needle or a laser pulse prior to the cooling steps of vitrification improves survival rate and pregnancy outcome of vitrified human blastocysts. *Human Reproduction* 2006; 21: 3246–3252.

Ortega-Hrepich C, Stoop D, Guzmán I *et al.* A"freeze-all" embryos strategy after in vitro maturation: a novel approach in women with polycystic ovary syndrome? *Fertility and Sterility* 2013; 100: 1003–1007.

Panagiotidis Y, Vanderzwalmen P, Prapas Y *et al.* Open versus closed vitrification of blastocysts from an oocyte-donation programme: a prospective randomized study. *Reproductive BioMedicine Online* 2013; 26: 470–476.

Parmegiani L, Accorsi A, Cognigni GE *et al.* Sterilization of liquid nitrogen with ultraviolet irradiation for safe vitrification of human oocytes or embryos. *Fertility and Sterility* 2010; 4: 1525–1528.

Parmegiani L, Cognigni G, Bernardi S *et al.* Efficiency of aseptic open vitrification and hermetical cryostorage of human oocytes. *Reproductive BioMedicine Online* 2011; 23: 505–512.

Papatheodorou A, Vanderzwalmen P, Panagiotidis Y *et al.* Open versus closed oocyte vitrification system: a prospective randomized sibling-oocyte study. *Reproductive BioMedicine Online* 2013; 26: 595–602.

Quinn P. Suppression of ice in aqueous solutions and its application to vitrification in assisted reproductive technology. In Ri-Cheng C, Quinn P (eds) *Fertility*

Cryopreservation. Cambridge University Press, Cambridge, 2010, pp. 10–15.

Rall W, Fahy G. Ice-free cryopreservation of mouse embryos at −196 degrees C by vitrification. *Nature* 1985; 313: 573–575.

Seki S, Mazur P. Effect of warming rate on the survival of vitrified mouse oocytes and on the recrystallization of intracellular ice. *Biology of Reproduction* 2008; 79: 727–737.

Seki S, Mazur P. The dominance of warming rate over cooling rate in the survival of mouse oocytes subjected to a vitrification procedure. *Cryobiology* 2009; 59: 75–82.

Shaw-Jackson C, Bertrand E, Becker B *et al.* Vitrification of blastocysts derived from fair to poor quality cleavage stage embryos can produce high pregnancy rates after warming. *Journal of Assisted Reproduction and Genetics* 2013; 30: 1035–1042.

Shu Y, Watt J, Gebhardt J *et al.* The value of fast blastocyst re-expansion in the selection of a viable thawed blastocyst for transfer. *Fertility and Sterility* 2008; 91: 401–406.

Stachecki J, Garrisi J, Sabino S *et al.* A new safe, simple and successful vitrification method for bovine and human blastocysts. *Reproductive BioMedicine Online* 2008; 17: 360–367.

Stehlik E, Stehlik J, Katayama KP *et al.* Vitrification demonstrates significant improvement versus slow freezing of human blastocysts. *Reproductive BioMedicine Online* 2005; 11: 53–57.

Takahashi K, Mukaida T, Goto T *et al.* Perinatal outcome of blastocyst transfer with vitrification using cryoloop: a 4-year follow-up study. *Fertility and Sterility* 2005; 84: 88–92.

Van den Abbeel E, Camus M, Verheyen G *et al.* Slow controlled-rate freezing of sequentially cultured human blastocysts: an evaluation of two freezing strategies. *Human Reproduction* 2005; 20: 2929–2945.

Vanderzwalmen P, Bertin G, Debauche CH *et al.* Births after vitrification at morula and blastocyst stages: effect of artificial reduction of the blastocoelic cavity before vitrification. *Human Reproduction* 2002; 17: 744–751.

Vanderzwalmen P, Bertin G, Debauche CH *et al.* Vitrification of human blastocysts with the Hemi-Straw carrier: application of assisted hatching after thawing. *Human Reproduction* 2003; 18: 1504–1511.

Vanderzwalmen P, Ectors F, Grobet L *et al.* Aseptic vitrification of blastocysts from infertile patients, egg donors and after IVM. *Reproductive BioMedicine Online* 2010; 19: 700–707.

Vanderzwalmen P, Zech NH, Ectors F *et al.* Blastocyst transfer after aseptic vitrification of zygotes: an approach to overcome an impaired uterine environment. *Reproductive BioMedicine Online* 2012; 25: 591–599.

Vanderzwalmen P, Ectors F, Grobet L *et al.* Adaptation of a universal procedure for cryopreservation of different developmental stages: is it conceivable? In Varghese AC, Sjöblom P, Jayaprakasan K (eds) *Practical Guide to Setting Up an IVF Lab, Embryo Culture Systems and Running the Unit.* Jaypee Brothers Medical Publishers, New Delhi, 2013a, pp. 118–131 and 2101–2110.

Vanderzwalmen P, Connan D, Grobet L *et al.* Lower intracellular concentration of cryoprotectants after vitrification than after slow freezing despite exposure to higher concentration of cryoprotectant solutions. *Human Reproduction* 2013b; 28: 2101–2110.

Van Landuyt L, Stoop D, Verheyen G *et al.* Outcome of closed blastocyst vitrification in relation to blastocyst quality: evaluation of 759 warming cycles in a single-embryo transfer policy. *Human Reproduction* 2011; 26: 527–534.

Wikland M, Hardarson T, Hillensjo T *et al.* Obstetric outcomes after transfer of vitrified blastocysts. *Human Reproduction* 2010; 25: 1699–1707.

Wirleitner B, Vanderzwalmen P, Bach M *et al.* The time aspect in storing vitrified blastocysts: its impact on survival rate, implantation potential and babies born. *Human Reproduction* 2013; 28: 2950–2957.

Yan J, Suzuki J, Yu XM *et al.* Effects of duration of cryo-storage of mouse oocytes on cryo-survival, fertilization and embryonic development following vitrification. *Journal of Assisted Reproduction and Genetics* 2011; 28: 643–649.

Zech N, Lejeune B, Zech H *et al.* Vitrification of hatching and hatched human blastocysts: effect of an opening in the zona pellucida before vitrification. *Reproductive BioMedicine Online* 2005; 11: 355–361.

Part A

Open Vitrification Method

Case 1

2 years 2° infertility Diagnosis: Hypogonadotropic hypogonadism

Female partner

Age 32, nurse

Tubal status: patent

MH: secondary amenorrhea

BMI: 16.9

Smoker, no alcohol consumption

Osteopenia

Dyspareunia

Basal FSH: 0.1 IU/L

Basal LH: 0.1 IU/L

Basal estradiol: 22.0 pg/mL

Basal AMH: 12.08 ng/mL

Midluteal progesterone: 0.3 ng/mL

Midluteal prolactin: 6.2 ng/mL

Male partner

Age 35, lawyer

History/examination: NAD

Non-smoker, no alcohol consumption

Previous treatments

2011 split IVF/ICSI	Not pregnant
2012 vitrified/warmed cycle	Missed abortion, no heart activity

Fresh cycle: 2012

Semen assessment: normozoospermia

Volume	9.0 mL
Abstinence	4 days
Concentration	68×10^6/mL
Progressive motility	60%
Non-progressive motility	10%
Immotile	30%
Normal forms	13%

Stimulation protocol	Antagonist protocol (recombinant FSH)
Days of stimulation	20
Total dose	2587.5 IU
Estradiol at ovulation induction	705 ng/mL
Number of follicles ≥ 12 mm	26
Total number of COCs	26
Metaphase II	26
Injected/inseminated	26
Fertilization rate	73%
Cleavage rate	90%
Blastocyst rate	53%
Culture medium	EmbryoAssist/BlastAssist

Fresh transfer

Quality of embryo(s)	No fresh transfer because of OHSS
Outcome	
Vitrification	4 compacting embryos (day 4), 3 blastocysts (day 5)

Vitrified/warmed cycle: 2012

Stimulation	HSP
Endometrium	8.5 mm
Quality before vitrification	Morula
Warming day	4
Survival	Yes
Assisted hatching	Yes
Transfer day	5
Quality	5aa
Duration of cryostorage	2 months
Time between warming and transfer	19h

Outcome: Not pregnant

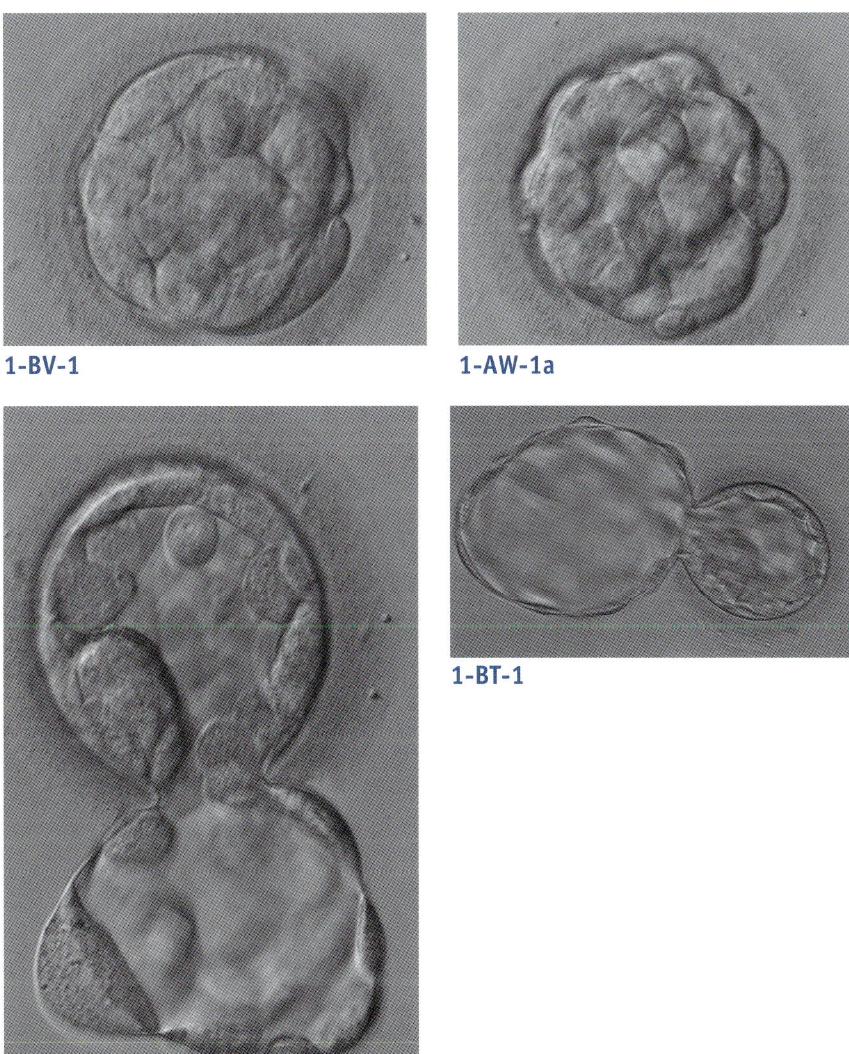

1-BV-1

1-AW-1a

1-BT-1

1-AW-1b

1-BV-1   Day 4 morula before vitrification
1-AW-1a   Same morula immediately after warming
1-AW-1b   Overnight culture to day 5 blastocyst (17 h post warming)
1-BT-1   Blastocyst 5aa before transfer

Case 2

2.5 years 2° infertility   Diagnosis: Male factor infertility

Female partner

Age 33, unskilled worker
Tubal status: patent
MH: 5/28
BMI: 21.3
Non-smoker, no alcohol
   consumption
Basal FSH: 4.4 IU/L
Basal LH: 4.2 IU/L

Basal estradiol: 58.2 pg/mL
Basal AMH: 2.24 ng/mL
Midluteal progesterone: 20.6 ng/mL
Midluteal prolactin: 31.3 ng/mL

Male partner

Age 38, unskilled worker
History/examination: NAD
Non-smoker, no alcohol consumption

Previous treatments

None

Fresh cycle: 2009 ICSI
Semen assessment: asthenoteratozoospermia

Volume	3.2 mL
Abstinence	3 days
Concentration	12×10^6/mL
Progressive motility	12%
Non-progressive motility	0%
Immotile	88%
Normal forms	2%

Stimulation protocol	Agonist protocol (recombinant FSH)
Days of stimulation	8
Total dose	1125 IU
Estradiol at ovulation induction	2976 ng/mL
Number of follicles $\geq$ 12 mm	11
Total number of COCs	8
Metaphase II	8
Injected/inseminated	8
Fertilization rate	75%
Cleavage rate	100%
Blastocyst rate	100%
Culture medium	GM501

Fresh transfer

Quality of embryo(s)	5aa
Outcome	Not pregnant
Vitrification	5 blastocysts

Previous vitrified/warmed cycles

2010	Missed abortion (no heart activity)
2011	Not pregnant
2011	Live birth, healthy girl
2013	Biochemical pregnancy

Vitrified/warmed cycle: 2013

Stimulation	NC
Endometrium	9 mm
Quality before vitrification	5aa
Warming day	5
Survival	Yes
Assisted hatching	No
Transfer day	5
Quality	Non re-expanded 5aa
Duration of cryostorage	4 years
Time between warming and transfer	6h

Outcome: Missed abortion (no heart activity)

Remarks: Cytoplasmic fragments were removed using a biopsy pipette

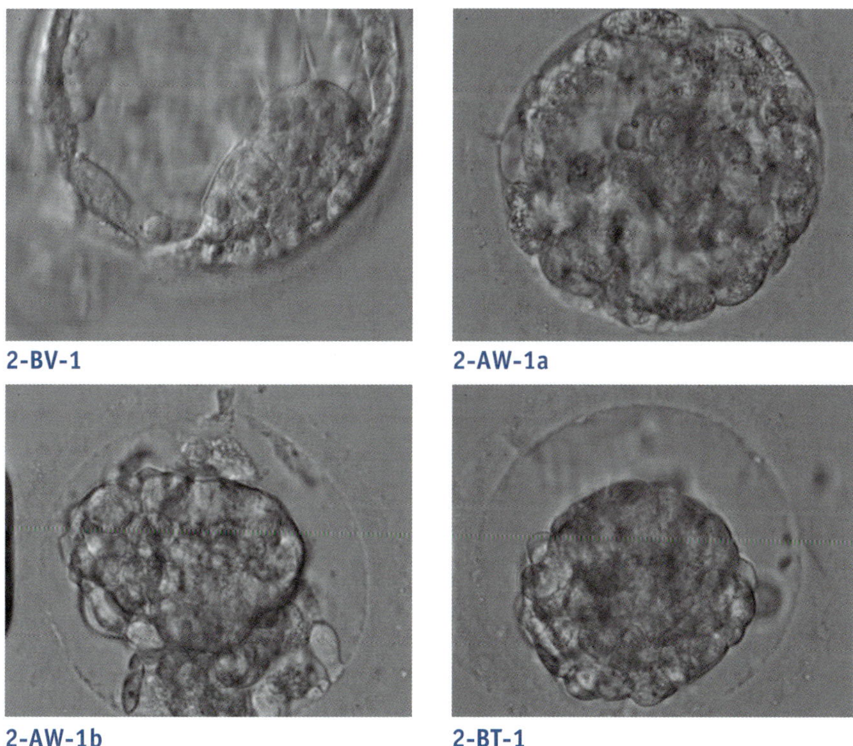

2-BV-1

2-AW-1a

2-AW-1b

2-BT-1

2-BV-1   Day 5 blastocyst (5aa) before vitrification, hatching site (8 o'clock position) out of focus
2-AW-1a Immediate but temporary re-expansion after warming
2-AW-1b Collapsed blastocyst showing fragment exclusion (5 hours after warming)
2-BT-1   Fragment-free collapsed blastocyst, hatching site at the 3 o'clock position

Case 3

2 years 1° infertility   Diagnosis: Endometriosis, PCO

Female partner

Age 28, nurse
Tubal status: patent
MH: dysmenorrhea
BMI: 19.3
Smoker, no alcohol
  consumption

Basal AMH: 8.4 ng/mL
Basal FSH: 3.5 IU/L
Basal LH: 3.7 IU/L
Basal estradiol: 32.1 pg/mL

Male partner

Age 32, stove setter
History/examination: NAD
Non-smoker, no alcohol consumption

Previous treatments

2012 ICSI   Not pregnant

Fresh cycle: 2013 IVF
Semen assessment: normozoospermia

Volume	3.2 mL
Abstinence	15 days
Concentration	95×10^6/mL
Total sperm number	304×10^6/mL
Progressive motility	57%
Non-progressive motility	5%
Immotile	38%
Normal forms	16%

Stimulation protocol	Antagonist protocol (recombinant FSH)
Days of stimulation	11
Total dose	975 IU
Estradiol at ovulation induction	1832 ng/mL
Number of follicles ≥ 12 mm	>25
Total number of COCs	27
Metaphase II	24
Injected/inseminated	24
Fertilization rate	88%
Cleavage rate	100%
Blastocyst rate	83%
Culture medium	EmbryoAssist/BlastAssist

Fresh transfer

Quality of embryo(s)	
Outcome	No fresh transfer because of OHSS
Vitrification	14 compacting embryos (day 4), 5 blastocysts (day 5)

Vitrified/warmed cycle: 2013

Stimulation	HSP
Endometrium	9 mm
Quality before vitrification	5ab
Warming day	5
Survival	Yes
Assisted hatching	No
Transfer day	5
Quality	5ab
Duration of cryostorage	2 months
Time between warming and transfer	3

Outcome: Live birth, healthy boy

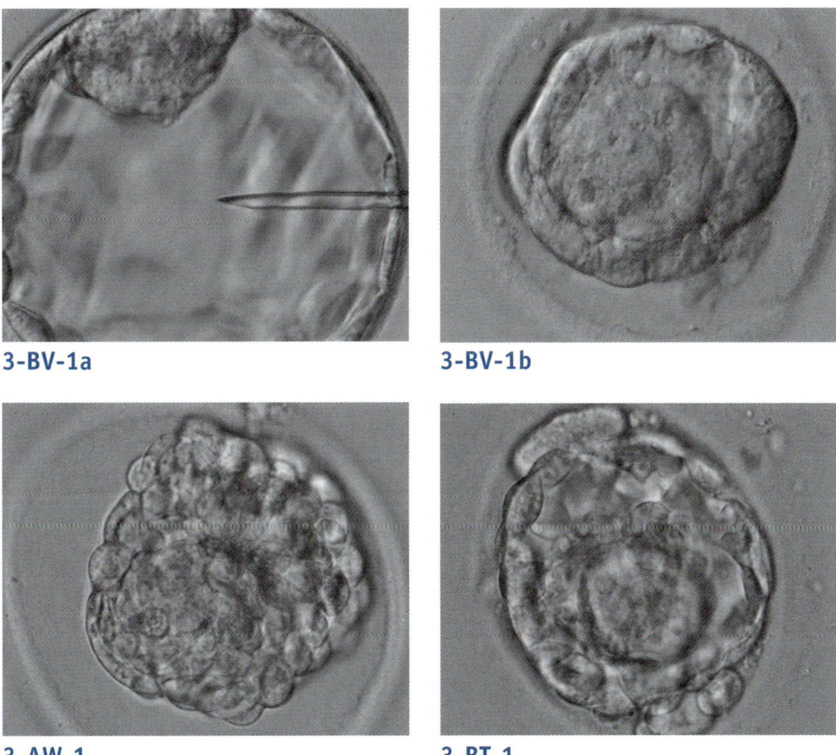

3-BV-1a

3-BV-1b

3-AW-1

3-BT-1

3-BV-1a Blastocyst 5ab prepared for artificial shrinkage of the blastocoel
3-BV-1b Artificially shrunken blastocyst, spontaneous hatching site at the 4 o'clock position
3-AW-1 Warmed blastocyst with hatching site at 1 o'clock position
3-BT-1 Re-expanded blastocyst with excluded fragments

Female partner

Age 36, civil servant
Tubal status: patent
MH: 5/28
BMI: 28.2
Smoker, no alcohol consumption
Normal female karyotype
History of thrombosis
Basal FSH: 7.8 IU/L
Basal LH: 6.3 IU/L

Basal estradiol: 46.2 pg/mL
Basal AMH: 3.83 ng/mL
Midluteal progesterone: <0.2 ng/mL
Midluteal prolactin: 27.2 ng/mL

Male partner

Age 46, civil servant
History/examination: NAD
Non-smoker, no alcohol consumption
Normal male karyotype

Previous treatments

2012 ICSI   Not pregnant

Fresh cycle: 2012 ICSI
Semen assessment: oligoasthenoteratozoospermia

Volume	1.8 mL
Abstinence	3 days
Concentration	14×10^6/mL
Progressive motility	14%
Non-progressive motility	4%
Immotile	82%
Normal forms	2%

Stimulation protocol	Agonist protocol (HMG)
Days of stimulation	13
Total dose	2587.5 IU
Estradiol at ovulation induction	1550 ng/mL
Number of follicles ≥ 12 mm	12
Total number of COCs	11
Metaphase II	11
Injected/inseminated	11
Fertilization rate	73%
Cleavage rate	100%
Blastocyst rate	63%
Culture medium	GM501

Fresh transfer

Quality of embryo(s)	4aa
Outcome	Not pregnant
Vitrification	3 blastocysts

Previous vitrified/warmed cycles

2012	Not pregnant

Vitrified/warmed cycle: 2013

Stimulation	NC
Endometrium	7.5 mm
Quality before vitrification	2 (day 4)
Warming day	4
Survival	Yes
Assisted hatching	Yes
Transfer day	4
Quality at transfer	3ab
Duration of cryostorage	10 months
Time between warming and transfer	3h

Outcome: Live birth, healthy monochorionic diamniotic twins

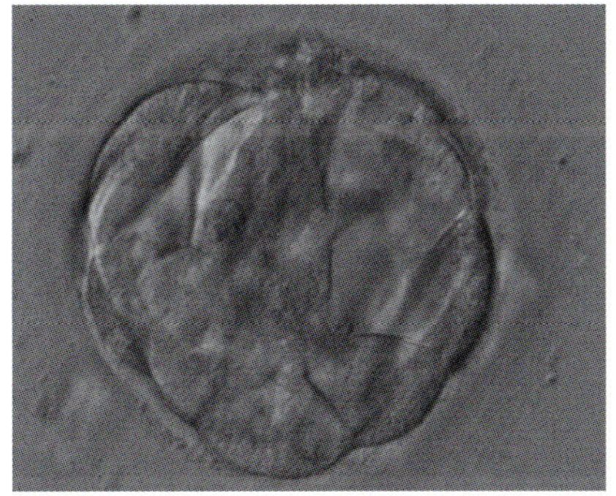

4-BV-1

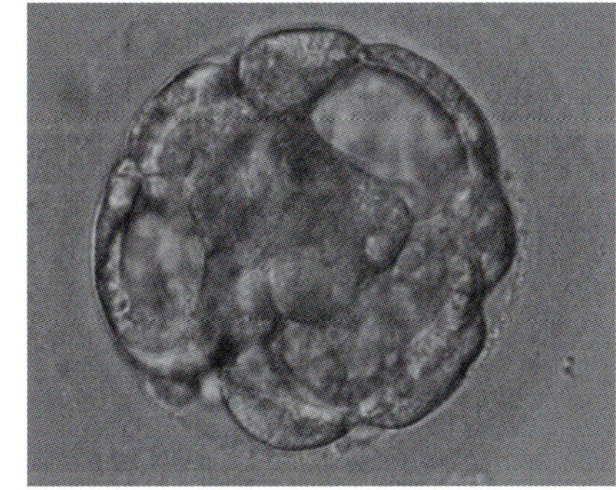

4-AW-1

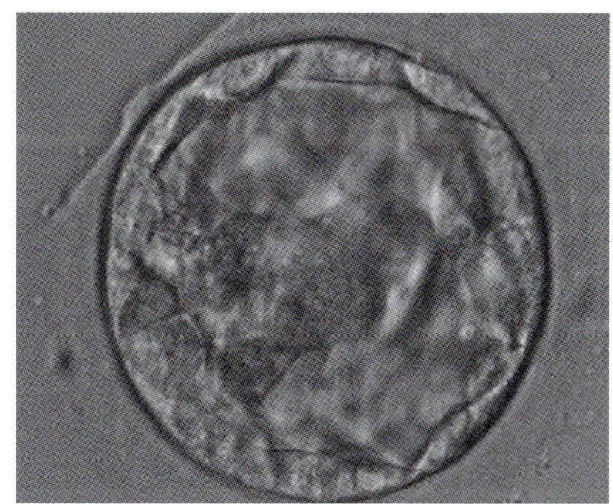

4-BT-1

4-BV-1   Early blastocyst
4-AW-1   Early blastocyst
4-BT-1   Viable full blastocyst with artificial zona thinning (9 to 11 o'clock position)

Female partner

Age 25, employee
Tubal status: patent
MH: 6/30
BMI: 24.0
Smoker, no alcohol consumption
Hypothyreosis
History of thrombosis
Basal FSH: 6.2 IU/L
Basal LH: 4.7 IU/L

Basal estradiol: 28.2 pg/mL
Basal AMH: 4.29 ng/mL
Midluteal progesterone: 12.0 ng/mL
Midluteal prolactin: 19.2 ng/mL
TSH: 2.78 IU/mL

Male partner

Age 31, lorry driver
History/examination: history
  of orchitis
Smoker, no alcohol consumption

Previous treatments

None

Fresh cycle: 2011 ICSI
Semen assessment: asthenoteratozoospermia

Volume	3.3 mL
Abstinence	6 days
Concentration	22×10^6/mL
Progressive motility	18%
Non-progressive motility	18%
Immotile	64%
Normal forms	3%

Stimulation protocol	Agonist protocol (recombinant FSH)
Days of stimulation	9
Total dose	1236 IU
Estradiol at ovulation induction	1150 ng/mL
Number of follicles ≥ 12 mm	18
Total number of COCs	14
Metaphase II	11
Injected/inseminated	11
Fertilization rate	91%
Cleavage rate	100%
Blastocyst rate	100%
Culture medium	EmbryoAssist/BlastAssist

Fresh transfer

Quality of embryo(s)	4aa
Outcome	Biochemical pregnancy
Vitrification	8 blastocysts

Previous vitrified/warmed cycles

2011	Not pregnant

Vitrified/warmed cycle: 2013

Stimulation	NC
Endometrium	11 mm
Quality before vitrification	4ab, 4ab
Warming day	5
Survival	Yes, Partial
Assisted hatching	Yes, Yes
Transfer day	5
Quality	5ab, 4ab
Duration of cryostorage	7 months
Time between warming and transfer	3h

Outcome: Live birth, healthy dichorionic diamniotic twins (boys)

Remark: Blastocyst #2 was considered for disposal because of beginning degeneration

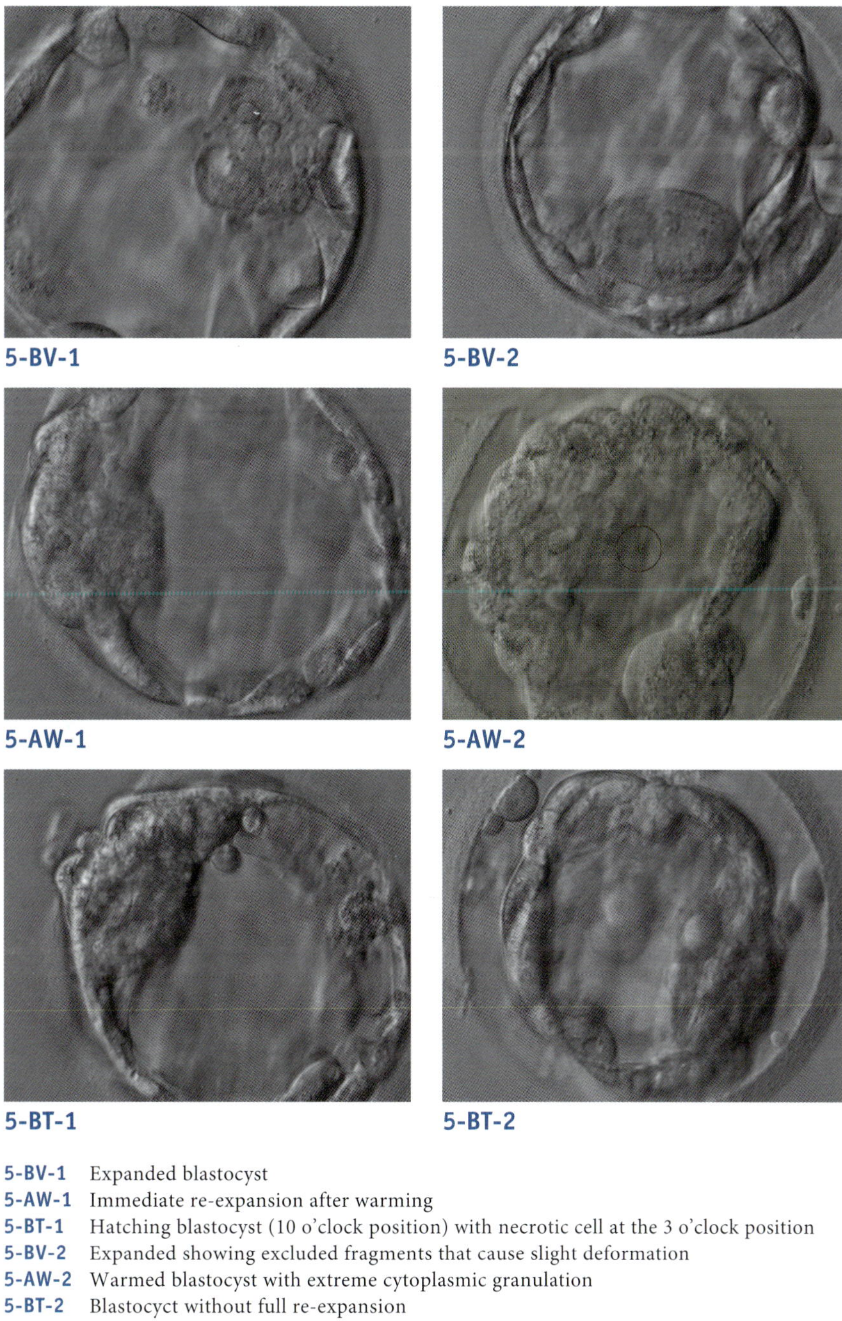

5-BV-1   Expanded blastocyst
5-AW-1   Immediate re-expansion after warming
5-BT-1   Hatching blastocyst (10 o'clock position) with necrotic cell at the 3 o'clock position
5-BV-2   Expanded showing excluded fragments that cause slight deformation
5-AW-2   Warmed blastocyst with extreme cytoplasmic granulation
5-BT-2   Blastocyct without full re-expansion

Case 6

Female partner

Age 27, machinist
Tubal status: patent
MH: oligomenorrhea, anovulation
BMI: 21.5
Non-smoker, no alcohol consumption
Basal FSH: 4.3 IU/L
Basal LH: 16.9 IU/L

Basal estradiol: 71.0 pg/mL
Basal AMH: 23.5 ng/mL
Basal AMH: 23.5 ng/mL
Midluteal progesterone: 17.6 ng/mL
TSH: 2.2 IU/L
Midluteal prolactin: 9.7 ng/mL

Male partner

Age 29, locksmith
History/examination: NAD
Non-smoker, no alcohol consumption

Previous treatments

2010 timed intercourse	Missed abortion (no FH activity)
2010 timed intercourse	Not pregnant

Fresh cycle: 2011 IVF (intracervical application of seminal plasma)
Semen assessment: Normozoospermia

Volume	4 mL
Abstinence	6 days
Concentration	64×10^6/mL
Progressive motility	59%
Non-progressive motility	6%
Immotile	36%
Normal forms	6%

Stimulation protocol	Antagonist protocol (recombinant FSH)
Days of stimulation	9
Total dose	1125 IU
Estradiol at ovulation induction	1874 ng/mL
Number of follicles ≥ 12 mm	>30
Total number of COCs	33
Metaphase II	33
Injected/inseminated	33
Fertilization rate	73%
Cleavage rate	100%
Blastocyst rate	46%
Culture medium	EmbryoAssist/BlastAssist

Fresh transfer

Quality of embryo(s)	4aa
Outcome	Missed abortion (positive FH activity)
Vitrification	1 morula and 8 blastocysts (day 5)

Vitrified/warmed cycle: 2013

Stimulation	HSP
Endometrium	8.5 mm
Quality before vitrification	4ab
Warming day	5
Survival	Yes
Assisted hatching	Yes
Transfer day	5
Quality	4aa
Duration of cryostorage	6 months
Time between warming and transfer	3h

Outcome: Live birth, boy with cerebral edema

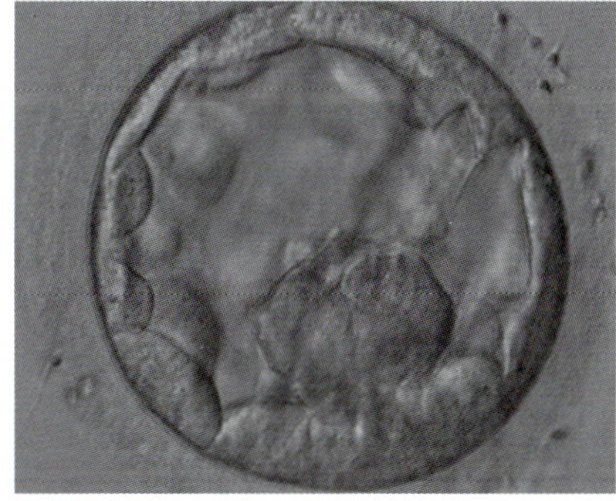 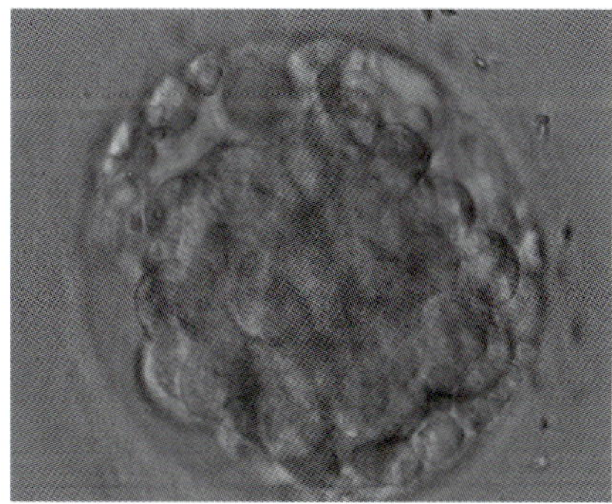 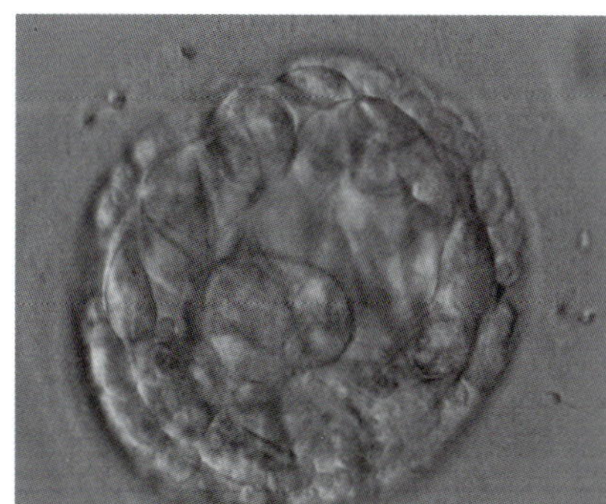

6-BV-1   **6-AW-1**   **6-BT-1**

6-BV-1 IVF-blastocyst with beginning expansion
6-AW-1 Same blastocyst without signs of re-expansion but excluded fragments
6-BT-1 Nearly re-expanded blastocysts (fragments interfere with complete re-expansion)

Female partner

Age 29, radiographer
Tubal status: patent
MH: 5/28
BMI: 18.2
Non-smoker, no alcohol
  consumption
Normal female karyotype

Basal FSH: 5.6 IU/L
Basal LH: 3.5 IU/L
Basal estradiol: 48.4 pg/mL
Basal AMH: 2.5 ng/mL
Midluteal prolactin: 4.4 ng/mL

Male partner

Age 32, manager
History/examination: NAD
Non-smoker, no alcohol
  consumption
Translocation carrier 46, XY, t (11;
  22) (p15.5; q13.1)

Previous treatments

2008 external ICSI × 3   Not pregnant
2009 external ICSI × 1   Biochemical pregnancy

Fresh cycle: 2010 ICSI
Semen assessment: asthenozoospermia

Volume	2 mL
Abstinence	3 days
Concentration	22×10^6/mL
Progressive motility	30%
Non-progressive motility	11%
Immotile	59%
Normal forms	8%

Stimulation protocol	Antagonist protocol (HMG)
Days of stimulation	12
Total dose	2250 IU
Estradiol at ovulation induction	1238 ng/mL
Number of follicles ≥ 12 mm	9
Total number of COCs	8
Metaphase II	8
Injected/inseminated	8
Fertilization rate	88%
Cleavage rate	100%
Blastocyst rate	71%
Culture medium	EmbryoAssist/BlastAssist

Fresh transfer

Quality of embryo(s)	4aa, 5aa
Outcome	Live birth, healthy girl
Vitrification	3 blastocysts

Vitrified/warmed cycle: 2013

Stimulation	HSP
Endometrium	8.5 mm
Quality before vitrification	4ab
Warming day	5
Survival	Yes
Assisted hatching	Yes
Transfer day	5
Quality	3ab
Duration of cryostorage	1.5 years
Time between warming and transfer	

Outcome: Live birth, healthy girl

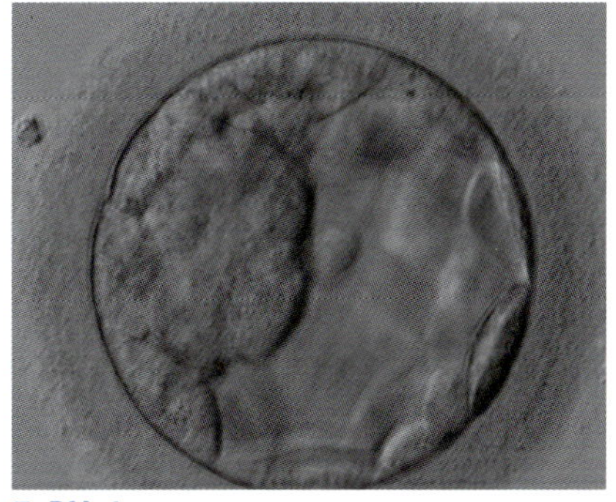

7-BV-1

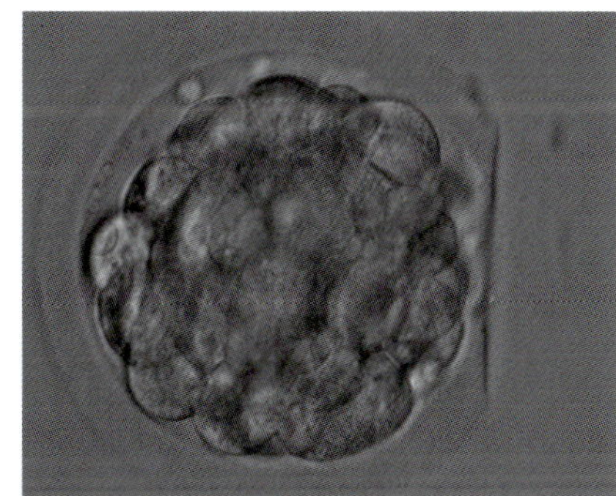

7-AW-1

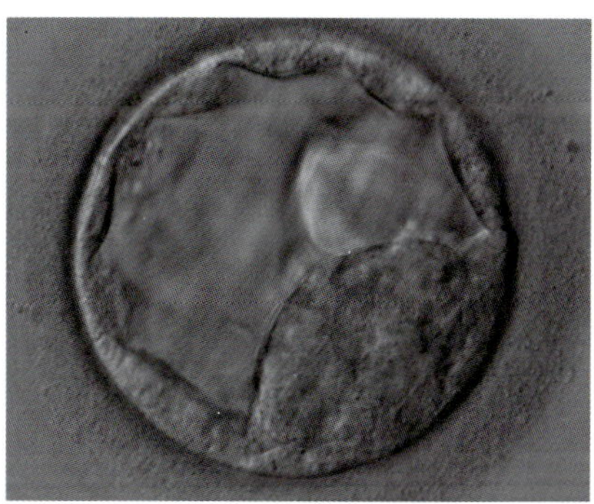

7-BT-1

7-BV-1 Full blastocyst with dark ZP
7-AW-1 Viable blastocyst
7-BT-1 Fully expanded blastocyst with dark and thick ZP

Female partner

Age 30, logistics manager
Tubal status: patent
MH: 5/28
BMI: 24.1
Non-smoker, no alcohol
 consumption
Basal FSH: 5.0 IU/L
Basal LH: 6.3 IU/L

Basal estradiol: 38.0 pg/mL
Basal AMH: 9.75 ng/mL
Midluteal progesterone: 31.0 ng/mL
Midluteal prolactin: 9.4 ng/mL

Male partner

Age 38, technician
History/examination: history
 of pulmonary embolism
Non-smoker, no alcohol
 consumption

Previous treatments

2007 timed intercourse × 4   Not pregnant

Fresh cycle: 2010 ICSI
Semen assessment: oligoteratozoospermia

Volume	4.4 mL
Abstinence	2 days
Concentration	1.2×10^6/mL
Progressive motility	85%
Non-progressive motility	0%
Immotile	15%
Normal forms	0%

Stimulation protocol	Antagonist protocol (recombinant FSH)
Days of stimulation	9
Total dose	1325 IU
Estradiol at ovulation induction	2301 ng/mL
Number of follicles ≥ 12 mm	13
Total number of COCs	13
Metaphase II	13
Injected/inseminated	13
Fertilization rate	54%
Cleavage rate	100%
Blastocyst rate	100%
Culture medium	EmbryoAssist/BlastAssist

Fresh transfer

Quality of embryo(s)	5aa
Outcome	Healthy live birth, boy
Vitrification	6 blastocysts

Vitrified/warmed cycle: 2013

Stimulation	HSP
Endometrium	9.0 mm
Quality before vitrification	4aa
Warming day	5
Survival	Yes, No
Assisted hatching	Yes, No
Transfer day	5
Quality	4aa
Duration of cryostorage	2 years
Time between warming and transfer	2h

Outcome: Live birth. Major malformation (cardiac anomaly, child death at age 5 months)

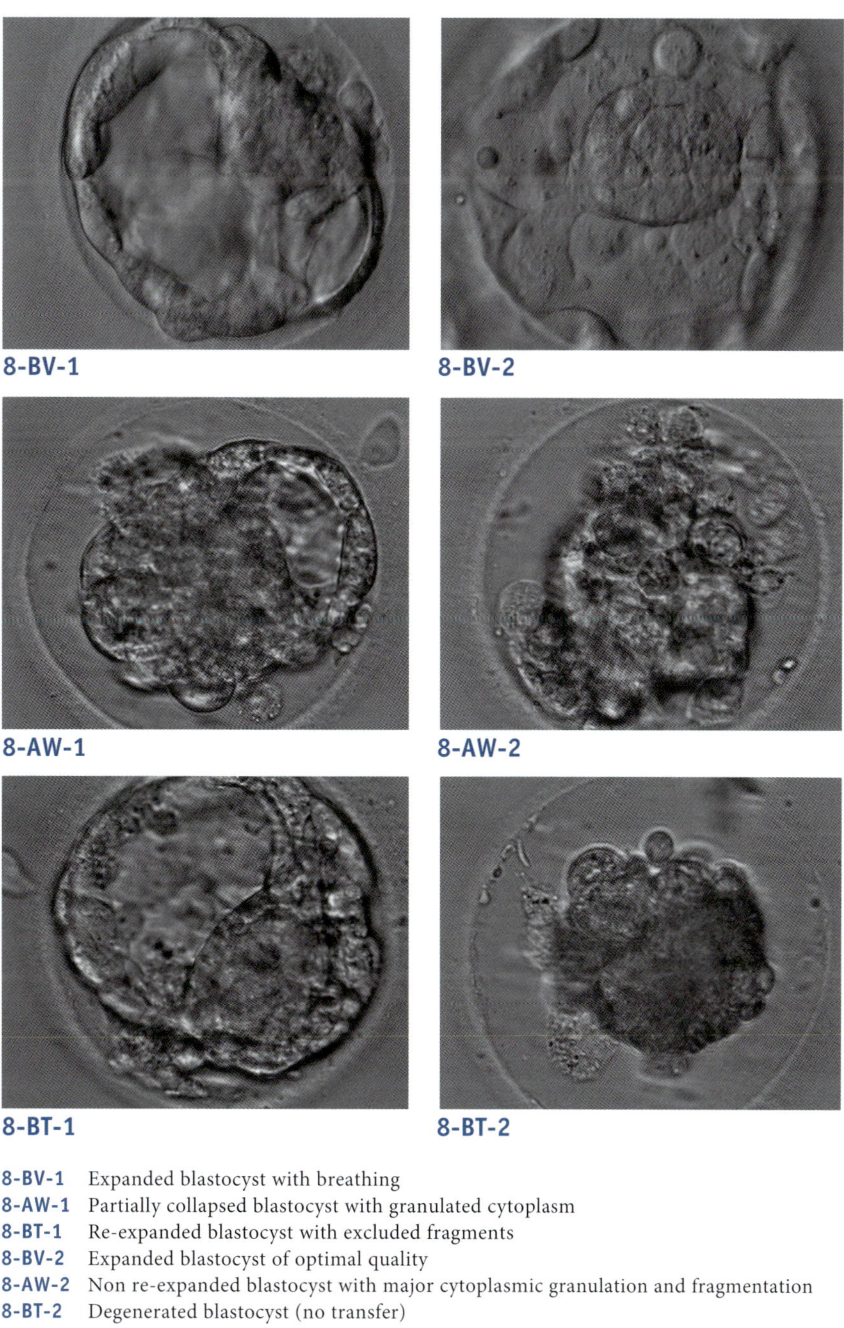

8-BV-1	Expanded blastocyst with breathing
8-AW-1	Partially collapsed blastocyst with granulated cytoplasm
8-BT-1	Re-expanded blastocyst with excluded fragments
8-BV-2	Expanded blastocyst of optimal quality
8-AW-2	Non re-expanded blastocyst with major cytoplasmic granulation and fragmentation
8-BT-2	Degenerated blastocyst (no transfer)

Female partner

Age 38, civil servant
Tubal status: patent
MH: 5/28
BMI: 26.3
Non-smoker, no alcohol
  consumption

Basal FSH: 6.5 IU/L
Basal LH: 6.1 IU/L
Basal estradiol: 40.0 pg/mL
Normal male karyotype
Basal AMH: 3.86 ng/mL

Male partner

Age 38, gardener
History/examination: NAD
Non-smoker, no alcohol consumption

Previous treatments

2007 ICSI	Not pregnant
2008 ICSI × 2	Not pregnant

Fresh cycle: 2009 ICSI, intracervical application of seminal plasma

Semen assessment: severe oligoasthenoteratozoospermia

Volume	1.2 mL
Abstinence	3 days
Concentration	1.1×10^6/mL
Progressive motility	22%
Non-progressive motility	0%
Immotile	78%
Normal forms	3%

Stimulation protocol	Agonist protocol (HMG)
Days of stimulation	11
Total dose	1650 IU
Estradiol at ovulation induction	1602 ng/mL
Number of follicles ≥ 12 mm	24
Total number of COCs	22
Metaphase II	13
Injected/inseminated	13
Fertilization rate	85%
Cleavage rate	91%
Blastocyst rate	36%
Culture medium	EmbryoAssist/BlastAssist

Fresh transfer

Quality of embryo(s)	3ab, 4ab
Outcome	Live birth, healthy boy
Vitrification	2 blastocysts

Vitrified/warmed cycle: 2013

Stimulation	NC
Endometrium	7.5 mm
Quality before vitrification	4aa, 3ab
Warming day	5
Survival	Yes, Yes
Assisted hatching	Yes, Yes
Transfer day	5
Quality	5aa, 3ab
Duration of cryostorage	2 years
Time between warming and transfer	3h

Outcome: Live birth, healthy dichorionic, diamniotic twins (2 girls)

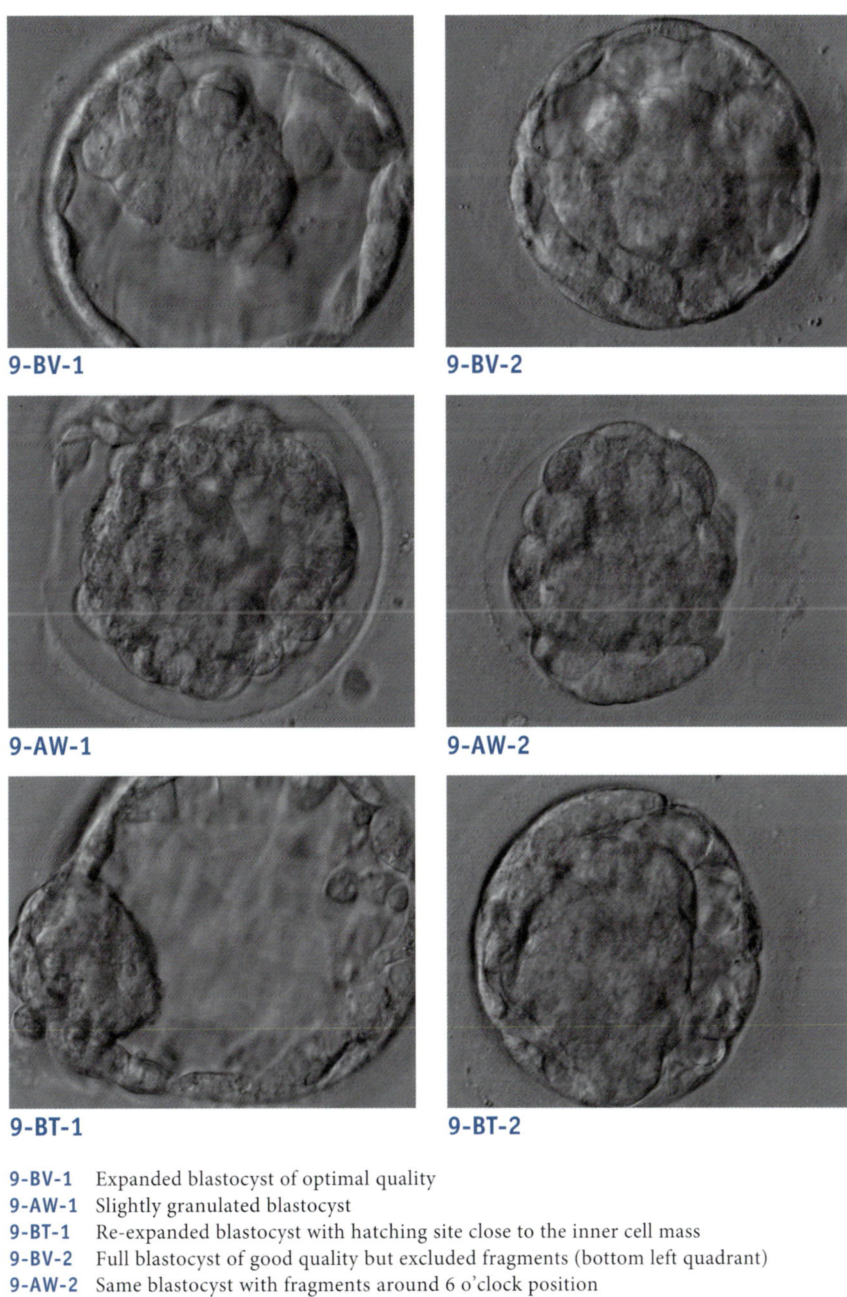

9-BV-1   Expanded blastocyst of optimal quality
9-AW-1   Slightly granulated blastocyst
9-BT-1   Re-expanded blastocyst with hatching site close to the inner cell mass
9-BV-2   Full blastocyst of good quality but excluded fragments (bottom left quadrant)
9-AW-2   Same blastocyst with fragments around 6 o'clock position
9-BT-2   Re-expanded full blastocyst

Female partner

Age 42, teacher

Tubal status: patent

MH: amenorrhea

BMI: 26.9

Non-smoker, no alcohol
  consumption

Small uterine myomas

Basal FSH: 5.2 IU/L

Basal LH: 6.4 IU/L

Basal AMH: 8.22 ng/mL

Normal male karyotype

Male partner

Age 40, diplomat

History/examination: NAD

Non-smoker, no alcohol consumption

Previous treatments

2010 external ICSI × 3   Not pregnant

Fresh cycle: 2011 ICSI

Semen assessment: teratozoospermia

Volume	3.0 mL
Abstinence	3 days
Concentration	25×10^6/mL
Progressive motility	32%
Non-progressive motility	0%
Immotile	68%
Normal forms	2%

Stimulation protocol	External antagonist protocol (HMG)
Days of stimulation	12
Total dose	1800 IU
Estradiol at ovulation induction	>4800 ng/mL
Number of follicles ≥ 12 mm	>35
Total number of COCs	38
Metaphase II	29
Injected/inseminated	29
Fertilization rate	86%
Cleavage rate	96%
Blastocyst rate	32%
Culture medium	EmbryoAssist/BlastAssist

Fresh transfer

Quality of embryo(s)	No transfer because of OHSS
Outcome	
Vitrification	3 compacting embryos, 1 morula, 4 blastocysts (all day 5)

Previous vitrified/warmed cycle

Quality of embryo(s)	5aa, 5aa
Outcome	Not pregnant

Vitrified/warmed cycle: 2012

Stimulation	HSP
Endometrium	9.5 mm
Quality before vitrification	Morula, compacting embryos
Warming day	5
Survival	Yes
Assisted hatching	Yes
Transfer day	6
Quality	3bb, 5ab
Duration of cryostorage	5 months
Time between warming and transfer	22h

Outcome: Pregnant, intrauterine fetal death due to trisomy 21

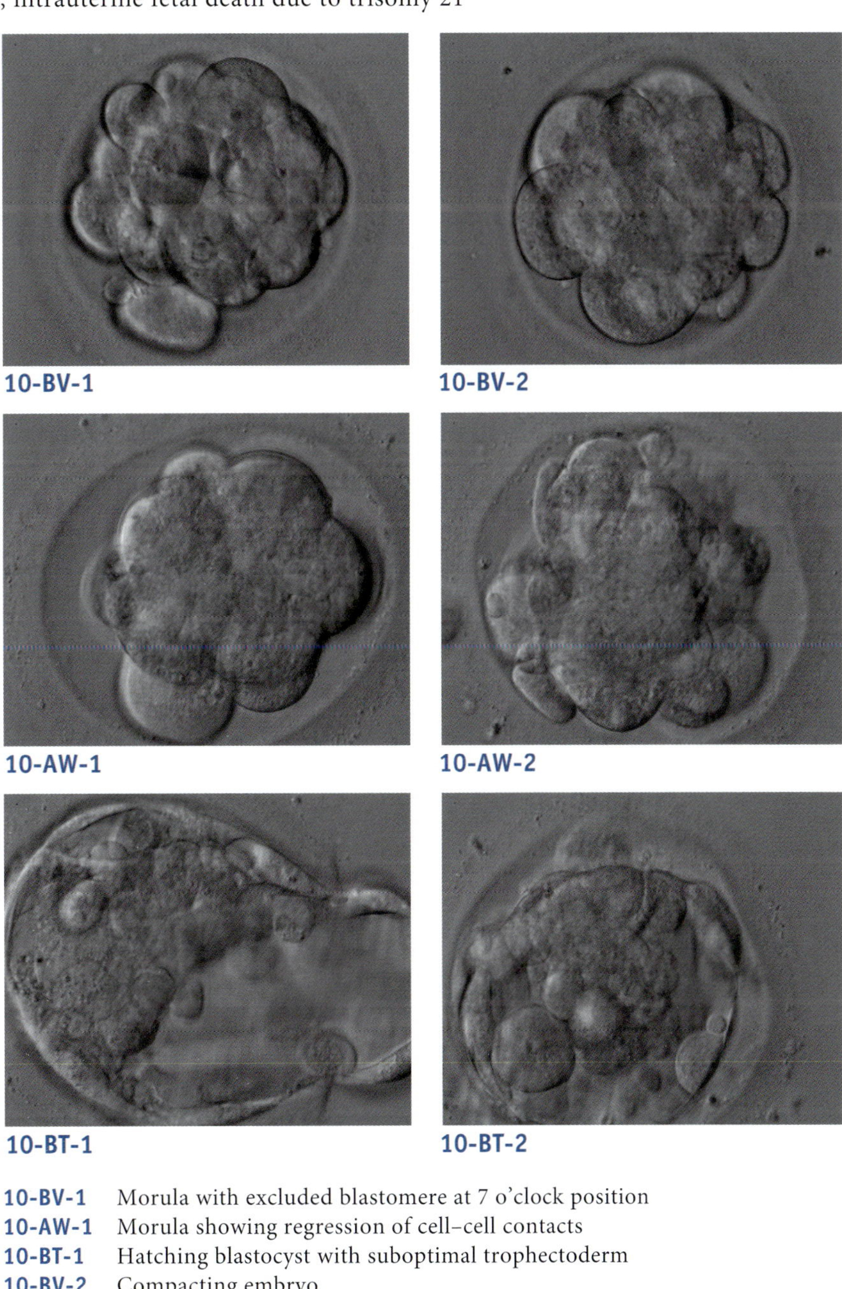

10-BV-1	Morula with excluded blastomere at 7 o'clock position
10-AW-1	Morula showing regression of cell–cell contacts
10-BT-1	Hatching blastocyst with suboptimal trophectoderm
10-BV-2	Compacting embryo
10-AW-2	Compacting embryo
10-BT-2	Partially re-expanded blastocyst with low quality trophectoderm and excluded blastomere in blastocoel (8 o'clock position)

Female partner

Age 34, hairdresser
Tubal status: patent
MH: 3–4/28
BMI: 28.2
Non-smoker, no alcohol
  consumption
Endometrioma
Basal FSH: 8.2 IU/L
Basal LH: 5.3 IU/L

Basal estradiol: 49.0 pg/mL
Basal AMH: 4.24 ng/mL
Midluteal progesterone: 6.7 ng/mL
Midluteal prolactin: 29.5 ng/mL

Male partner

Age 33, freelance merchant
History/examination: NAD
Non-smoker, no alcohol
  consumption

Previous treatments

None

Fresh cycle: 2013 ICSI (patient wish)

Semen assessment: normozoospermia

Volume	3.2 mL
Abstinence	4 days
Concentration	100×10^6/mL
Progressive motility	76%
Non-progressive motility	2%
Immotile	32%
Normal forms	10%

Stimulation protocol	Agonist protocol (recombinant FSH)
Days of stimulation	13
Total dose	2000 IU
Estradiol at ovulation induction	1882 ng/mL
Number of follicles ≥ 12 mm	12
Total number of COCs	11
Metaphase II	9
Injected/inseminated	9
Fertilization rate	78%
Cleavage rate	100%
Blastocyst rate	57%
Culture medium	EmbryoAssist/BlastAssist

Fresh transfer

Quality of embryo(s)	5aa
Outcome	Not pregnant
Vitrification	1 blastocyst

Vitrified/warmed cycle: 2013

Stimulation	HSP
Endometrium	8.0 mm
Quality before vitrification	5ab
Warming day	5
Survival	Yes
Assisted hatching	Yes
Transfer day	5
Quality	5ab
Duration of cryostorage	3 months
Time between warming and transfer	3h

Outcome: Not pregnant

Remark: Please note that prior to vitrification blastocoel was artificially shrunk.

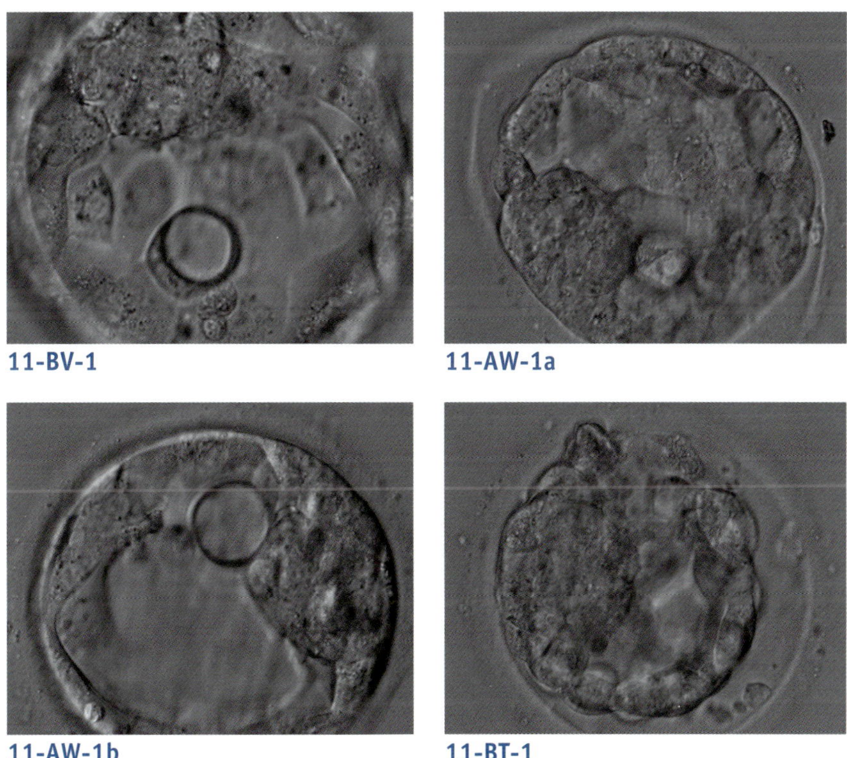

11-BV-1

11-AW-1a

11-AW-1b

11-BT-1

11-BV-1   Hatching blastocyst with hatching site out of focus (11 o'clock position)
11-AW-1a Starting re-expansion of collapsed blastocyst
11-AW-1b Re-expanded blastocyst with vacuolized blastomere in blastocoel (vacuole was removed by a single laser shot)
11-BT-1   Laser shot caused blastocyst collapse

Case 12

4 years 2° infertility   Diagnosis: Tubal infertility

Female partner

Age 29, clinician
Tubal status: bilateral
  tubectomy
MH: 5–6/30–31
BMI: 17.6
Non-smoker, no alcohol
  consumption
History of 2 ectopic
  pregnancies

Basal FSH: 7.7 IU/L
Basal LH: 7.5 IU/L
Basal estradiol: 24.7 pg/mL
Basal AMH: 8.97 ng/mL
Midluteal progesterone: 8.9 ng/mL
Midluteal prolactin: 18.8 ng/mL

Male partner

Age 40, technician
History/examination: NAD
Non-smoker, no alcohol consumption

Previous treatments

2012 ICSI	Not pregnant
	Impaired ICSI fertilization (<30%)

Fresh cycle: 2012 ICSI with ionophore treatment
Semen assessment: normozoospermia

Volume	4.4 mL
Abstinence	3 days
Concentration	68×10^6/mL
Progressive motility	44%
Non-progressive motility	4%
Immotile	52%
Normal forms	6%

Stimulation protocol	Antagonist protocol (recombinant FSH)
Days of stimulation	9
Total dose	1225 IU
Estradiol at ovulation induction	1085 ng/mL
Number of follicles ≥ 12 mm	14
Total number of COCs	15
Metaphase II	12
Injected/inseminated	12
Fertilization rate	75%
Cleavage rate	100%
Blastocyst rate	100%
Culture medium	EmbryoAssist/BlastAssist

Fresh transfer

Quality of embryo(s)	4ab
Outcome	Not pregnant
Vitrification	4 blastocysts

Vitrified/warmed cycle: 2012

Stimulation	HSP
Endometrium	8 mm
Quality before vitrification	4ab
Warming day	5
Survival	Yes
Assisted hatching	Yes
Transfer day	5
Quality	5ab
Duration of cryostorage	2 months
Time between warming and transfer	5h

Outcome: Ectopic pregnancy

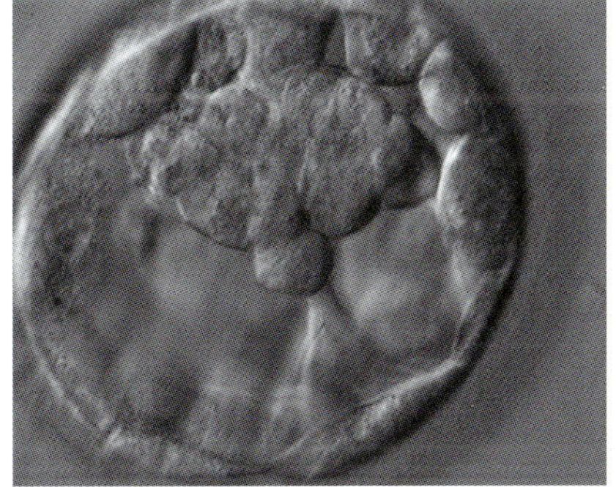

12-BV-1

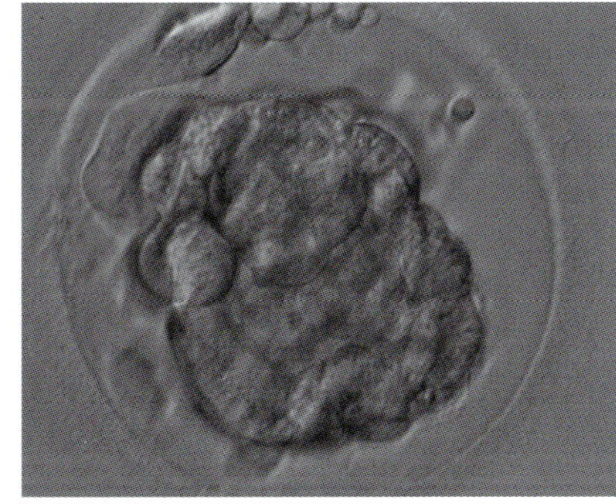

12-AW-1

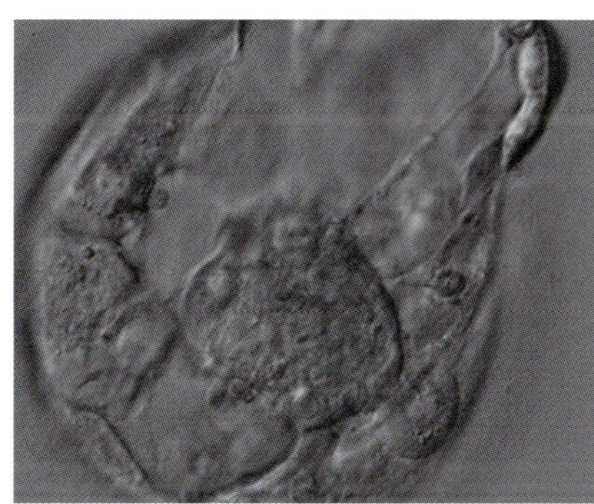

12-BT-1

12-BV-1 Expanded blastocyst (although zona is still thick)
12-AW-1 Warmed blastocyst showing excluded fragments
12-BT-1 Hatching blastocyst with cytoplasmic string spanning from inner cell mass to trophectoderm (upper right quadrant)

Case 13

2 years 2° infertility   Diagnosis: Tubal infertility

Female partner

Age 29, domestic aid
Tubal status: bilateral
  blockage
MH: 6/28–32
BMI: 26.7
Non-smoker, no alcohol
  consumption
History of chlamydia infection

Basal FSH: 4.7 IU/L
Basal LH: 4.6 IU/L
Basal estradiol: 81.9 pg/mL
Basal AMH: 7.48 ng/mL

Male partner

Age 32, mechanic
History/examination: NAD
Non-smoker, no alcohol consumption

Previous treatments

2008 timed intercourse	Biochemical pregnancy
2009 timed intercourse	Extrauterine pregnancy

Fresh cycle: 2011 IVF
Semen assessment: normozoospermia

Volume	5.2 mL
Abstinence	6 days
Concentration	122×10^6/mL
Progressive motility	68%
Non-progressive motility	0%
Immotile	32%
Normal forms	9%

Stimulation protocol	Agonist protocol (recombinant FSH)
Days of stimulation	10
Total dose	1200 IU
Estradiol at ovulation induction	1080 ng/mL
Number of follicles ≥ 12 mm	18
Total number of COCs	17
Metaphase II	
Injected/inseminated	17
Fertilization rate	35%
Cleavage rate	100%
Blastocyst rate	100%
Culture medium	Embryo Assist/Blast Assist

Fresh transfer

Quality of embryo(s)	No fresh transfer because of OHSS
Outcome	
Vitrification	6 blastocysts

Previous vitrified/warmed cycle

2011	Not pregnant

Vitrified/warmed cycle: 2012

Stimulation	HSP
Endometrium	8.0 mm
Quality before vitrification	2, 4ab
Warming day	5
Survival	Yes
Assisted hatching	Yes
Transfer day	5
Quality	3ab, 4ab
Duration of cryostorage	4 months
Time between warming and transfer	2h

Outcome: Dichorionic-diamniotic twin pregnancy, live birth, 1 healthy girl, 1 girl with atresia of duodenum

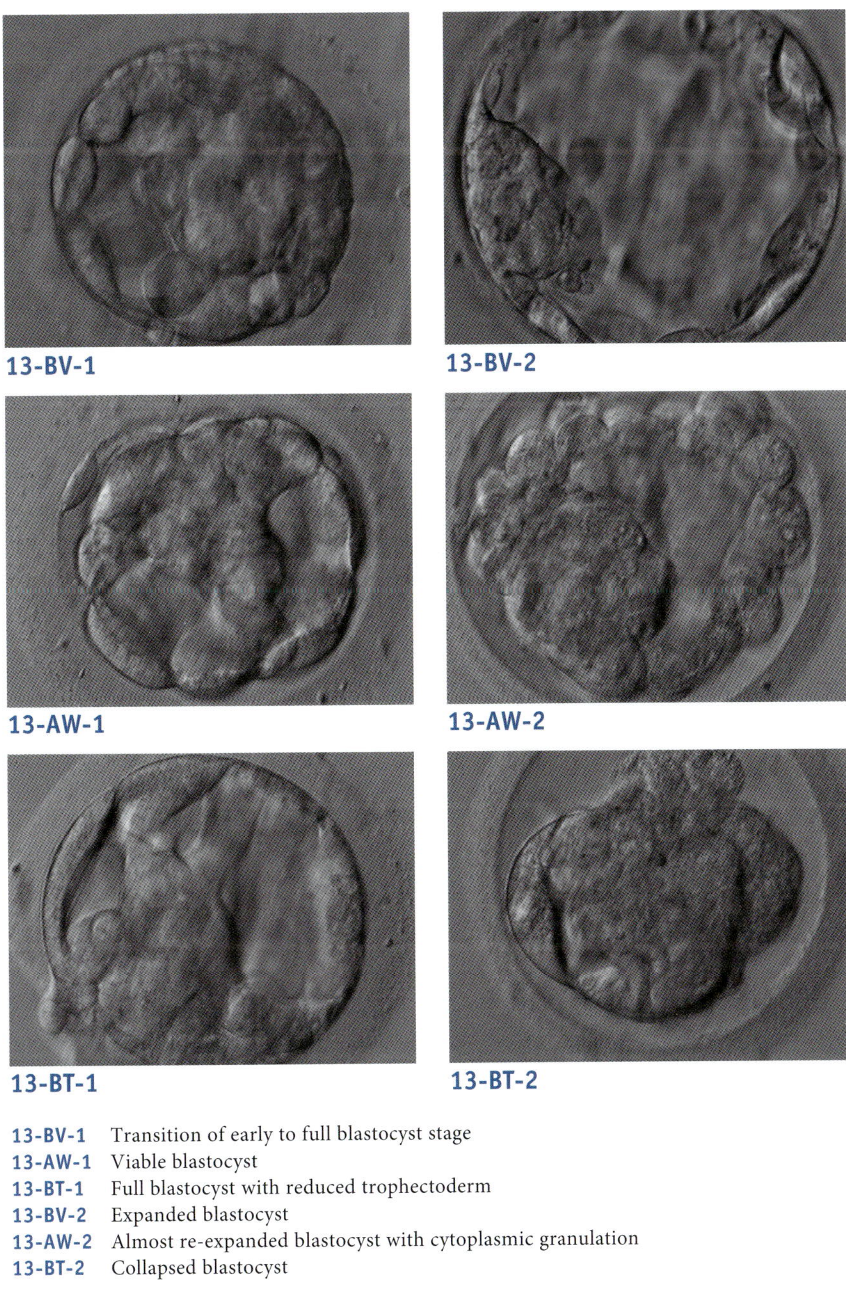

13-BV-1

13-BV-2

13-AW-1

13-AW-2

13-BT-1

13-BT-2

13-BV-1	Transition of early to full blastocyst stage
13-AW-1	Viable blastocyst
13-BT-1	Full blastocyst with reduced trophectoderm
13-BV-2	Expanded blastocyst
13-AW-2	Almost re-expanded blastocyst with cytoplasmic granulation
13-BT-2	Collapsed blastocyst

Female partner

Age 29, teacher
Tubal status: patent
MH: 5/28
BMI: 25.6
Smoker, no alcohol
  consumption
Normal female
  karyotype

Basal FSH: 7.9 IU/L
Basal LH: 3.6 IU/L
Basal estradiol: 34.6 pg/mL
Basal AMH: 4.56 ng/mL

Male partner

Age 36, teacher
History/examination: NAD
Non-smoker, no alcohol
  consumption
Normal male karyotype

Previous treatments

None

Fresh cycle: 2010 ICSI
Semen assessment: cryptozoospermia

Volume	3.4 mL
Abstinence	6 days
Concentration	0.001×10^{6}/mL
Progressive motility	16%
Non-progressive motility	7%
Immotile	77%
Normal forms	1%

Stimulation protocol	Antagonist protocol (recombinant FSH)
Days of stimulation	8
Total dose	1250 IU
Estradiol at ovulation induction	860 ng/mL
Number of follicles $\geq$ 12 mm	6
Total number of COCs	4
Metaphase II	4
Injected/inseminated	4
Fertilization rate	75%
Cleavage rate	100%
Blastocyst rate	
Culture medium	GM501

Fresh transfer

Quality of embryo(s)	8A (day 3)
Outcome	Live birth, healthy boy
Vitrification	1 morula (day 5)

Vitrified/warmed cycle: 2011

Stimulation	HSP
Endometrium	8 mm
Quality before vitrification	Morula
Warming day	5
Survival	Yes
Assisted hatching	Yes
Transfer day	5
Quality	1
Duration of cryostorage	21 months
Time between warming and transfer	2h

Outcome: Live birth, healthy girl

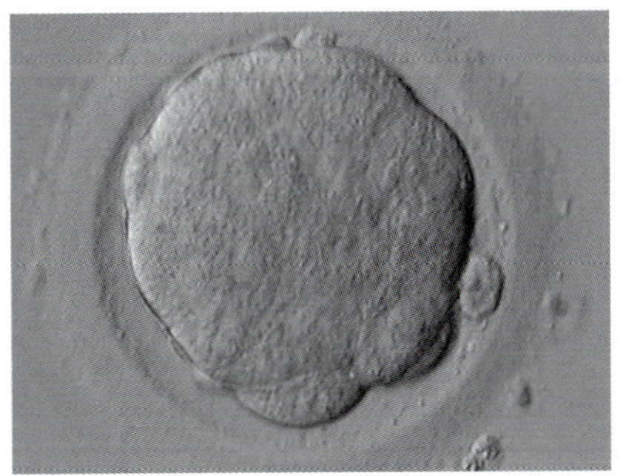

14-BV-1

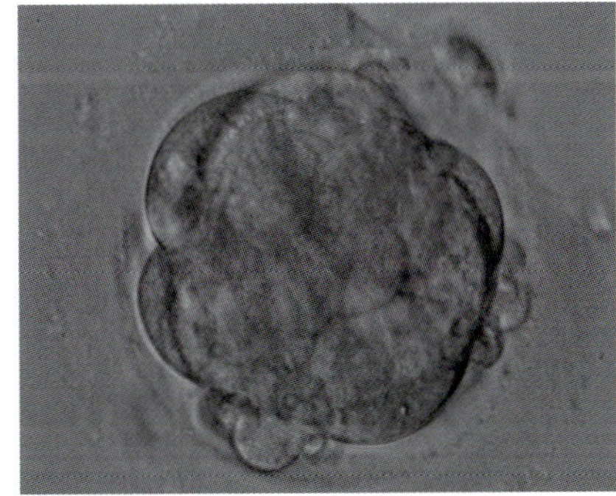

14-AW-1

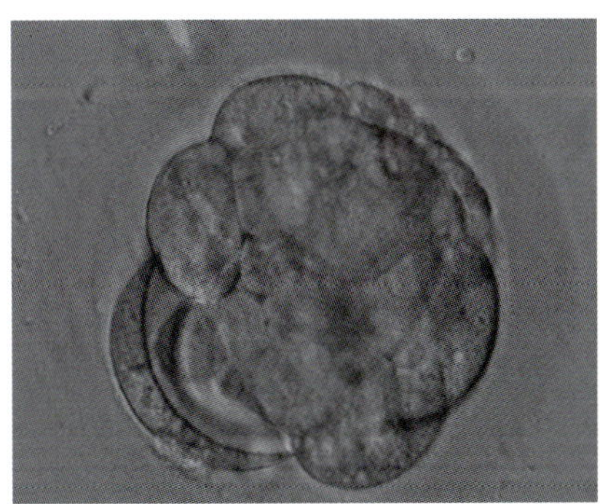

14-BT-1

14-BV-1 Day 5 morula of optimal quality
14-AW-1 Morula showing immediate survival
14-BT-1 Early blastocyst with blastocoel cavity forming in the bottom left quadrant

Female partner

Age 34, clinician
Tubal status: patent
MH: 5/28
BMI: 28.2
Smoker, no alcohol
  consumption

Hypothyreosis
Basal FSH: 6.1 IU/L
Basal LH: 5.1 IU/L
Basal estradiol: 39.6 pg/mL
Basal AMH: 9.48 ng/mL

Male partner

Age 36, clinician
History/examination: NAD
Non-smoker, no alcohol
  consumption
Normal male karyotype

Previous treatments

| 2008 ICSI | Not pregnant |
| 2008 vitrified/warmed cycle | Live birth, healthy boy |

Fresh cycle: 2011 ICSI
Semen assessment: oligoasthenoteratozoospermia

Volume	2.8 mL
Abstinence	4 days
Concentration	7×10^6/mL
Progressive motility	14%
Non-progressive motility	11%
Immotile	75%
Normal forms	2%

Stimulation protocol	Antagonist protocol (recombinant FSH)
Days of stimulation	11
Total dose	1000 IU
Estradiol at ovulation induction	1412 ng/mL
Number of follicles ≥ 12 mm	25
Total number of COCs	24
Metaphase II	22
Injected/inseminated	22
Fertilization rate	77%
Cleavage rate	100%
Blastocyst rate	29%
Culture medium	EmbryoAssist/BlastAssist

Fresh transfer

Quality of embryo(s)	
Outcome	No fresh transfer because of OHSS
Vitrification	2 early blastocysts, 1 full blastocyst, 2 expanded blastocysts

Vitrified/warmed cycle: 2013

Stimulation	NC
Endometrium	12.0 mm
Quality before vitrification	3aa
Warming day	5
Survival	Yes
Assisted hatching	Yes
Transfer day	5
Quality	4aa
Duration of cryostorage	2 months
Time between warming and transfer	4h

Outcome: Live birth, healthy boy

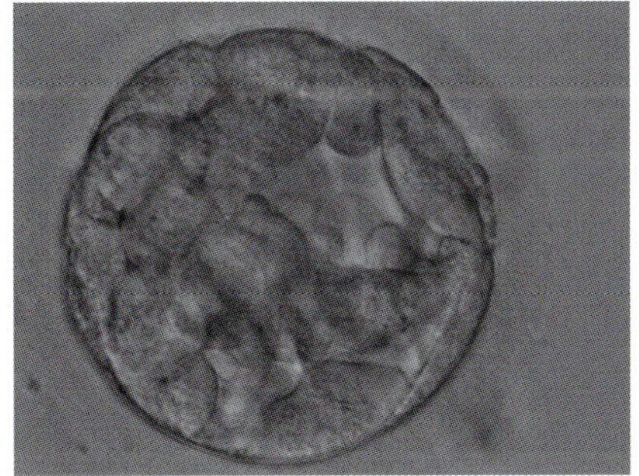

15-BV-1

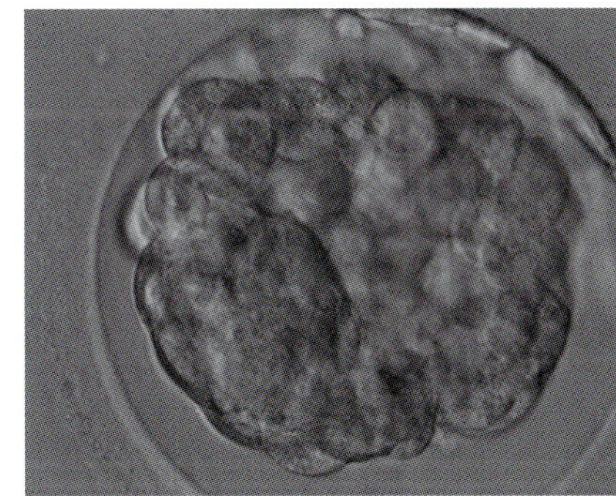

15-AW-1

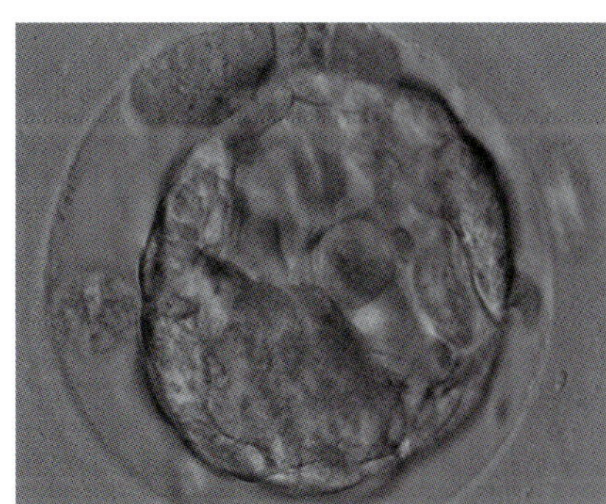

15-BT-1

15-BV-1 Blastocyst showing beginning expansion
15-AW-1 Same blastocyst 2h after warming
15-BT-1 Good quality blastocyst with minor fragmentation in blastocoel and perivitelline space

Female partner

Age 31, cashier

Tubal status: patent

MH: dysmenorrhea

BMI: 32.3

Non-smoker, no alcohol
 consumption

Adnexitis

Basal FSH: 6.6 IU/L

Basal LH: 2.0 IU/L

Basal estradiol: 48 pg/mL

Basal AMH: 5.51 ng/mL

Midluteal progesterone: 4.5 ng/mL

Midluteal prolactin: 13.7 ng/mL

Male partner

Age 33, worker

History/examination: NAD

Non-smoker, no alcohol
 consumption

Previous treatments

2008 timed intercourse × 3	Not pregnant
2009 insemination	Not pregnant

Fresh cycle: 2009 split IVF/ICSI

Semen assessment: normozoospermia

Volume	5.4 mL
Abstinence	3 days
Concentration	65×10^6/mL
Progressive motility	45%
Non-progressive motility	8%
Immotile	47%
Normal forms	9%

Stimulation protocol	Antagonist protocol (HMG)
Days of stimulation	10
Total dose	2100 IU
Estradiol at ovulation induction	2741 ng/mL
Number of follicles ≥ 12 mm	18
Total number of COCs	17
Metaphase II	17
Injected/inseminated	10 (ICSI), 7 (IVF)
Fertilization rate	70% (ICSI), failed IVF
Cleavage rate	86%
Blastocyst rate	100%
Culture medium	EmbryoAssist/BlastAssist

Fresh transfer

Quality of embryo(s)	5aa
Outcome	Live birth, healthy girl
Vitrification	4 blastocysts

Previous vitrified/warmed cycles

2012	Not pregnant

Vitrified/warmed cycle: 2012

Stimulation	HSP
Endometrium	14 mm
Quality before vitrification	4aa
Warming day	5
Survival	Partial
Assisted hatching	Yes
Transfer day	5
Quality	4bc
Duration of cryostorage	3 years
Time between warming and transfer	3

Outcome: Live birth, healthy boy

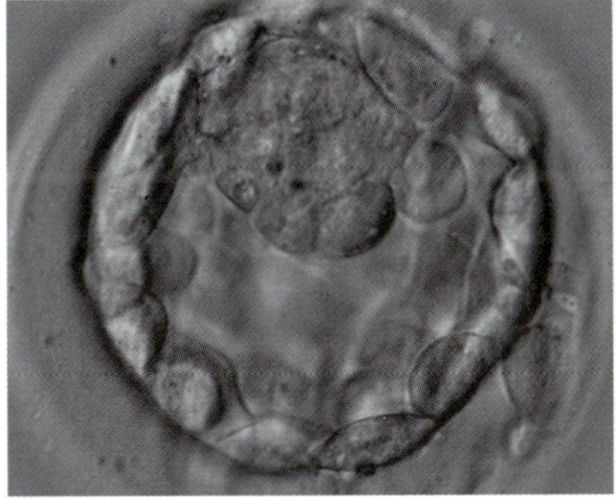 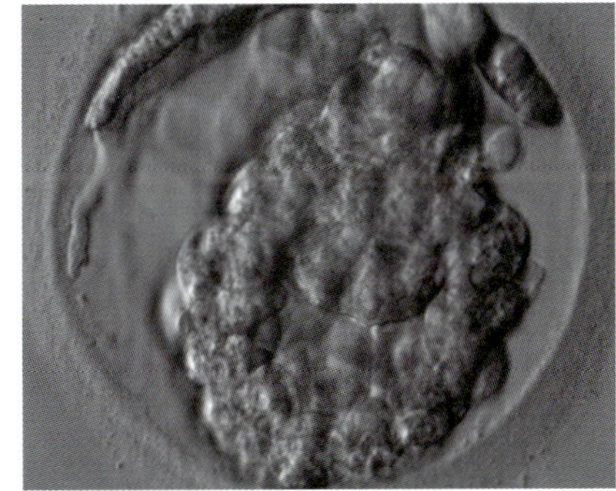 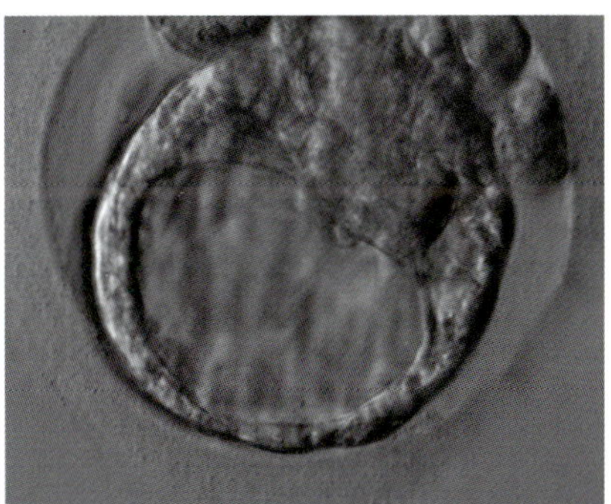

16-BV-1   16-AW-1   16-BT-1

16-BV-1 Expanded blastocyst starting to collapse in preparation for hatching
16-AW-1 Same blastocyst after warming, cytoplasm appears granulated
16-BT-1 Poor quality blastocyst showing excluded fragments (11 to 3 o'clock position)

Female partner

Age 39, saleswoman
Tubal status: patent
MH: 4/30–40
BMI: 18.04
Non-smoker, no alcohol
  consumption
Hyperprolactinemia
Basal FSH: 8.7 IU/L

Basal LH: 4.5 IU/L
Basal estradiol: 49.0 pg/mL
Basal AMH: 6.63 ng/mL
Midluteal progesterone: 11.6 ng/mL
Midluteal prolactin: 77.4 ng/mL
TSH: 2.70 IU/L

Male partner

Age 46, mechanic
History/examination: NAD
Smoker, no alcohol consumption
Normal male karyotype

Previous treatments

2008 ICSI	Not pregnant
2009 Vitrified/warmed cycle	Not pregnant

Fresh cycle: 2012 ICSI
Semen assessment: teratozoospermia

Volume	5.2 mL
Abstinence	6 days
Concentration	75×10^{6}/mL
Progressive motility	45%
Non-progressive motility	10%
Immotile	45%
Normal forms	1%

Stimulation protocol	Agonist protocol (recombinant FSH)
Days of stimulation	12
Total dose	1800 IU
Estradiol at ovulation induction	1291 ng/mL
Number of follicles ≥ 12 mm	8
Total number of COCs	12
Metaphase II	9
Injected/inseminated	8
Fertilization rate	100%
Cleavage rate	100%
Blastocyst rate	50%
Culture medium	EmbryoAssist/BlastAssist

Fresh transfer

Quality of embryo(s)	4aa, 5aa
Outcome	Missed abortion
Vitrification	1 compacting embryo, 2 blastocysts (all day 5)

Vitrified/warmed cycle: 2012

Stimulation	NC
Endometrium	7 mm
Quality before vitrification	4ab
Warming day	5
Survival	Partly
Assisted hatching	Yes
Transfer day	5
Quality	4ab
Duration of cryostorage	3.5 years
Time between warming and transfer	5h

Outcome: Termination of pregnancy (trisomy 21)

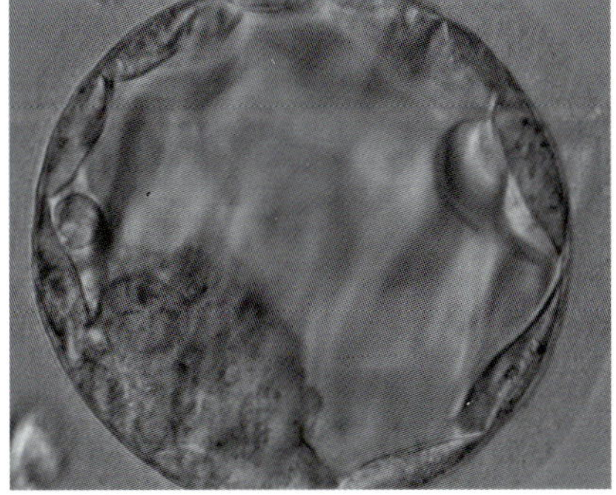
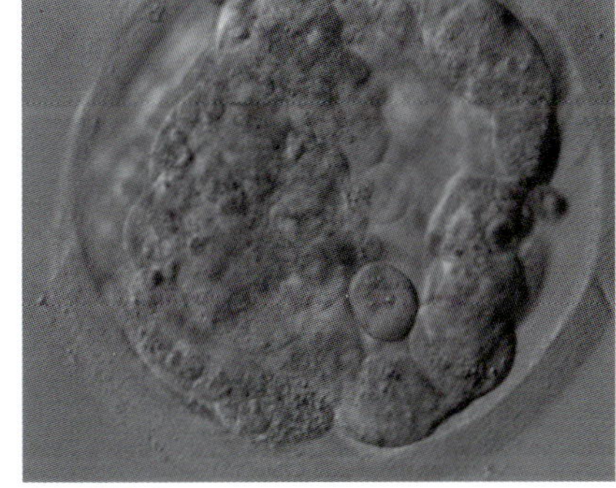
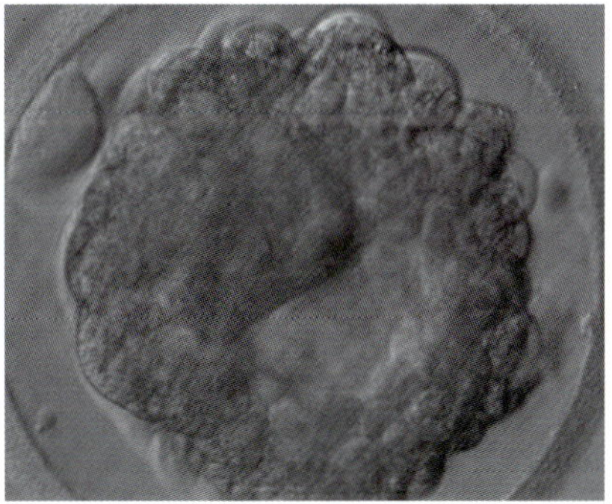

17-BV-1 **17-AW-1** **17-BT-1**

17-BV-1 Expanded blastocyst with thick ZP
17-AW-1 Warmed blastocyst with extensive cytoplasmic granulation
17-BT-1 Not fully re-expanded blastocyst with extensive cytoplasmic granulation

Female partner

Age 40, civil servant
Tubal status: patent
MH: 4/21–35
BMI: 20.4
Non-smoker, no alcohol
  consumption
Basal FSH: 7.1 IU/L
Basal LH: 7.1 IU/L

Basal estradiol: 29.9 pg/mL
Basal AMH: 2.52 ng/mL
Midluteal progesterone: 11.4 ng/mL
Midluteal prolactin: 27.0 ng/mL

Male partner

Age 44, EU politician
History/examination: NAD
Non-smoker, no alcohol
  consumption
Normal male karyotype

Previous treatments

2012 timed intercourse   Not pregnant

Fresh cycle: 2013 ICSI
Semen assessment: asthenoteratozoospermia

Volume	3.3 mL
Abstinence	7 days
Concentration	172×10^6/mL
Progressive motility	17%
Non-progressive motility	1%
Immotile	82%
Normal forms	2%

Stimulation protocol	Antagonist protocol (HMG)
Days of stimulation	11
Total dose	1800 IU
Estradiol at ovulation induction	2036 ng/mL
Number of follicles ≥ 12 mm	14
Total number of COCs	12
Metaphase II	12
Injected/inseminated	11
Fertilization rate	73%
Cleavage rate	100%
Blastocyst rate	38%
Culture medium	EmbryoAssist/BlastAssist

Fresh transfer

Quality of embryo(s)	Fully compacted embryo (day 4)
Outcome	Not pregnant
Vitrification	Fully compacted embryo (day 4), 2 morulae, 1 blastocyst (day 5)

Vitrified/warmed cycle: 2013

Stimulation	HSP
Endometrium	8.5 mm
Quality before vitrification	Fully compacted embryo
Warming day	4
Survival	Yes
Assisted hatching	Yes
Transfer day	5
Quality	5ba
Duration of cryostorage	2 months
Time between warming and transfer	19h

Outcome: Live birth, healthy girl

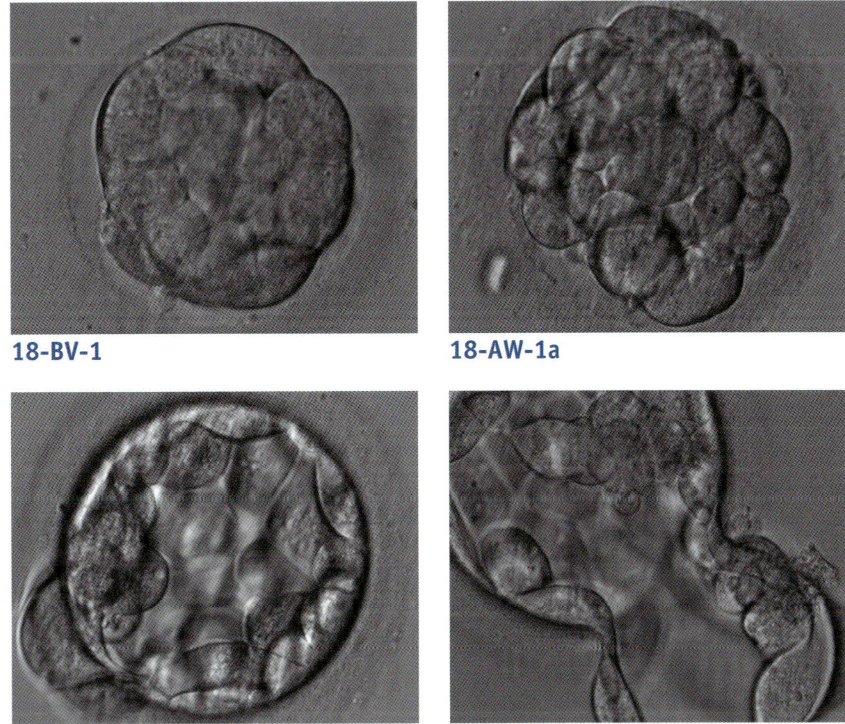

18-BV-1

18-AW-1a

18-AW-1b

18-BT-1

18-BV-1 Transition from fully compacted stage to morula
18-AW-1a Immediate survival
18-AW-1b Full blastocyst with hatching site close to inner cell mass (16h past warming)
18-BT-1 Hatching blastocyst

Female partner

Age 40, judge
Tubal status: patent
MH: 5–6/28–30
BMI: 20.2
Non-smoker, no alcohol
    consumption
Induced abortion (1992)

Basal FSH: 7.2 IU/L
Basal LH: 5.1 IU/L
Basal estradiol: 20.0 pg/mL
Basal estradiol: 20.0 pg/mL
Basal AMH: 3.22 ng/mL

Male partner

Age 37, university assistant
History/examination: history
    of multiple prostatitis
Non-smoker, no alcohol
    consumption
HIV positive

Previous treatments

None

Not pregnant

Fresh cycle: 2013 ICSI
Semen assessment: severe oligoasthenoteratozoospermia

Volume	3.7 mL
Abstinence	5 days
Concentration	0.4×10^6/mL
Progressive motility	0%
Non-progressive motility	10%
Immotile	90%
Normal forms	1%

Stimulation protocol	Agonist protocol (HMG)
Days of stimulation	11
Total dose	1500 IU
Estradiol at ovulation induction	3058 ng/mL
Number of follicles ≥ 12 mm	>20
Total number of COCs	26
Metaphase II	19
Injected/inseminated	19
Fertilization rate	58%
Cleavage rate	73%
Blastocyst rate	Day 4 vitrification
Culture medium	EmbryoAssist/BlastAssist

Fresh transfer

Quality of embryo(s)	No transfer because of OHSS
Outcome	
Vitrification	1 early blastocyst, 2 morulae (day 4)

Vitrified/warmed cycle: 2013

Stimulation	HSP
Endometrium	9.0 mm
Quality before vitrification	1
Warming day	4
Survival	Yes
Assisted hatching	Yes
Transfer day	5
Quality	5bb
Duration of cryostorage	2 months
Time between warming and transfer	23h

Outcome: Not pregnant

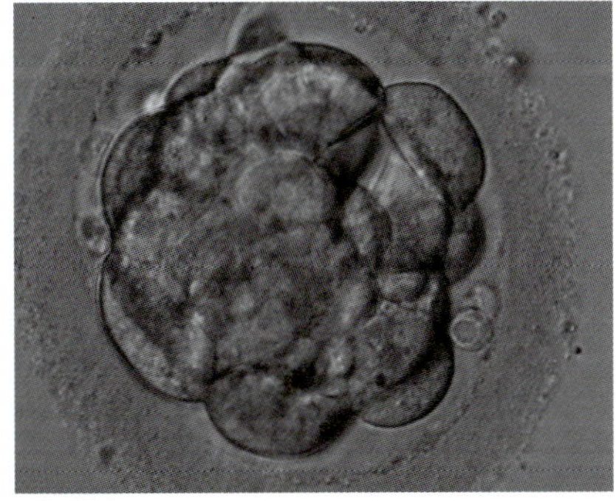

19-BV-1

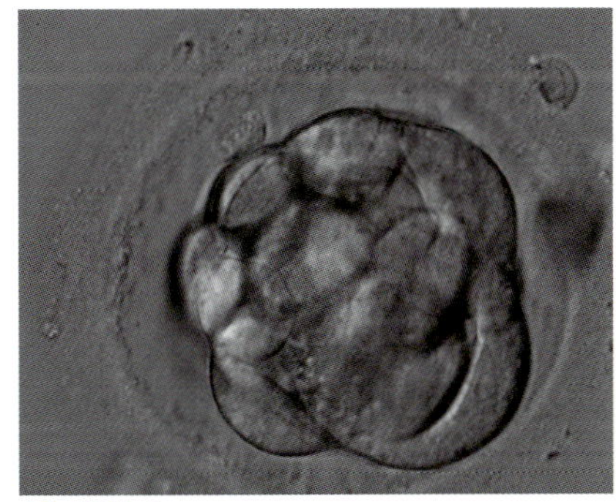

19-AW-1

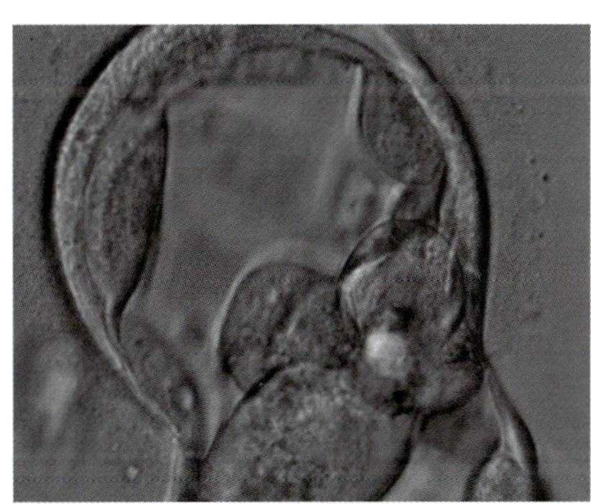

19-BT-1

19-BV-1 Early blastocyst with blastocoel formation at the 2 o'clock position
19-AW-1 Viable early blastocyst
19-BT-1 Hatching blastocyst

Case 20

1 year 1° infertility   **Diagnosis: Endometriosis, tubal infertility**

Female partner

Age 27, saleswoman
Tubal status: bilateral
  blockage
MH: 4–5/14–30
BMI: 28.2
Heavy smoker, no alcohol
  consumption

Basal FSH: 7.6 IU/L
Basal LH: 3.9 IU/L
Basal estradiol: 33.3 pg/mL
Basal AMH: 5.09 ng/mL

Male partner

Age 29, policeman
History/examination: NAD
Smoker, no alcohol
  consumption

Previous treatments

2013 IVF	Failed IVF

Fresh cycle: 2013 ICSI
Semen assessment: normozoospermia

Volume	2 mL
Abstinence	2.2 days
Concentration	48×10^6/mL
Progressive motility	43%
Non-progressive motility	4%
Immotile	53%
Normal forms	8%

Stimulation protocol	Antagonist protocol (HMG)
Days of stimulation	11
Total dose	2475 IU
Estradiol at ovulation induction	2010 ng/mL
Number of follicles ≥ 12 mm	11
Total number of COCs	10
Metaphase II	9
Injected/inseminated	9
Fertilization rate	67%
Cleavage rate	100%
Blastocyst rate	67%
Culture medium	GM501

Fresh transfer

Quality of embryo(s)	5aa
Outcome	Not pregnant
Vitrification	4 blastocysts

Vitrified/warmed cycle: 2013

Stimulation	HSP
Endometrium	10.0 mm
Quality before vitrification	5aa
Warming day	5
Survival	Yes
Assisted hatching	No
Transfer day	5
Quality	5aa
Duration of cryostorage	4 months
Time between warming and transfer	3h

Outcome: Live birth, healthy boy

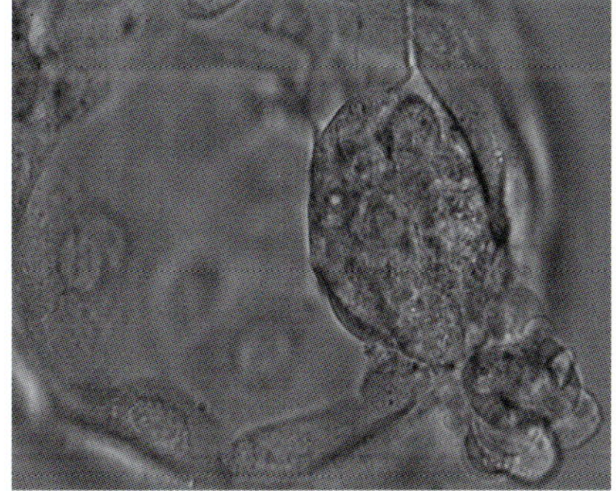

20-BV-1

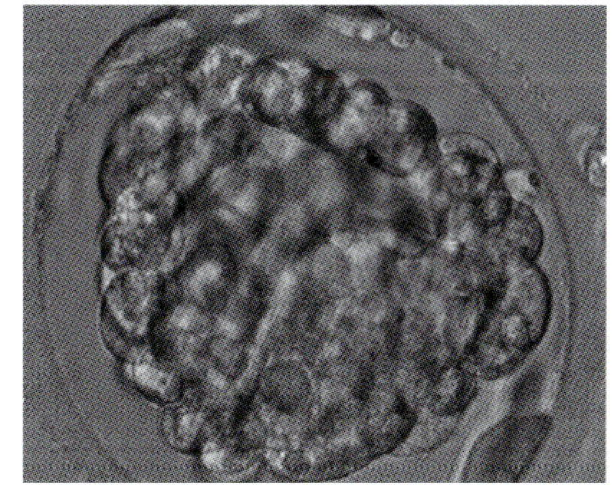

20-AW-1

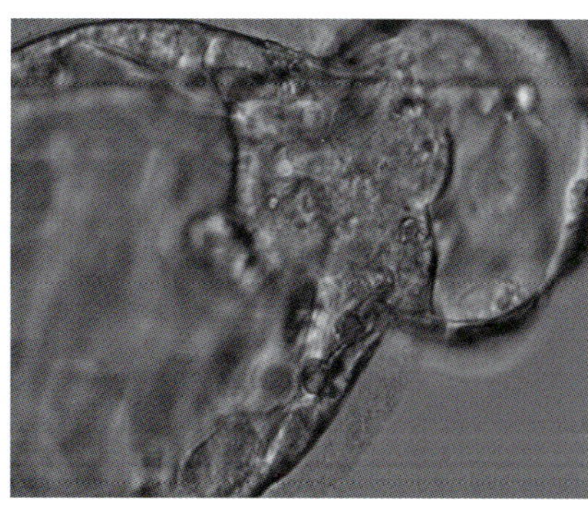

20-BT-1

20-BV-1 Expanded blastocyst hatching from the embryonic pole
20-AW-1 Viable warmed blastocyst
20-BT-1 Hatching blastocyst

Female partner

Age 39, teacher
Tubal status: bilateral
  blockage
MH: 7/27
BMI: 21.3
Non-smoker, no alcohol
  consumption
Myoma

Basal FSH: 6.8 IU/L
Basal LH: 5.6 IU/L
Basal estradiol: 71.4 pg/mL
Basal AMH: 3.52 ng/mL
Midluteal progesterone: 13.6 ng/mL
Midluteal prolactin: 18.7 ng/mL

Male partner

Age 38, engineer
History/examination: NAD
Non-smoker, no alcohol
  consumption
Normal male karyotype

Previous treatments

None

Fresh cycle: 2010 IVF
Semen assessment: normoozoospermia

Volume	4.0 mL
Abstinence	2 days
Concentration	96×10^6/mL
Progressive motility	45%
Non-progressive motility	10%
Immotile	45%
Normal forms	14%

Stimulation protocol	Agonist protocol (HMG)
Days of stimulation	11
Total dose	1725 IU
Estradiol at ovulation induction	3345 ng/mL
Number of follicles ≥ 12 mm	14
Total number of COCs	14
Metaphase II	
Injected/inseminated	14
Fertilization rate	86%
Cleavage rate	100%
Blastocyst rate	67%
Culture medium	EmbryoAssist/BlastAssist

Fresh transfer

Quality of embryo(s)	5aa
Outcome	Live birth, healthy girl
Vitrification	5 blastocysts

Vitrified/warmed cycle: 2013

Stimulation	NC
Endometrium	10.0 mm
Quality before vitrification	4aa
Warming day	5
Survival	Yes
Assisted hatching	Yes
Transfer day	5
Quality	5aa
Duration of cryostorage	3 years
Time between warming and transfer	3h

Outcome: Live birth, healthy boy

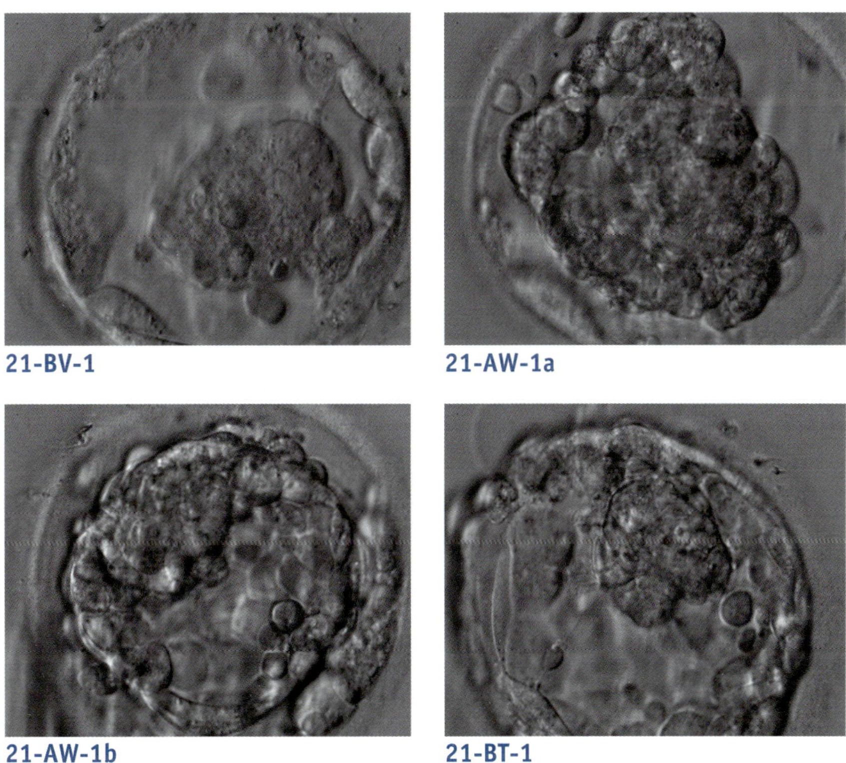

21-BV-1

21-AW-1a

21-AW-1b

21-BT-1

21-BV-1   Expanded blastocyst
21-AW-1a Non re-expanded blastocyst with moderate cytoplasmic granulation
21-AW-1b Beginning re-expansion
21-BT-1   Hatching blastocyst with hatching site out of focus (11 o'clock position)

Female partner

Age 39, worker
Tubal status: patent
MH: 21–28 days
BMI: 25.0
Non-smoker, no alcohol
 consumption
Uterus arcuatus,
 PCO-like ovaries
Basal FSH: 5.3 IU/L

Basal LH: 5.7 IU/L
Basal estradiol: 68 pg/mL
Basal AMH: 17.16 ng/mL
Midluteal progesterone: <0.2 ng/mL
Midluteal prolactin: 16.0 ng/mL
Anovulation

Male partner

Age 38, cook
History/examination: NAD
Smoker, no alcohol
 consumption

Previous treatments

None

Fresh cycle: 2011 ICSI
Semen assessment: oligoasthenoteratozoospermia

Volume	1.2 mL
Abstinence	1 day
Concentration	3×10^6/mL
Progressive motility	15%
Non-progressive motility	10%
Immotile	75%
Normal forms	2%

Stimulation protocol	Antagonist protocol (HMG)
Days of stimulation	11
Total dose	1325 IU
Estradiol at ovulation induction	759 ng/mL
Number of follicles ≥ 12 mm	7
Total number of COCs	5
Metaphase II	3
Injected/inseminated	3
Fertilization rate	100%
Cleavage rate	100%
Blastocyst rate	67%
Culture medium	EmbryoAssist/BlastAssist

Fresh transfer

Quality of embryo(s)	Day 3 embryo with beginning compaction
Outcome	Not pregnant
Vitrification	2 blastocysts (day 5)

Vitrified/warmed cycle: 2013

Stimulation	NC
Endometrium	13 mm
Quality before vitrification	4ab
Warming day	5
Survival	Yes
Assisted hatching	Yes
Transfer day	5
Quality	4ab
Duration of cryostorage	7 months
Time between warming and transfer	3h

Outcome: Live birth, healthy boy

Remarks: Please note vacuole in ICM and cytoplasmic strings in blastocoel (22-BV-1)

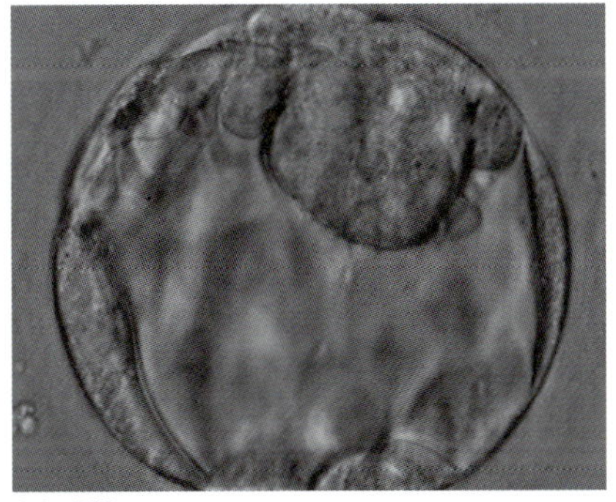

22-BV-1

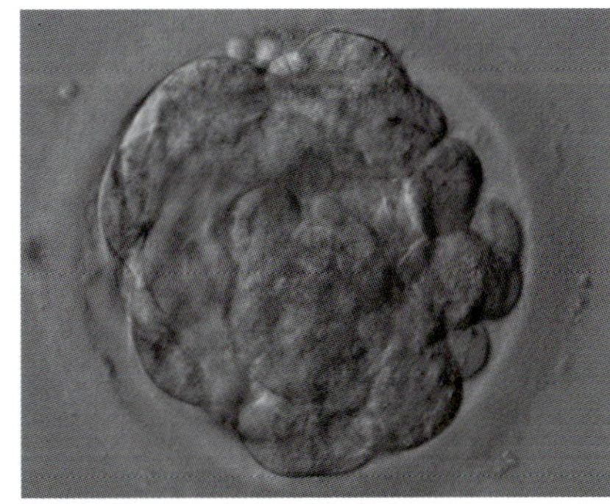

22-AW-1

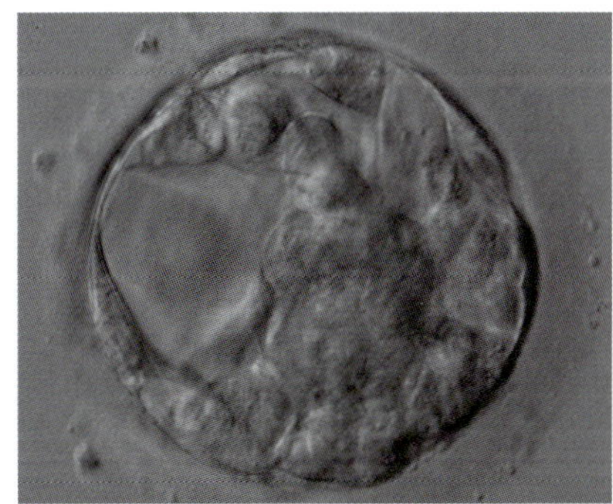

22-BT-1

22-BV-1   Blastocyst (4ab) showing beginning of expansion
22-AW-1   Warmed blastocyst
22-BT-1   Re-expanded blastocyst

Female partner

Age 34, nurse
Tubal status: patent
MH: 5/28
BMI: 23.0
Non-smoker, no alcohol
  consumption
Basal FSH: 12.1 IU/L
Basal LH: 4.4 IU/L

Basal estradiol: 56.5 pg/mL
Basal AMH: 2.77 ng/mL
Midluteal progesterone: 20.1 ng/mL
Midluteal prolactin: 13.3 ng/mL

Male partner

Age 34, technician
History/examination: NAD
Non-smoker, no alcohol
  consumption

Previous treatments

2006 insemination	Not pregnant
2007 ICSI	Not pregnant
2007 Vitrified/warmed cycle × 2	Not pregnant

Fresh cycle: 2013 ICSI
Semen assessment: oligoasthenozoospermia

Volume	2 mL
Abstinence	17 days
Concentration	10×10^6/mL
Progressive motility	15%
Non-progressive motility	15%
Immotile	70%
Normal forms	7%

Stimulation protocol	Antagonist protocol (recombinant FSH)
Days of stimulation	10
Total dose	1425 IU
Estradiol at ovulation induction	3887 ng/mL
Number of follicles ≥ 12 mm	14
Total number of COCs	7
Metaphase II	7
Injected/inseminated	7
Fertilization rate	43%
Cleavage rate	67%
Blastocyst rate	Day 3 transfer
Culture medium	EmbryoAssist/BlastAssist

Fresh transfer

Quality of embryo(s)	8A
Outcome	Not pregnant
Vitrification	Early blastocyst (day 5)

Vitrified/warmed cycle: 2013

Stimulation	HSP
Endometrium	8.5 mm
Quality before vitrification	1
Warming day	5
Survival	Yes
Assisted hatching	Yes
Transfer day	5
Quality	3bb
Duration of cryostorage	10 months
Time between warming and transfer	3h

Outcome: Not pregnant

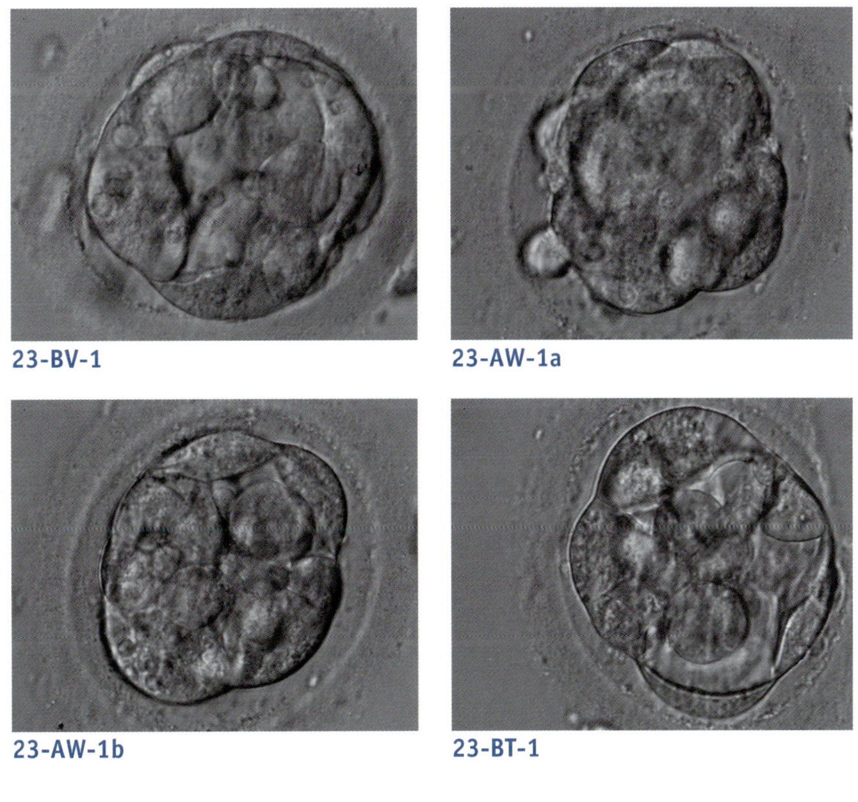

23-BV-1

23-AW-1a

23-AW-1b

23-BT-1

23-BV-1   Early blastocyst
23-AW-1a Viable early blastocyst
23-AW-1b Viable early blastocyst with excluded blastomere in beginning blastocoel
23-BT-1   Full blastocyst with excluded blastomere below inner cell mass

Female partner

Age 28, hairdresser
Tubal status: patent
MH: amenorrhea
BMI: 20.6
Non-smoker, no alcohol
  consumption
Penicillin allergy
Basal FSH: 5.3 IU/L
Basal LH: 5.1 IU/L

Basal estradiol: 31.9 pg/mL
Basal AMH: 11.30 ng/mL
Midluteal progesterone: 0.2 ng/mL
Midluteal prolactin: 4.9 ng/mL
TSH: 2.58 IU/L
Androstenedione: 2.53 ng/mL

Male partner

Age 29, lorry driver
History/examination: NAD
Non-smoker, no alcohol
  consumption

Previous treatments

None

Fresh cycle: 2011 ICSI
Semen assessment: teratozoospermia

Volume	4 mL
Abstinence	8 days
Concentration	36×10^6/mL
Progressive motility	50%
Non-progressive motility	0%
Immotile	50%
Normal forms	2%

Stimulation protocol	Antagonist protocol (recombinant FSH)
Days of stimulation	19
Total dose	1275 IU
Estradiol at ovulation induction	616 ng/mL
Number of follicles ≥ 12 mm	8
Total number of COCs	16
Metaphase II	8
Injected/inseminated	8
Fertilization rate	38%
Cleavage rate	100%
Blastocyst rate	Cryopreservation day 4
Culture medium	EmbryoAssist/BlastAssist

Fresh transfer

Quality of embryo(s)	No fresh transfer because of OHSS
Outcome	
Vitrification	2 compacting embryos and 1 morula (day 4)

Vitrified/warmed cycle: 2012

Stimulation	HSP
Endometrium	8.7 mm
Quality before vitrification	Morula (day 4)
Warming day	4
Survival	Partial
Assisted hatching	Yes
Transfer day	4
Quality	1
Duration of cryostorage	3 months
Time between warming and transfer	3h

Outcome: Live birth, boy, malformations (mild form of Goldenhar syndrome)

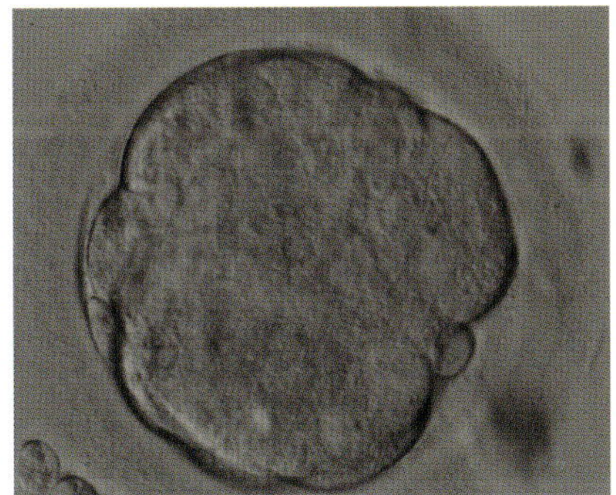

24-BV-1

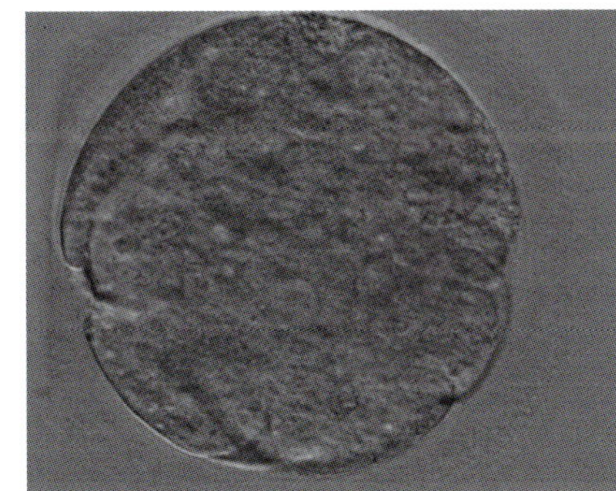

24-AW-1

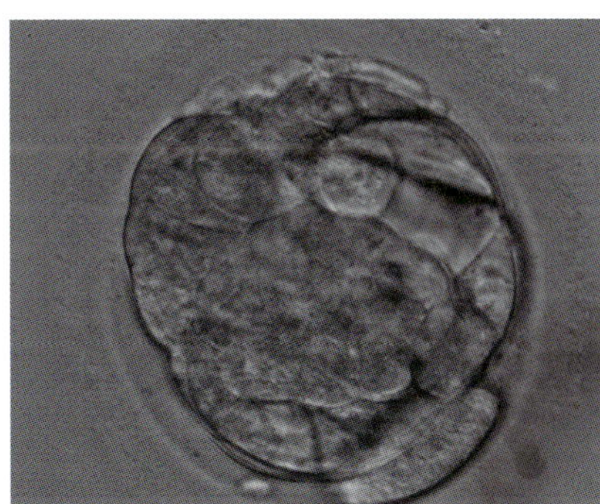

24-BT-1

24-BV-1 Beginning morula
24-AW-1 Warmed morula with signs of degeneration (extensive granulation, almost no membranes visible)
24-BT-1 Viable early blastocyst (1) with excluded fragments

Female partner

Age 31, pharmacist
Tubal status: patent
MH: 5/28
BMI: 23.8
Non-smoker, no alcohol
  consumption

Basal FSH: 5.6 IU/L
Basal LH: 4.1 IU/L
Basal estradiol: 32.1 pg/mL
Basal AMH: 4.31 ng/mL

Male partner

Age 40, clinician
History/examination: NAD
Non-smoker, no alcohol
  consumption

Previous treatments

2009 external ICSI × 2	Not pregnant
2010 external ICSI × 1	Not pregnant
2010 external frozen/thawed transfer × 2	Not pregnant

Fresh cycle: 2011 ICSI

Semen assessment: asthenoteratozoospermia

Volume	6 mL
Abstinence	4 days
Concentration	22×10^6/mL
Progressive motility	18%
Non-progressive motility	14%
Immotile	68%
Normal forms	3%

Stimulation protocol	Antagonist protocol (recombinant FSH+HMG)
Days of stimulation	10
Total dose	2500 IU
Estradiol at ovulation induction	2278 ng/mL
Number of follicles ≥ 12 mm	15
Total number of COCs	20
Metaphase II	15
Injected/inseminated	15
Fertilization rate	87%
Cleavage rate	100%
Blastocyst rate	31%
Culture medium	EmbryoAssist/BlastAssist

Fresh transfer

Quality of embryo(s)	4aa
Outcome	Not pregnant
Vitrification	2 blastocysts, 1 morula

Vitrified/warmed cycle: 2012

Stimulation	HSP
Endometrium	10.5 mm
Quality before vitrification	5ab, morula
Warming day	5
Survival	Yes, Yes
Assisted hatching	Yes, Yes
Transfer day	5
Quality	5aa, 1
Duration of cryostorage	11 months
Time between warming and transfer	2h

Outcome: Live birth, healthy boy

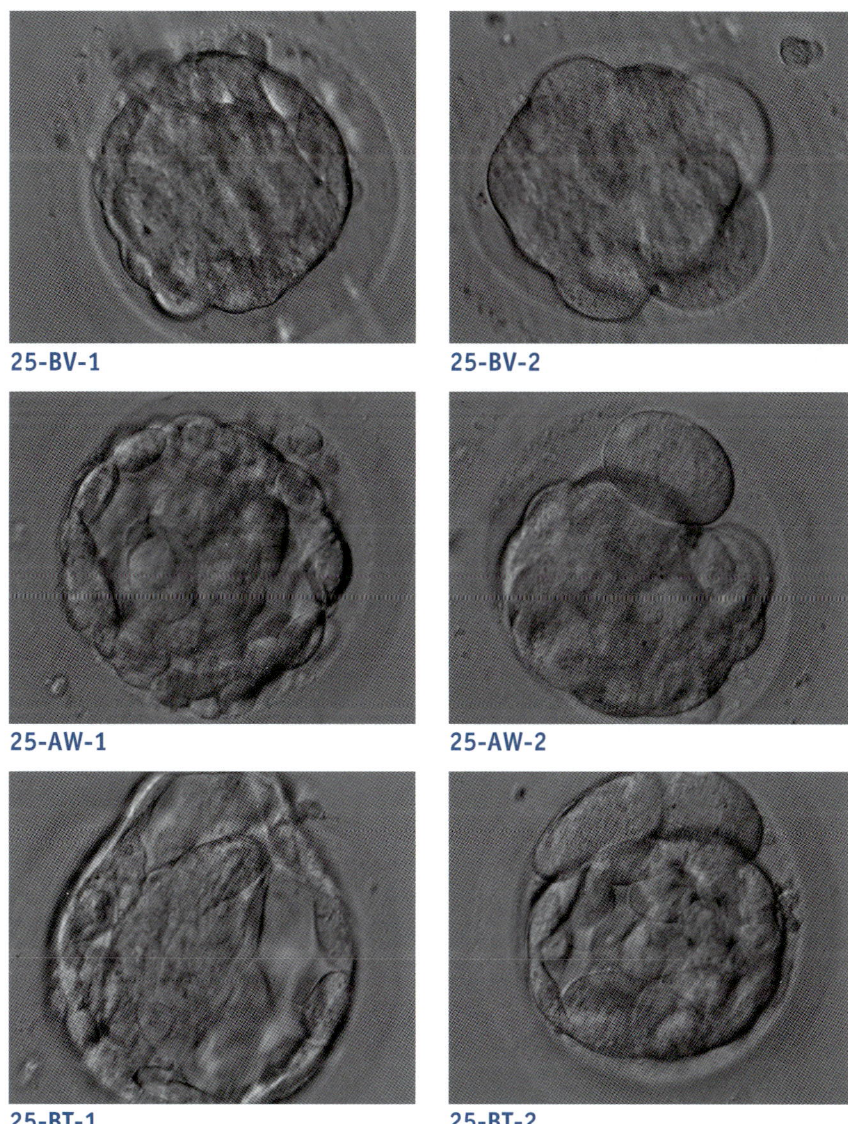

25-BV-1   25-BV-2

25-AW-1   25-AW-2

25-BT-1   25-BT-2

25-BV-1   Hatching blastocyst that collapsed during hatching process (hatching site at 11 o'clock position)
25-AW-1   Partly re-expanded blastocyst
25-BT-1   Hatching of blastocyst through artificial gap
25-BV-2   Beginning morula
25-AW-2   Morula with excluded blastomere
25-BT-2   Early blastocyst with 2 excluded blastomeres

Female partner

Age 26, saleswoman
Tubal status: patent
MH: 5/28, dysmenorrhea
BMI: 23.7
Smoker, no alcohol
  consumption
Normal female karyotype

Basal FSH: 6.7 IU/L
Basal LH: 3.5 IU/L
Basal estradiol: 30.7 pg/mL
Basal AMH: 10.34 ng/mL
Midluteal progesterone: 11.3 ng/mL
Midluteal prolactin: 32.4 ng/mL

Male partner

Age 30, farmer
History/examination: carrier
  of Delta-F-508 mutation
  (cystic fibrosis)
Non-smoker, no alcohol
  consumption

Previous treatments

None

Fresh cycle: 2011 ICSI
Semen assessment: cryptozoospermia

Volume	3.3 mL
Abstinence	2 days
Concentration	0.001×10^6/mL
Progressive motility	5%
Non-progressive motility	0%
Immotile	95%
Normal forms	0%

Stimulation protocol	Agonist protocol (recombinant FSH)
Days of stimulation	11
Total dose	1650 IU
Estradiol at ovulation induction	3921 ng/mL
Number of follicles ≥ 12 mm	30
Total number of COCs	28
Metaphase II	24
Injected/inseminated	23
Fertilization rate	83%
Cleavage rate	95%
Blastocyst rate	74%
Culture medium	EmbryoAssist/BlastAssist

Fresh transfer

Quality of embryo(s)	No transfer because of OHSS
Outcome	
Vitrification	12 blastocysts

Previous vitrified/warmed cycles

2011 ×3   Not pregnant
2012 ×1   Not pregnant

Vitrified/warmed cycle: 2012

Stimulation	NC
Endometrium	9.5 mm
Quality before vitrification	3ab
Warming day	5
Survival	Yes
Assisted hatching	Yes
Transfer day	5
Quality	3ab
Duration of cryostorage	1 year
Time between warming and transfer	3h

Outcome: Biochemical pregnancy

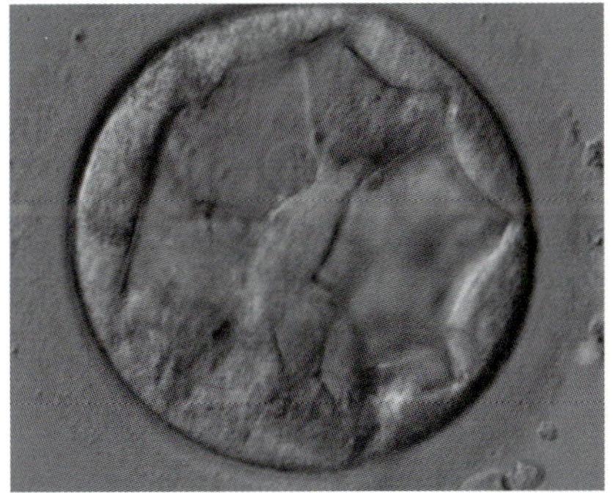 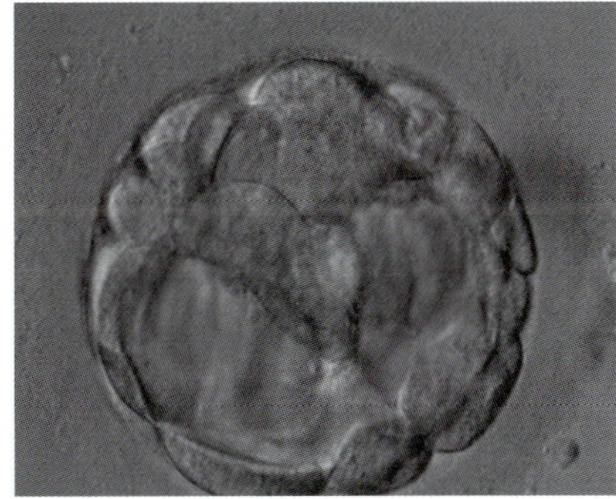 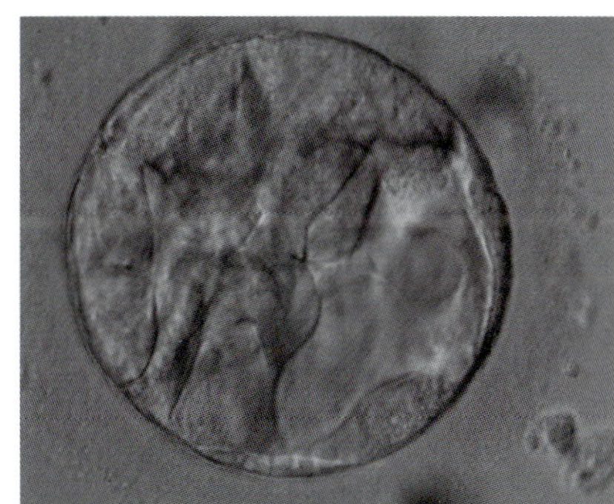

26-BV-1　　　　　　26-AW-1　　　　　　26-BT-1

26-BV-1 Full blastocyst
26-AW-1 Full blastocyst showing immediate re-expansion
26-BT-1 Full blastocyst with trophectoderm consisting of few cells

Case 27

12 years 2° infertility   **Diagnosis: Endometriosis, tubal infertility**

Female partner

Age 38, nurse
Tubal status: bilateral
  tubectomy
MH: 6–7/28
BMI: 19.3
Smoker, no alcohol
  consumption
3 ectopic pregnancies

Basal FSH: 6.9 IU/L
Basal LH: 11.7 IU/L
Basal estradiol: 43.5 pg/mL
Basal AMH: 8.86 ng/mL
Midluteal prolactin: 20.8 ng/mL

Male partner

Age 39, clinician
History/examination: NAD
Smoker, no alcohol consumption

Previous treatments

2010 external IVF ×2	Not pregnant, low fertilization
2011 external ICSI ×2	Not pregnant, low fertilization

Fresh cycle: 2012 ICSI with ionophore treatment
Semen assessment: asthenozoospermia

Volume	8.5 mL
Abstinence	10 days
Concentration	95×10^6/mL
Progressive motility	10%
Non-progressive motility	10%
Immotile	80%
Normal forms	6%

Stimulation protocol	Agonist protocol (HMG)
Days of stimulation	10
Total dose	1125 IU
Estradiol at ovulation induction	3663 ng/mL
Number of follicles ≥ 12 mm	23
Total number of COCs	18
Metaphase II	15
Injected/inseminated	14
Fertilization rate	86%
Cleavage rate	100%
Blastocyst rate	75%
Culture medium	EmbryoAssist/BlastAssist

Fresh transfer

Quality of embryo(s)	No transfer because of OHSS
Outcome	
Vitrification	6 blastocysts

Vitrified/warmed cycle: 2013

Stimulation	HSP
Endometrium	8.5 mm
Quality before vitrification	4aa
Warming day	5
Survival	Yes
Assisted hatching	Yes
Transfer day	5
Quality	4aa
Duration of cryostorage	3 months
Time between warming and transfer	2h

Outcome: Live birth, healthy boy

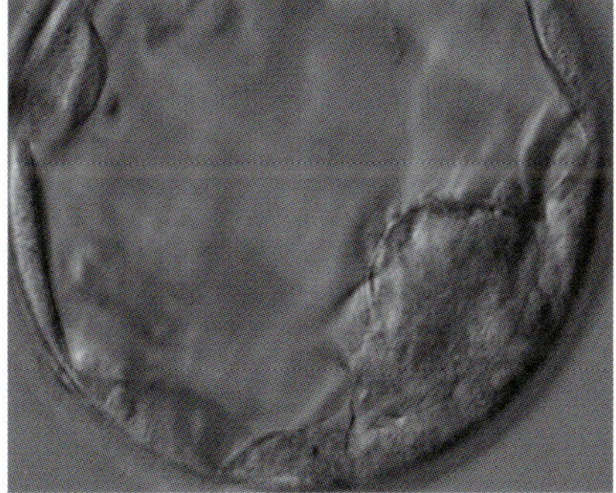

27-BV-1

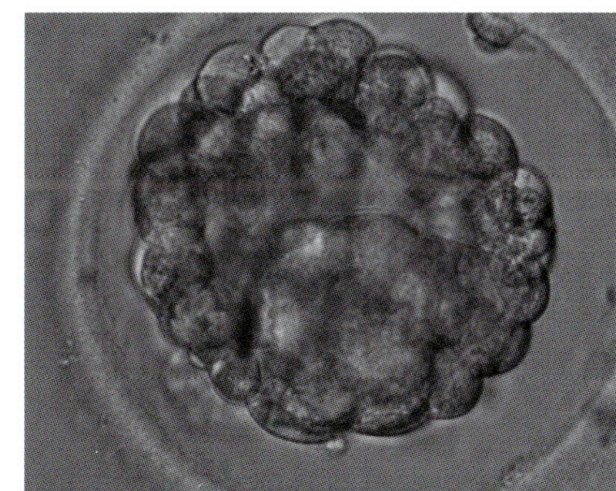

27-AW-1

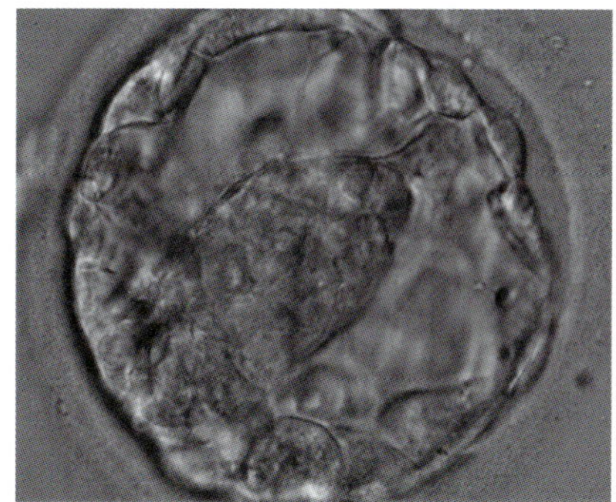

27-BT-1

27-BV-1 Expanded blastocyst with cytoplasmic strings out of focus
27-AW-1 Expanded blastocyst with moderate cytoplasmic granulation
27-BT-1 Hatching blastocyst with hatching site out of focus (9 o'clock position)

Female partner

Age 28, civil servant

Tubal status: unilateral tubectomy

MH: 4–5/27

BMI: 29.0

Non-smoker, no alcohol
  consumption

Normal female karyotype

Adipositas

Basal FSH: 11.0 IU/L

Basal LH: 4.5 IU/L

Basal estradiol: 25.3 pg/mL

Basal AMH: 0.73 ng/mL

TSH: 1.33 IU/L

Male partner

Age 29, civil servant

History/examination: NAD

Non-smoker, no alcohol consumption

Normal male karyotype

Previous treatments

2010 ICSI	Not pregnant
2010 vitrified/warmed cycle	Not pregnant
2011 ICSI	Not pregnant
2011 ICSI	Live birth, healthy boy
2012 insemination	Not pregnant

Fresh cycle: 2012 ICSI (patient wish)

Semen assessment: normozoospermia

Volume	3.0 mL
Abstinence	3 days
Concentration	52×10^6/mL
Progressive motility	52%
Non-progressive motility	6%
Immotile	42%
Normal forms	9%

Stimulation protocol	Agonist protocol (HMG)
Days of stimulation	10
Total dose	2475 IU
Estradiol at ovulation induction	2769 ng/mL
Number of follicles $\geq$ 12 mm	14
Total number of COCs	13
Metaphase II	12
Injected/inseminated	12
Fertilization rate	83%
Cleavage rate	100%
Blastocyst rate	88%
Culture medium	EmbryoAssist/BlastAssist

Fresh transfer

Quality of embryo(s)	5aa
Outcome	Not pregnant
Vitrification	2 morulae, 4 blastocysts (day 4), 1 blastocyst (day 5)

Vitrified/warmed cycle: 2013

Stimulation	HSP
Endometrium	12.0 mm
Quality before vitrification	1
Warming day	5
Survival	Yes
Assisted hatching	Yes
Transfer day	5
Quality	3bb
Duration of cryostorage	7 months
Time between warming and transfer	3h

Outcome: Ectopic pregnancy

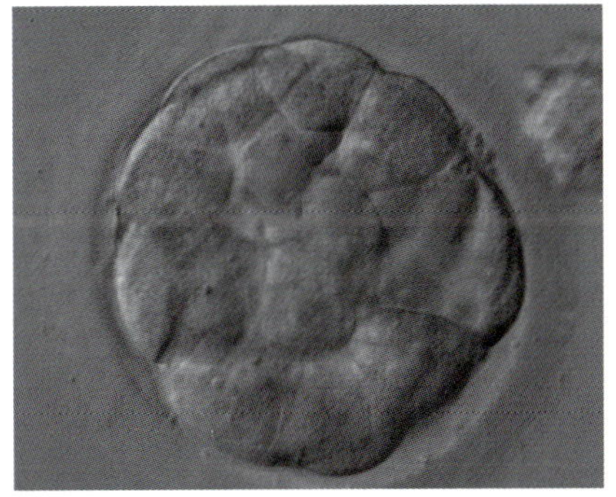

28-BV-1

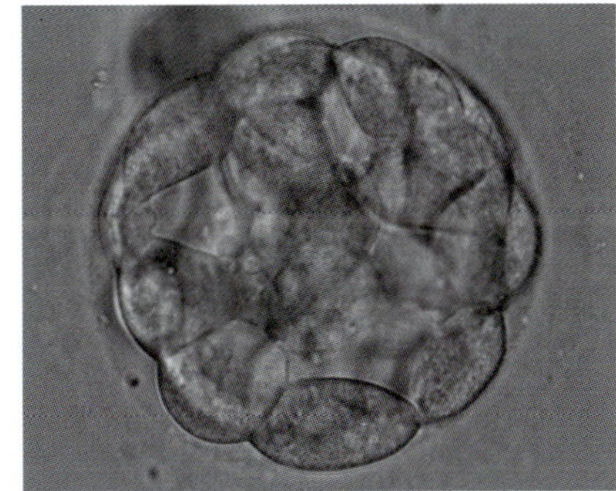

28-AW-1

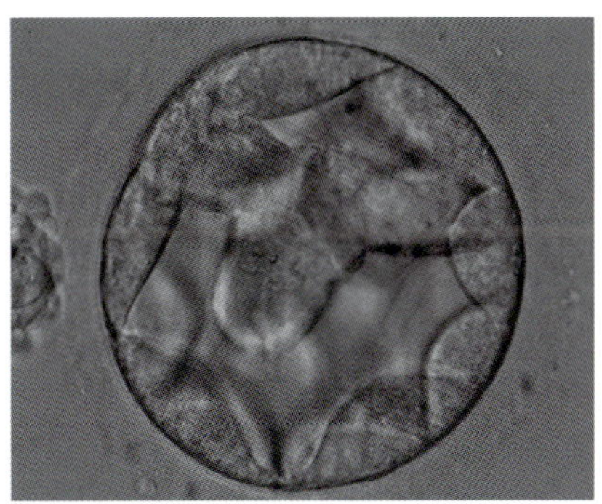

28-BT-1

28-BV-1 Early blastocyst
28-AW-1 Early blastocyst
28-BT-1 Full blastocyst with moderate quality

Case 29

2 years 2° infertility   Diagnosis: Unexplained infertility

Female partner

Age 30, office administrator
Tubal status: patent
MH: 5/28
BMI: 22.3
Non-smoker, no alcohol
  consumption
Cervical stenosis

Basal FSH: 5.9 IU/L
Basal LH: 7.6 IU/L
Basal estradiol: 48.8 pg/mL
Basal AMH: 2.86 ng/mL
Midluteal progesterone: 6.4 ng/mL
Midluteal prolactin: 14.5 ng/mL

Male partner

Age 28, employee
History/examination: NAD
Non-smoker, no alcohol
  consumption

Previous treatments

None

Fresh cycle: 2012 ICSI (patient wish)
Semen assessment: normozoospermia

Volume	6.8 mL
Abstinence	4 days
Concentration	154×10^6/mL
Progressive motility	46%
Non-progressive motility	5%
Immotile	49%
Normal forms	%

Stimulation protocol	Antagonist protocol (HMG)
Days of stimulation	8
Total dose	1350 IU
Estradiol at ovulation induction	1097 ng/mL
Number of follicles ≥ 12 mm	10
Total number of COCs	6
Metaphase II	5
Injected/inseminated	5
Fertilization rate	40%
Cleavage rate	100%
Blastocyst rate	Cryopreservation day 4
Culture medium	EmbryoAssist/BlastAssist

Fresh transfer

Quality of embryo(s)	No fresh transfer manageable because of cervical stenosis
Outcome	
Vitrification	1 compacting embryo and 1 early blastocyst (day 4)

Vitrified/warmed cycle: 2013

Stimulation	HSP
Endometrium	9.5 mm
Quality before vitrification	II (day 4)
Warming day	4
Survival	Yes
Assisted hatching	Yes
Transfer day	4
Quality	3ba
Duration of cryostorage	2 months
Time between warming and transfer	3h

Outcome: Live birth, healthy boy

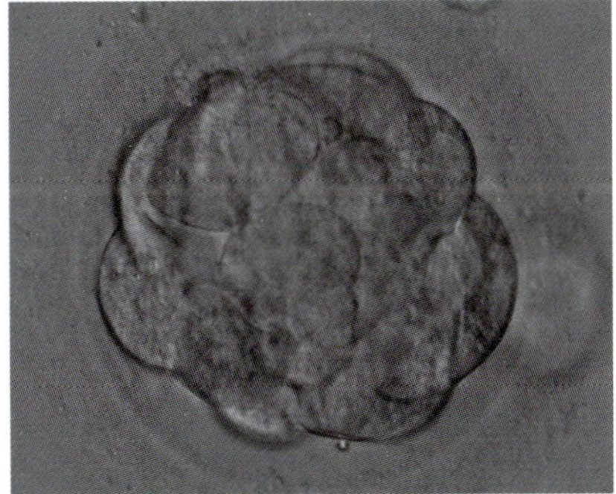

29-BV-1

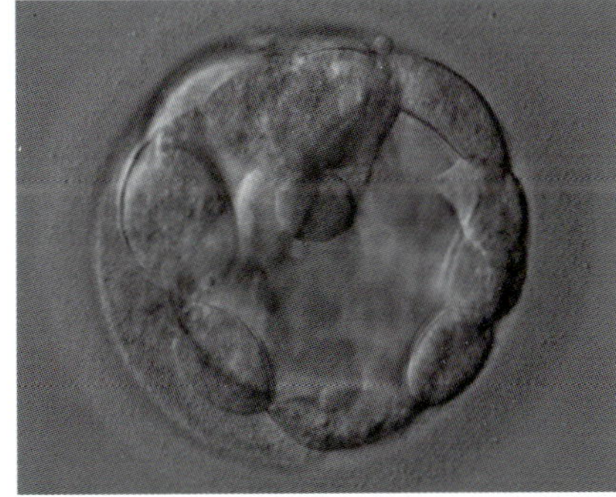

29-AW-1

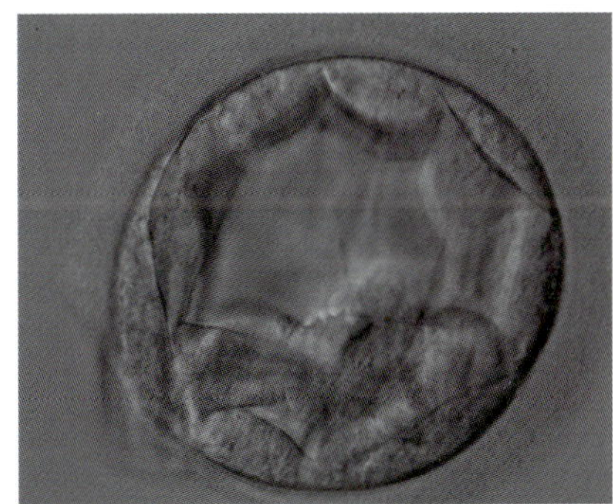

29-BT-1

29-BV-1   Early blastocyst
29-AW-1   Early blastocyst with lysed blastomeres in the bottom left area of the PVS
29-BT-1   Full blastocyst (lysed cells close to hatching site)

Female partner

Age 31, police officer
Tubal status: patent
MH: cycle length 42 days
BMI: 23.3
Non-smoker, no alcohol
  consumption
PCO-like ovaries, anovulation
Hypothyreosis

Basal FSH: 4.8 IU/L
Basal LH: 2.4 IU/L
Basal estradiol: 26.0 pg/mL
Basal AMH: 5.23 ng/mL
Midluteal progesterone: 0.3 ng/mL
Midluteal prolactin: 32.9 ng/mL

Male partner

Age 32, businessman
History/examination: NAD
Non-smoker, no alcohol
  consumption

Previous treatments

None

Fresh cycle: 2011 ICSI
Semen assessment: asthenoteratozoospermia

Volume	6.4 mL
Abstinence	3 days
Concentration	18×10^6/mL
Progressive motility	11%
Non-progressive motility	22%
Immotile	67%
Normal forms	3%

Stimulation protocol	Antagonist protocol (recombinant FSH)
Days of stimulation	10
Total dose	1400 IU
Estradiol at ovulation induction	1916 ng/mL
Number of follicles ≥ 12 mm	15
Total number of COCs	15
Metaphase II	12
Injected/inseminated	12
Fertilization rate	66.7%
Cleavage rate	100%
Blastocyst rate	63%
Culture medium	GM501

Fresh transfer

Quality of embryo(s)	No fresh transfer because of OHSS
Outcome	
Vitrification	3 compacting embryos, 1 early blastocyst (day 4), 1 blastocyst (day 5)

Vitrified/warmed cycle: 2013

Stimulation	HSP
Endometrium	8.5 mm
Quality before vitrification	4ab
Warming day	5
Survival	Yes
Assisted hatching	Yes
Transfer day	5
Quality	4ab
Duration of cryostorage	3 months
Time between warming and transfer	3

Outcome: Live birth, healthy girl

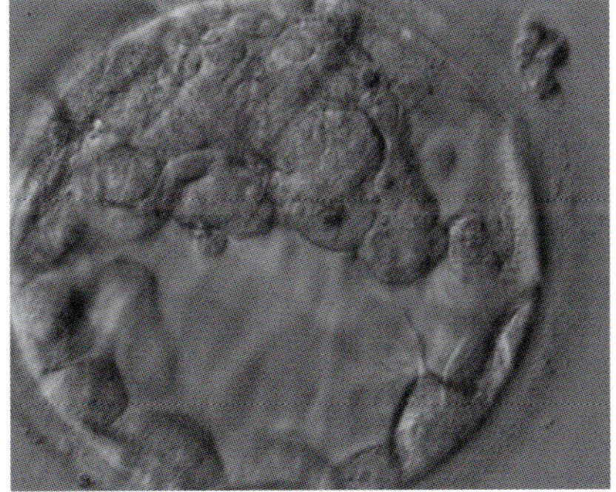
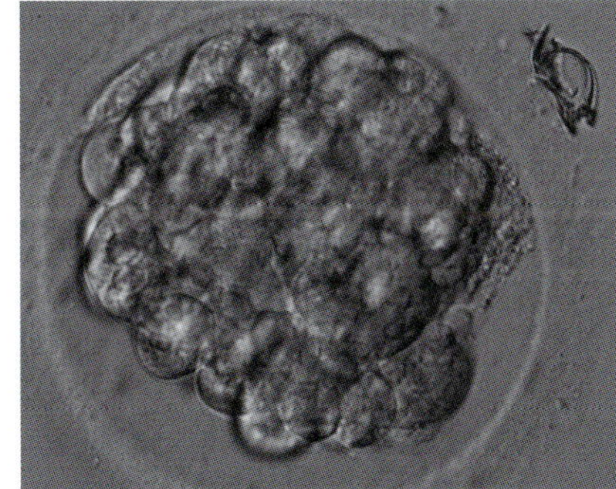
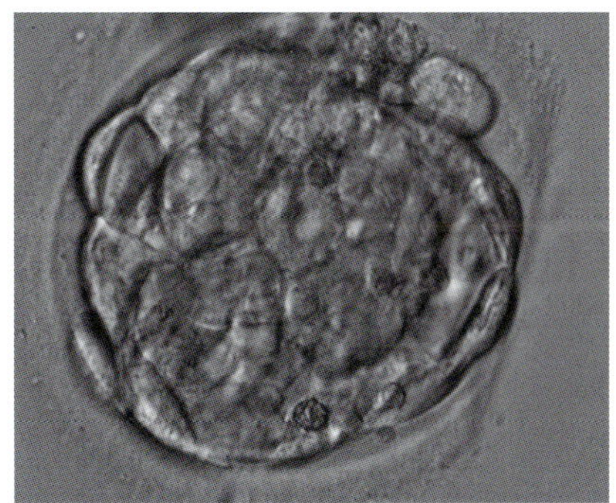

30-BV-1

30-AW-1

30-BT-1

30-BV-1 Expanded blastocyst (4ab)
30-AW-1 Warmed blastocyst with plastic remnants from the culture dish (2 o'clock position)
30-BT-1 Re-expanded blastocyst with excluded fragments (top section of image)

Female partner

Age 36, cleaner
Tubal status: patent
MH: 5/21–35
BMI: 24.5
Non-smoker, no alcohol
  consumption
3 spontaneous live births,
  1 stillbirth

Basal FSH: 6.0 IU/L
Basal LH: 1.3 IU/L
Basal estradiol: 32.0 pg/mL
Basal AMH: 1.68 ng/mL
Midluteal progesterone: 14.0 ng/mL
Midluteal prolactin: 13.6 ng/mL

Male partner

Age 41, taxi driver
History/examination: unilateral
  orchiectomy
Smoker, no alcohol
  consumption

Previous treatments

None

Fresh cycle: 2011 ICSI
Semen assessment: asthenoteratozoospermia

Volume	5.2 mL
Abstinence	7 days
Concentration	32×10^6/mL
Progressive motility	9%
Non-progressive motility	6%
Immotile	85%
Normal forms	3%

Stimulation protocol	Agonist protocol (recombinant FSH)
Days of stimulation	13
Total dose	1825 IU
Estradiol at ovulation induction	1488 ng/mL
Number of follicles ≥ 12 mm	7
Total number of COCs	6
Metaphase II	6
Injected/inseminated	6
Fertilization rate	100%
Cleavage rate	100%
Blastocyst rate	17%
Culture medium	EmbryoAssist/BlastAssist

Fresh transfer

Quality of embryo(s)	3aa
Outcome	Not pregnant
Vitrification	2 compacting embryos (day 5)

Vitrified/warmed cycle: 2013

Stimulation	NC
Endometrium	9.0 mm
Quality before vitrification	Morula
Warming day	5
Survival	Yes
Assisted hatching	Yes
Transfer day	5
Quality	1
Duration of cryostorage	7 months
Time between warming and transfer	6h

Outcome: Biochemical pregnancy

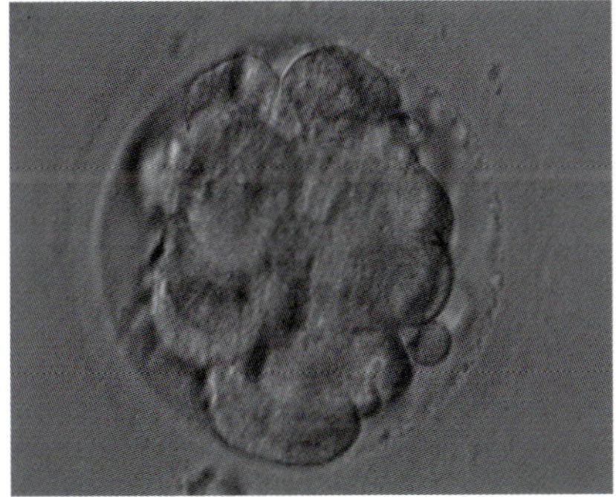

31-BV-1

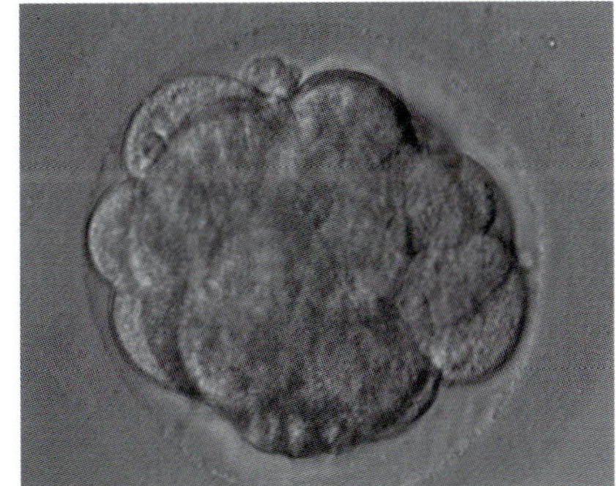

31-AW-1

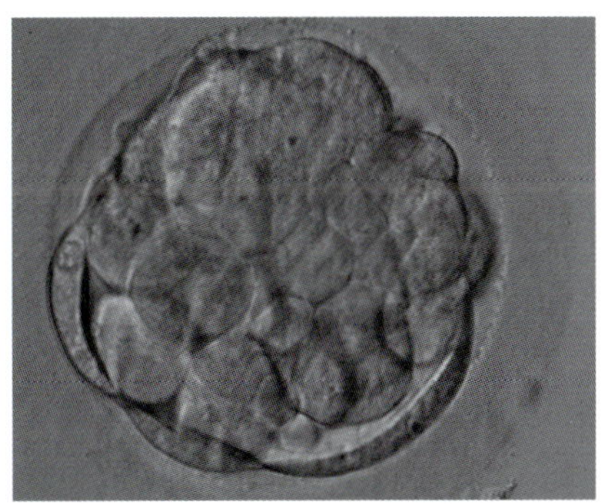

31-BT-1

31-BV-1 Compacting embryo
31-AW-1 Viable compacting embryo with cytoplasmic pitting
31-BT-1 Early blastocyst

Case 32

5 years 2° infertility   Diagnosis: Male factor infertility

Female partner

Age 37, bank assistant
Tubal status: patent
MH: 3–5/28–34
BMI: 37.5
Non-smoker, no alcohol
  consumption
Adipositas

Basal FSH: 6.4 IU/L
Basal LH: 2.7 IU/L
Basal estradiol: 39.5 pg/mL
Basal AMH: 3.99 ng/mL
Midluteal progesterone: 0.2 ng/mL
Midluteal prolactin: 10.4 ng/mL

Male partner

Age 34, bank assistant
History/examination: NAD
Non-smoker, no alcohol
  consumption

Previous treatments

None

Fresh cycle: 2013 ICSI
Semen assessment: teratozoospermia

Volume	1.0 mL
Abstinence	3 days
Concentration	112×10^6/mL
Progressive motility	35%
Non-progressive motility	5%
Immotile	60%
Normal forms	3%

Stimulation protocol	Antagonist protocol (HMG)
Days of stimulation	10
Total dose	2550 IU
Estradiol at ovulation induction	1391 ng/mL
Number of follicles ≥ 12 mm	15
Total number of COCs	15
Metaphase II	11
Injected/inseminated	10
Fertilization rate	90%
Cleavage rate	89%
Blastocyst rate	56%
Culture medium	EmbryoAssist/BlastAssist

Fresh transfer

Quality of embryo(s)	4aa
Outcome	Missed abortion
Vitrification	2 blastocysts

Vitrified/warmed cycle: 2014

Stimulation	HSP
Endometrium	12.0 mm
Quality before vitrification	5aa
Warming day	5
Survival	Yes
Assisted hatching	Yes
Transfer day	5
Quality	5aa
Duration of cryostorage	7 months
Time between warming and transfer	5h

Outcome: Pregnant, missed abortion (no heart activity)

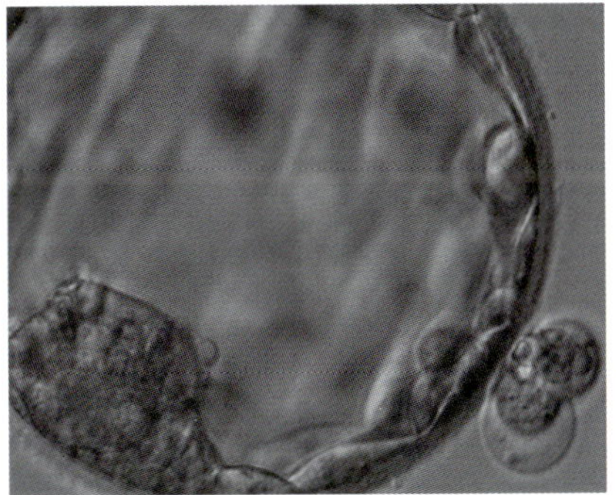 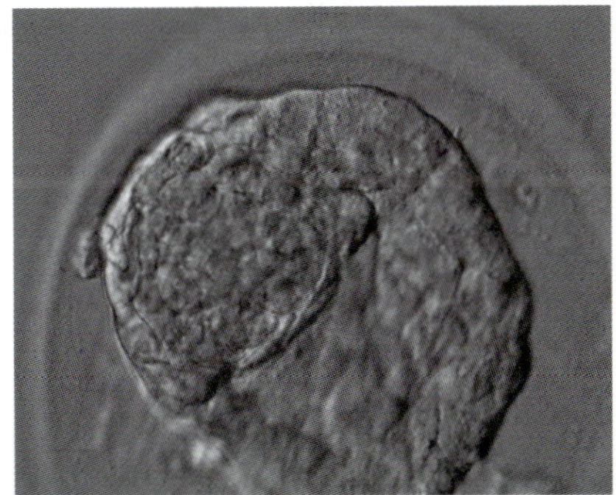 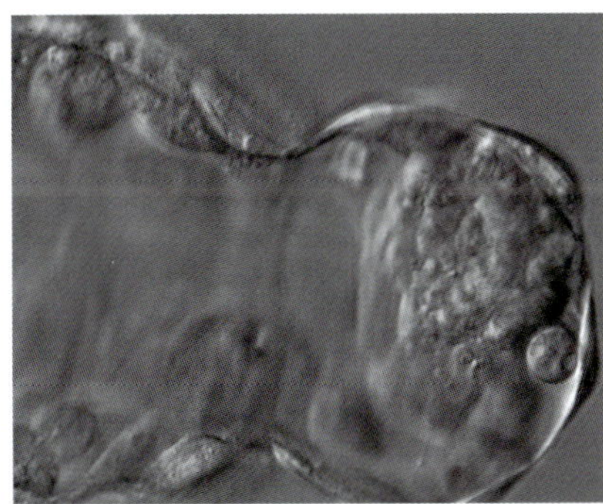

32-BV-1   **32-AW-1**   **32-BT-1**

32-BV-1   Blastocyst hatching at 4 o'clock position
32-AW-1   Warmed blastocyst
32-BT-1   Blastocyst hatching from the site of the inner cell mass

Female partner

Age 38, kindergartener
Tubal status: patent
MH: 5/28
BMI: 24.2
Smoker, no alcohol consumption
Basal FSH: 6.8 IU/L
Basal LH: 4.5 IU/L
Basal estradiol: 30.0 pg/mL
Basal AMH: 2.74 ng/mL

Male partner

Age 40, teacher
History/examination: NAD
Non-smoker, no alcohol consumption

Previous treatments

None

Fresh cycle: 2008 ICSI
Semen assessment: oligoasthenoteratozoospermia

Volume	3.2 mL
Abstinence	7 days
Concentration	7×10^6/mL
Progressive motility	12%
Non-progressive motility	24%
Immotile	64%
Normal forms	2%

Stimulation protocol	Agonist protocol (HMG)
Days of stimulation	9
Total dose	1500 IU
Estradiol at ovulation induction	2229 ng/mL
Number of follicles ≥ 12 mm	10
Total number of COCs	9
Metaphase II	8
Injected/inseminated	8
Fertilization rate	75%
Cleavage rate	83%
Blastocyst rate	80%
Culture medium	EmbryoAssist/BlastAssist

Fresh transfer

Quality of embryo(s)	Morula, 3ab
Outcome	Not pregnant
Vitrification	2 blastocysts

Vitrified/warmed cycle: 2013

Stimulation	NC
Endometrium	8.0 mm
Quality before vitrification	3ab
Warming day	5
Survival	Yes
Assisted hatching	Yes
Transfer day	5
Quality	2
Duration of cryostorage	3 years
Time between warming and transfer	2h

Outcome: Missed abortion, no heart activity

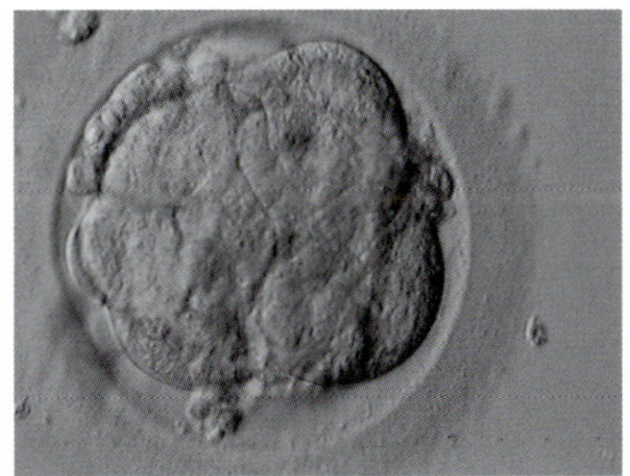

33-BV-1

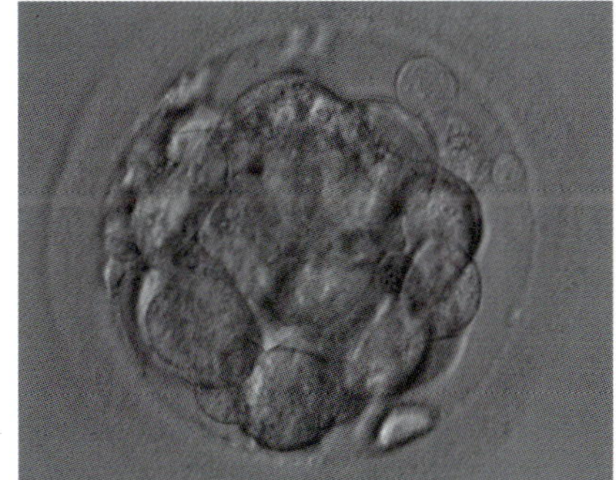

33-AW-1

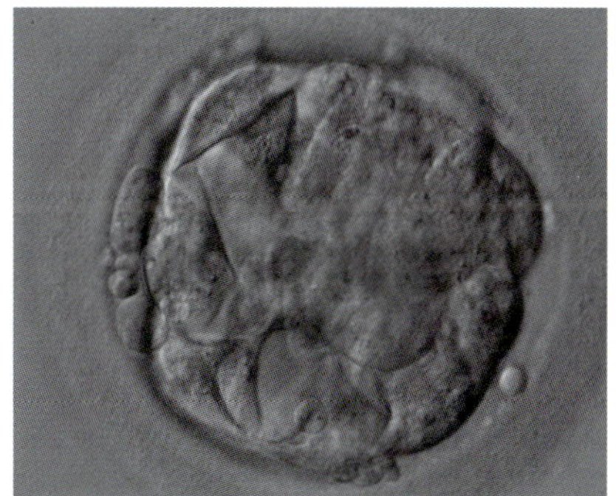

33-BT-1

33-BV-1 Early blastocyst (blastocoel out of view)
33-AW-1 Early blastocyst without re-expansion
33-BT-1 Re-expanded early blastocyst (location of inner cell mass can be estimated)

Female partner

Age 31, cook
Tubal status: patent
MH: 5/28
BMI: 21.9
Smoker, no alcohol consumption
Normal female karyotype
History of thrombosis
Basal FSH: 6.0 IU/L
Basal LH: 4.1 IU/L
Basal estradiol: 29.6 pg/mL
Basal AMH: 3.3 ng/mL

Male partner

Age 32, interpreter
History/examination: mumps in puberty
Non-smoker, no alcohol consumption
Normal male karyotype

Previous treatments

None

Fresh cycle: 2010 ICSI
Semen assessment: severe oligoasthenoteratozoospermia

Volume	6 mL
Abstinence	8 days
Concentration	0.7×10^6/mL
Progressive motility	12%
Non-progressive motility	7%
Immotile	81%
Normal forms	0%

Stimulation protocol	Agonist protocol (recombinant FSH)
Days of stimulation	11
Total dose	1650 IU
Estradiol at ovulation induction	1669 ng/mL
Number of follicles ≥ 12 mm	15
Total number of COCs	14
Metaphase II	13
Injected/inseminated	13
Fertilization rate	85%
Cleavage rate	100%
Blastocyst rate	64%
Culture medium	GM501

Fresh transfer

Quality of embryo(s)	5aa
Outcome	Not pregnant
Vitrification	6 blastocysts

Vitrified/warmed cycle: 2012

Stimulation	NC
Endometrium	10.0 mm
Quality before vitrification	5aa
Warming day	5
Survival	Yes
Assisted hatching	Yes
Transfer day	5
Quality	5aa
Duration of cryostorage	21 months
Time between warming and transfer	2h

Outcome: Live birth, healthy boy

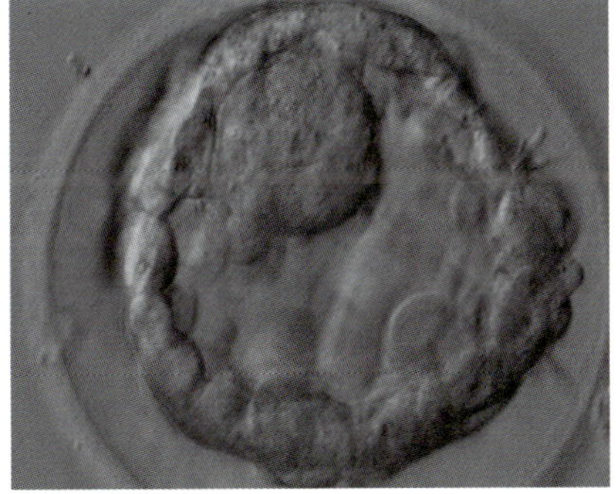

34-BV-1

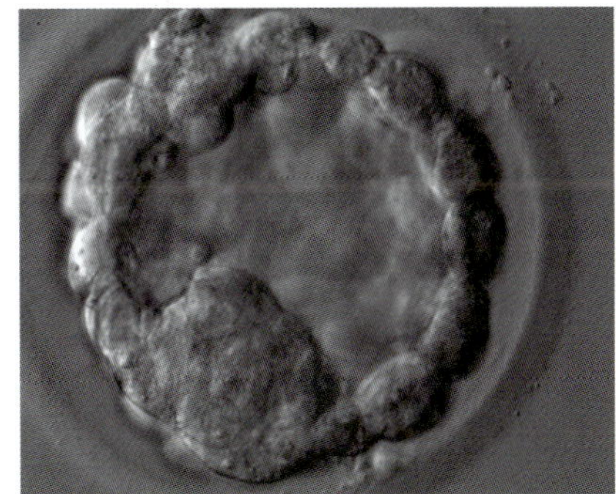

34-AW-1

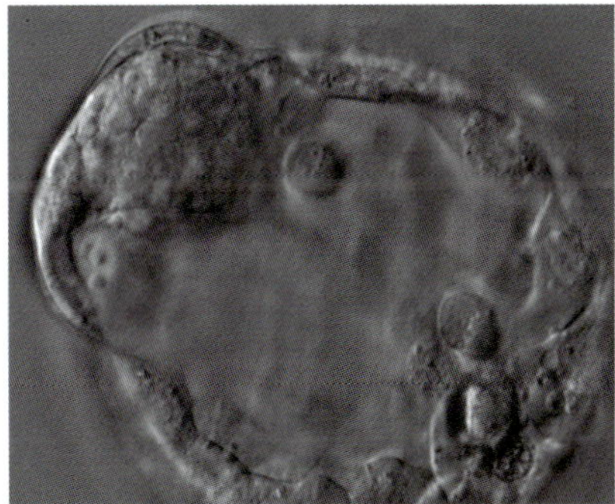

34-BT-1

34-BV-1 Breathing blastocyst (hatching site indicated at 4 o'clock position)
34-AW-1 Not fully re-expanded blastocyst
34-BT-1 Hatching blastocyst with necrotic foci in trophectoderm

Female partner

Age 34, nurse
Tubal status: patent
MH: 4–5/28–33
BMI: 20.9
Non-smoker, no alcohol
  consumption
Basal FSH: 8.4 IU/L
Basal LH: 5.2 IU/L
Basal estradiol: 34.9 pg/mL

Basal AMH: 4.17 ng/mL
Midluteal progesterone: 6.4 ng/mL
Midluteal prolactin: 27.8 ng/mL

Male partner

Age 70, technician
History/examination: Erectile dysfunction
Non-smoker, no alcohol consumption

Previous treatments

None

Fresh cycle: 2011 ICSI

Semen assessment: asthenoteratozoospermia

Volume	2 mL
Abstinence	4 days
Concentration	30×10^6/mL
Progressive motility	15%
Non-progressive motility	0%
Immotile	85%
Normal forms	3%

Stimulation protocol	Agonist protocol (HMG)
Days of stimulation	10
Total dose	1575 IU
Estradiol at ovulation induction	2220 ng/mL
Number of follicles $\geq$ 12 mm	9
Total number of COCs	9
Metaphase II	7
Injected/inseminated	7
Fertilization rate	57%
Cleavage rate	100%
Blastocyst rate	100%
Culture medium	EmbryoAssist/BlastAssist

Fresh transfer

Quality of embryo(s)	4ab
Outcome	Live birth, healthy boy
Vitrification	2 blastocysts

Vitrified/warmed cycle: 2013

Stimulation	HSP
Endometrium	9.0 mm
Quality before vitrification	4ab
Warming day	5
Survival	Yes
Assisted hatching	Yes
Transfer day	5
Quality	4aa
Duration of cryostorage	2.5 years
Time between warming and transfer	2h

Outcome: Not pregnant

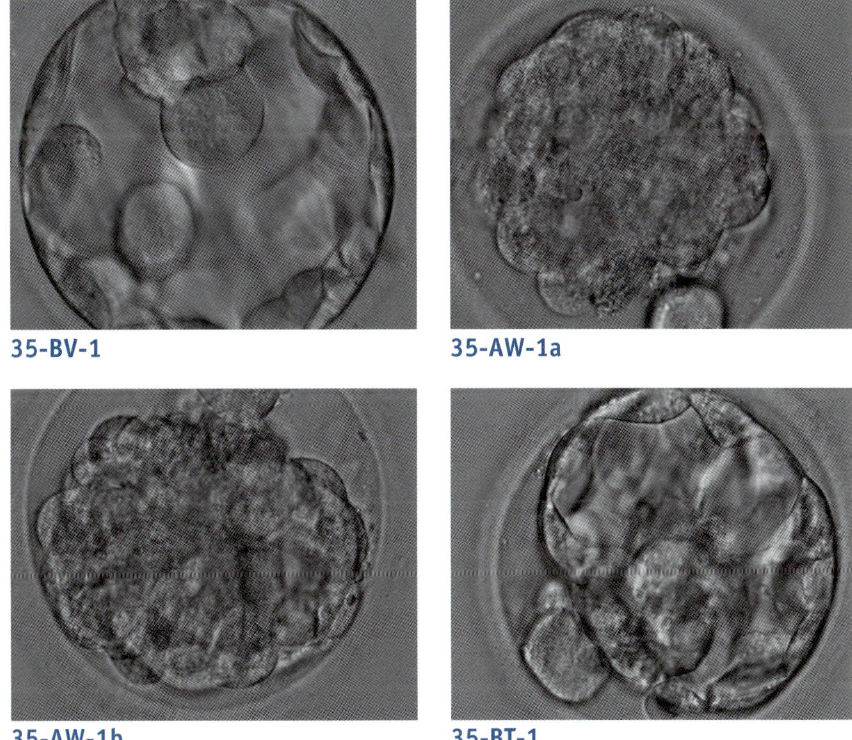

35-BV-1

35-AW-1a

35-AW-1b

35-BT-1

35-BV-1	Expanded blastocyst with inner cell mass at 12 o'clock position (excluded blastomere attached to inner cell mass)
35-AW-1a	Warmed blastocyst with extensive cytoplasmic granulation
35-AW-1b	Same blastocyst as 35-BV-1a within half an hour
35-BT-1	Re-expanded blastocyst with one excluded blastomere on top of inner cell mass and another in the perivitelline space

Case 36

7 years 2° infertility   **Diagnosis: PCO, male factor infertility**

Female partner

Age 33, worker
Tubal status: patent
MH: 4–5/30–33
BMI: 24.7
Non-smoker, no alcohol
   consumption
Normal female karyotype
Induced abortion ×2

Basal FSH: 7.1 IU/L
Basal LH: 7.4 IU/L
Basal estradiol: 31.2 pg/mL
Basal AMH: 9.43 ng/mL
Midluteal progesterone: 7.4 ng/mL
Midluteal prolactin: 12.5 ng/mL
TSH: 0.94 IU/L

Male partner

Age 43, worker
History/examination: NAD
Non-smoker, no alcohol consumption
Normal male karyotype

Previous treatments

None

Fresh cycle: 2008 ICSI
Semen assessment: teratozoospermia

Volume	3.0 mL
Abstinence	4 days
Concentration	17×10^6/mL
Progressive motility	56%
Non-progressive motility	0%
Immotile	44%
Normal forms	1%

Stimulation protocol	Antagonist protocol (recombinant FSH)
Days of stimulation	10
Total dose	1125 IU
Estradiol at ovulation induction	5831 ng/mL
Number of follicles ≥ 12 mm	18
Total number of COCs	10
Metaphase II	10
Injected/inseminated	10
Fertilization rate	100%
Cleavage rate	90%
Blastocyst rate	Day 4 vitrification
Culture medium	EmbryoAssist/BlastAssist

Fresh transfer

Quality of embryo(s)	No transfer because of OHSS
Outcome	
Vitrification	8 compacting embryos (day 4)

Previous vitrified/warmed cycles

2008	Not pregnant
2009	Stillbirth

Vitrified/warmed cycle: 2013

Stimulation	HSP
Endometrium	9.5 mm
Quality before vitrification	Compacting embryo, beginning morula
Warming day	4
Survival	Yes, Yes
Assisted hatching	Yes, Yes
Transfer day	4
Quality	Compacting embryo, 3bb
Duration of cryostorage	5 years
Time between warming and transfer	4h

Outcome: Live birth, dichorionic diamniotic twins, one girl with minor malformation (ventricular septum defect)

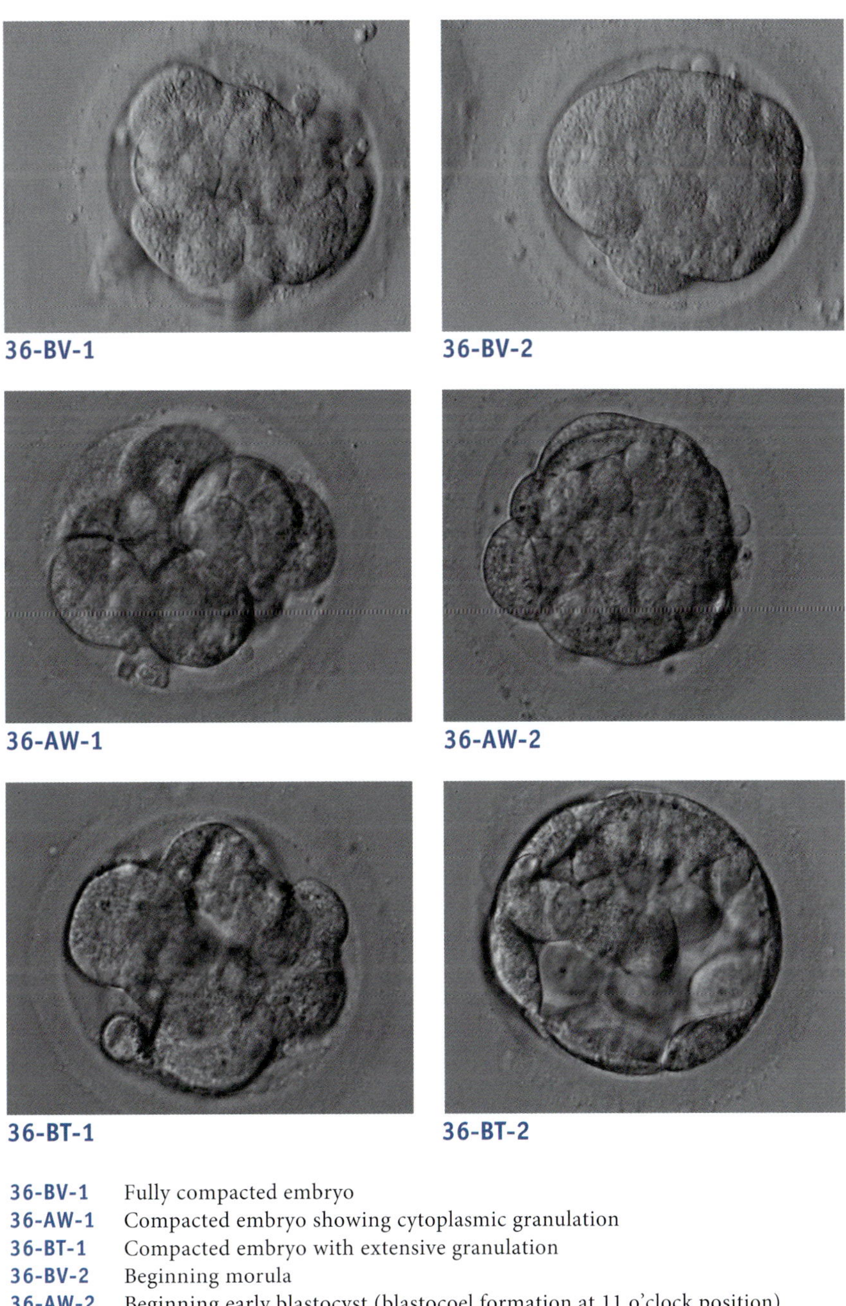

36-BV-1   36-BV-2

36-AW-1   36-AW-2

36-BT-1   36-BT-2

36-BV-1	Fully compacted embryo
36-AW-1	Compacted embryo showing cytoplasmic granulation
36-BT-1	Compacted embryo with extensive granulation
36-BV-2	Beginning morula
36-AW-2	Beginning early blastocyst (blastocoel formation at 11 o'clock position)
36-BT-2	Full blastocyst

Female partner

Age 29, factory employee
Tubal status: patent
MH: 5/28
BMI: 24.7
Smoker, no alcohol
  consumption

Basal FSH: 3.5 IU/L
Basal LH: 3.8 IU/L
Basal estradiol: 133 pg/mL
Basal AMH: 3.32 ng/mL

Male partner

Age 36, plumber
History/examination: cryptorchism
Non-smoker, no alcohol consumption
Normal male karyotype

Previous treatments

2008 ICSI   Live birth, healthy boy
2010 vitrified/warmed cycle   Not pregnant

Fresh cycle: 2011 ICSI
Semen assessment: severe oligoasthenoteratozoospermia

Volume	2.1 mL
Abstinence	5 days
Concentration	1×10^6/mL
Progressive motility	12%
Non-progressive motility	8%
Immotile	80%
Normal forms	1%

Stimulation protocol	Agonist protocol (recombinant FSH)
Days of stimulation	10
Total dose	1500 IU
Estradiol at ovulation induction	990 ng/mL
Number of follicles ≥ 12 mm	7
Total number of COCs	7
Metaphase II	6
Injected/inseminated	6
Fertilization rate	83%
Cleavage rate	100%
Blastocyst rate	60%
Culture medium	GM501

Fresh transfer

Quality of embryo(s)	4ab
Outcome	Not pregnant
Vitrification	1 morula, 1 early blastocyst

Vitrified/warmed cycle: 2011

Stimulation	HSP
Endometrium	14 mm
Quality before vitrification	M, 1
Warming day	5
Survival	Yes, Yes
Assisted hatching	Yes, Yes
Transfer day	5
Quality	1, 3aa
Duration of cryostorage	2 months
Time between warming and transfer	3

Outcome: Live birth, healthy dichorionic diamniotic twins (boy and girl)

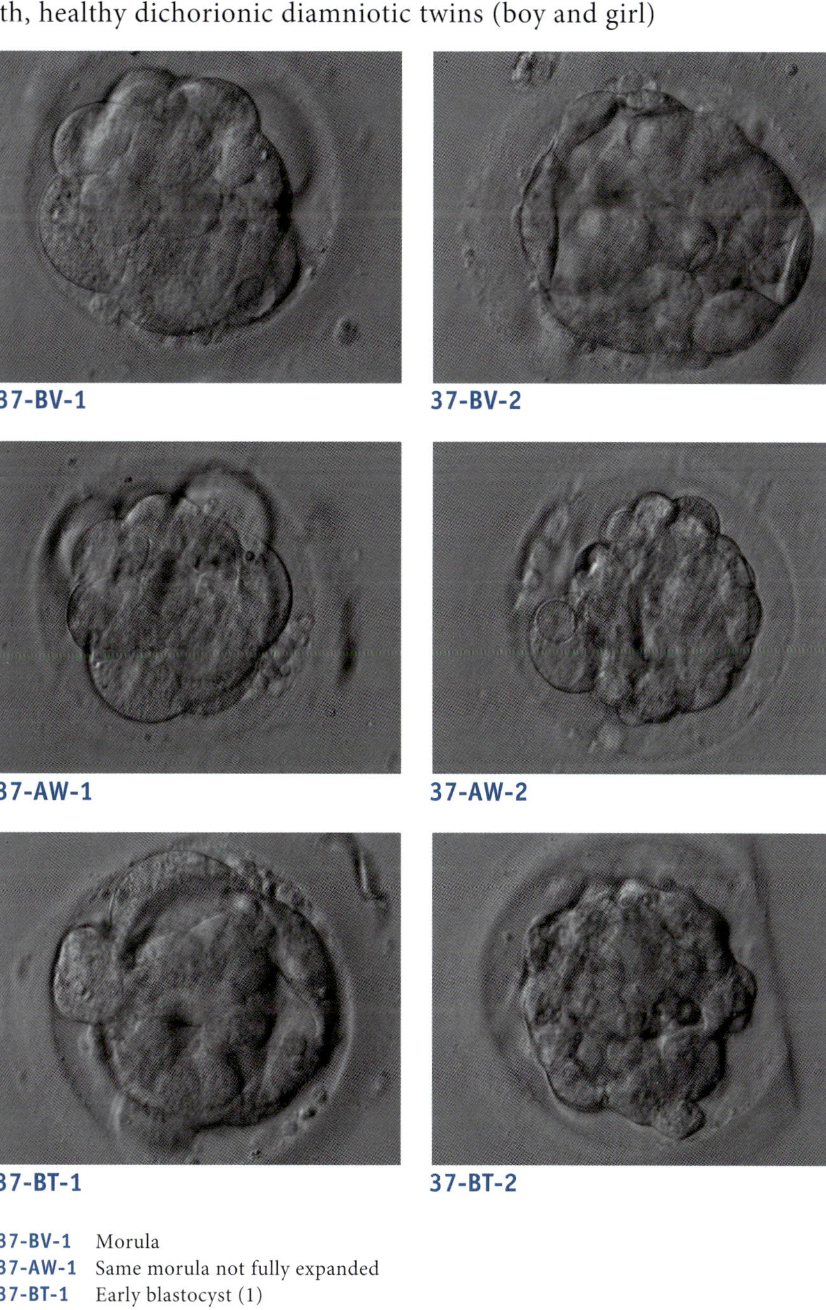

37-BV-1 37-BV-2

37-AW-1 37-AW-2

37-BT-1 37-BT-2

37-BV-1	Morula
37-AW-1	Same morula not fully expanded
37-BT-1	Early blastocyst (1)
37-BV-2	Early blastocyst (1)
37-AW-2	Early blastocyst showing vacuolized blastomere at 9 o'clock position
37-BT-2	Full blastocyst (3aa) without re-expansion

Case 38

5 years 2° infertility Diagnosis: HIV, male factor infertility

Female partner

Age 35, secretary
Tubal status: patent
MH: 5/28
BMI: 20.4
Non-smoker, no alcohol
  consumption
HIV

Basal FSH: 5.2 IU/L
Basal LH: 4.5 IU/L
Basal estradiol: 109.0 pg/mL
Basal AMH: 7.72 ng/mL
Midluteal progesterone: 13.3 ng/mL

Male partner

Age 49, electrician
History/examination: NAD
Non-smoker, no alcohol
  consumption

Previous treatments

None

Fresh cycle: 2013 ICSI

Semen assessment: severe oligoasthenoteratozoospermia

Volume	0.8 mL
Abstinence	5 days
Concentration	1.0×10^6/mL
Progressive motility	22%
Non-progressive motility	18%
Immotile	60%
Normal forms	1%

Stimulation protocol	Agonist protocol (HMG)
Days of stimulation	
Total dose	1700 IU
Estradiol at ovulation induction	4200 ng/mL
Number of follicles ≥ 12 mm	>30
Total number of COCs	35
Metaphase II	30
Injected/inseminated	30
Fertilization rate	77%
Cleavage rate	100%
Blastocyst rate	30%
Culture medium	EmbryoAssist/BlastAssist

Fresh transfer

Quality of embryo(s)	No transfer because of OHSS
Outcome	
Vitrification	4 blastocysts

Vitrified/warmed cycle: 2013

Stimulation	HSP
Endometrium	10.5 mm
Quality before vitrification	3ab
Warming day	5
Survival	Yes
Assisted hatching	Yes
Transfer day	5
Quality	5ab
Duration of cryostorage	10 months
Time between warming and transfer	5h

Outcome: Not pregnant

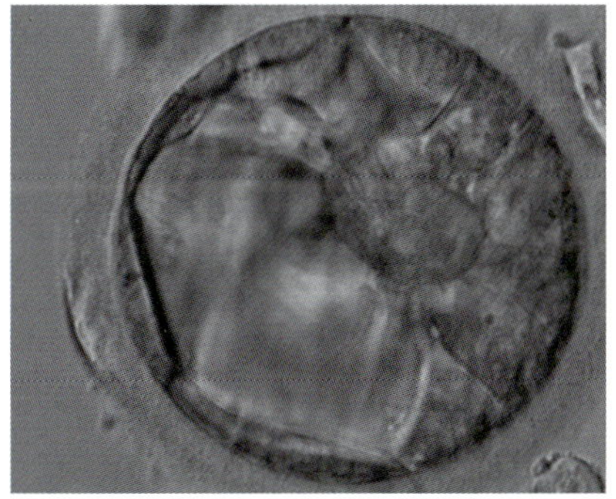

38-BV-1

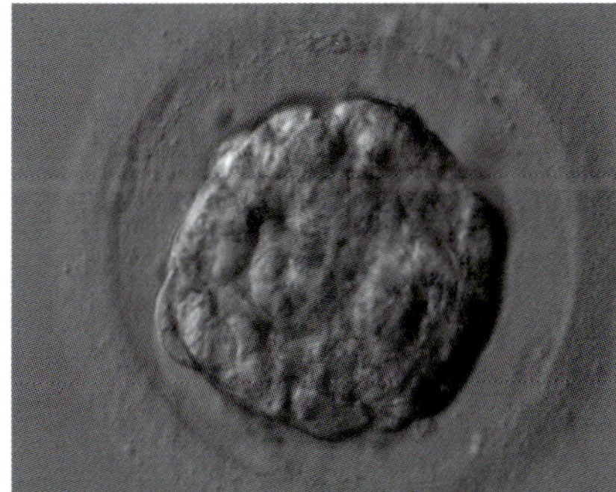

38-AW-1

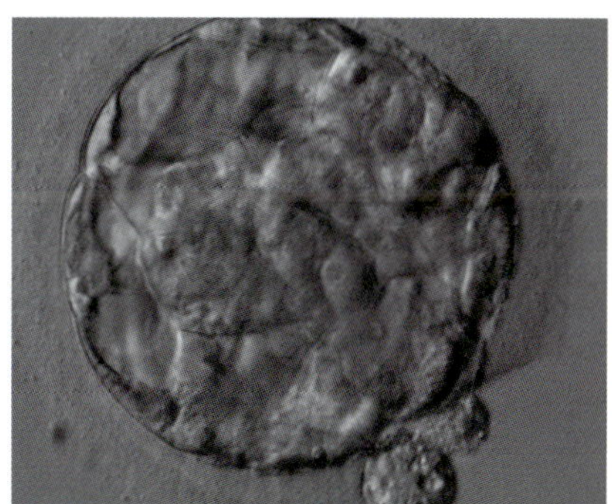

38-BT-1

38-BV-1 Full blastocyst with poor trophectoderm
38-AW-1 Viable blastocyst
38-BT-1 Hatching blastocyst

Female partner

Age 31, employee
Tubal status: patent
MH: 5/28
BMI: 29.4
Smoker, no alcohol consumption

Basal FSH: 8.0 IU/L
Basal LH: 13.1 IU/L

Basal estradiol: 66.6 pg/mL
Basal AMH: 11.59 ng/mL
Midluteal progesterone: 0.2 ng/mL
Midluteal prolactin: 6.8 ng/mL

Male partner

Age 41, worker
History/examination: double
  kidney unilateral
Smoker, no alcohol consumption

Previous treatments

2008 external insemination   Not pregnant

Fresh cycle: 2010 ICSI
Semen assessment: oligoasthenozoospermia

Volume	3.2 mL
Abstinence	3 days
Concentration	7×10^6/mL
Progressive motility	22%
Non-progressive motility	6%
Immotile	72%
Normal forms	4%

Stimulation protocol	Antagonist protocol (recombinant FSH)
Days of stimulation	9
Total dose	1125 IU
Estradiol at ovulation induction	1449 ng/mL
Number of follicles ≥ 12 mm	20
Total number of COCs	20
Metaphase II	16
Injected/inseminated	16
Fertilization rate	81%
Cleavage rate	100%
Blastocyst rate	62%
Culture medium	EmbryoAssist/BlastAssist

Fresh transfer

Quality of embryo(s)	5aa
Outcome	Live birth, healthy boy
Vitrification	5 blastocysts

Vitrified/warmed cycle: 2013

Stimulation	HSP
Endometrium	11.0 mm
Quality before vitrification	4aa
Warming day	5
Survival	Yes
Assisted hatching	Yes
Transfer day	5
Quality	5aa
Duration of cryostorage	3 years
Time between warming and transfer	3h

Outcome: Biochemical pregnancy

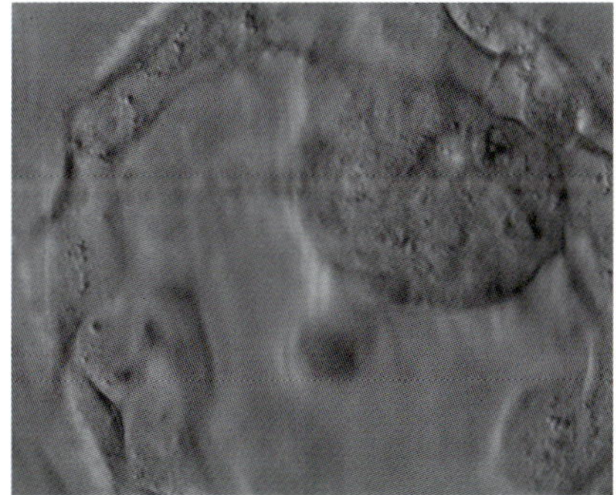

39-BV-1

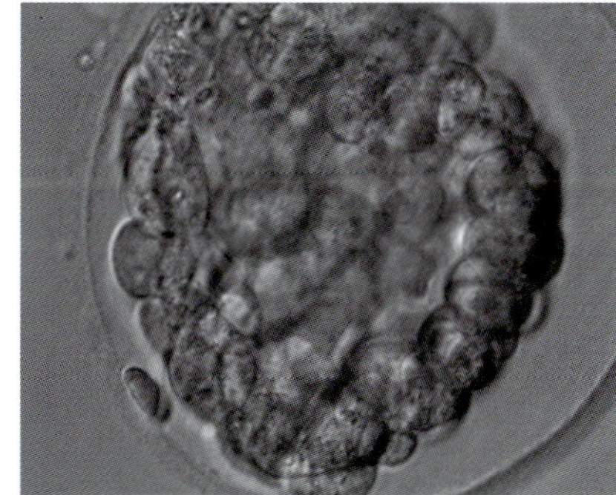

39-AW-1

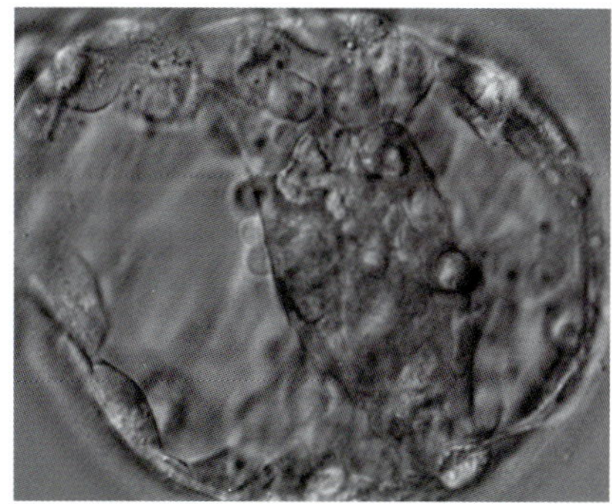

39-BT-1

39-BV-1 Expanded blastocyst with necrotic focus in inner cell mass
39-AW-1 Expanded blastocyst with cytoplasmic granulation
39-BT-1 Hatching blastocyst

Case 40

9 years 1° infertility   Diagnosis: Male factor infertility

Female partner

Age 34, employee
Tubal status: patent
MH: 4–5/28
BMI: 24.2
Non-smoker, no alcohol
  consumption
Basal FSH: 5.1 IU/L
Basal LH: 4.9 IU/L
Basal estradiol: 70.0 pg/mL

Basal AMH: 7.15 ng/mL
Midluteal progesterone: 2.2 ng/mL
Midluteal prolactin: 17.4 ng/mL
TSH: 2.5 IU/L

Male partner

Age 36, carpenter
History/examination: NAD
Non-smoker, no alcohol consumption

Previous treatments

None

Fresh cycle: 2010 ICSI
Semen assessment: asthenoteratozoospermia

Volume	1.0 mL
Abstinence	5 days
Concentration	200×10^6/mL
Progressive motility	3%
Non-progressive motility	3%
Immotile	94%
Normal forms	2%

Stimulation protocol	Agonist protocol (HMG)
Days of stimulation	10
Total dose	1800 IU
Estradiol at ovulation induction	2209 ng/mL
Number of follicles ≥ 12 mm	>25
Total number of COCs	26
Metaphase II	24
Injected/inseminated	24
Fertilization rate	88%
Cleavage rate	100%
Blastocyst rate	67%
Culture medium	EmbryoAssist/BlastAssist

Fresh transfer

Quality of embryo(s)	5aa
Outcome	Live birth, healthy boy
Vitrification	11 blastocysts

Vitrified/warmed cycle: 2013

Stimulation	HSP
Endometrium	7.5 mm
Quality before vitrification	5aa
Warming day	5
Survival	Yes
Assisted hatching	Yes
Transfer day	5
Quality	5ab
Duration of cryostorage	3 years
Time between warming and transfer	3h

Outcome: Live birth, healthy boy

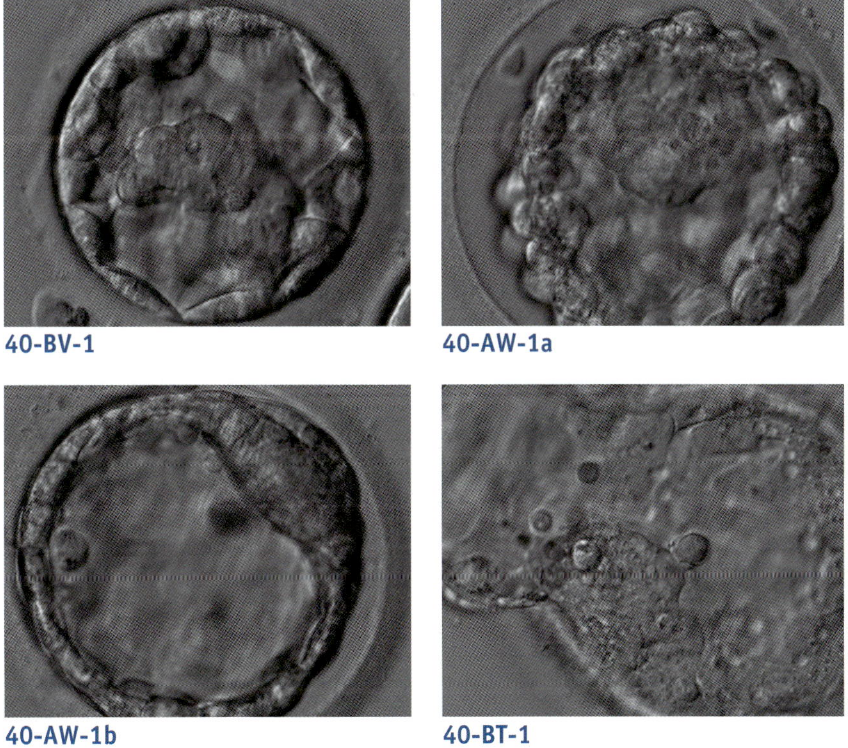

40-BV-1

40-AW-1a

40-AW-1b

40-BT-1

40-BV-1   Expanded blastocyst with necrotic focus in inner cell mass
40-AW-1a Viable blastocyst immediately after warming
40-AW-1b Re-expanded blastocyst (1h after 40-AW-1a)
40-BT-1   Hatching blastocyst with trophectoderm out of focus

Case 41

9 years 2° infertility **Diagnosis: Endometriosis, male factor infertility**

Female partner

Age 39, journalist
Tubal status: patent
MH: 4–5/27–28
BMI: 21.3
Non-smoker, no alcohol
  consumption
Dysmenorrhea
Recurrent cystectomy left ovary

Basal FSH: 6.3 IU/L
Basal LH: 3.5 IU/L
Basal estradiol: 71.2 pg/mL
Basal AMH: 2.79 ng/mL
Midluteal progesterone: 15.4 ng/mL
Midluteal prolactin: 31.8 ng/mL
TSH: 0.94 IU/L

Male partner

Age 40, technician
History/examination: NAD
Non-smoker, no alcohol consumption

Previous treatments

2008 timed intercourse ×4	Not pregnant
2009 ICSI	Low response, no fertilization
2009 ICSI	Not pregnant
2009 vitrified/warmed cycle	Live birth, healthy boy

Fresh cycle: 2012 ICSI

Semen assessment: severe oligoasthenoteratozoospermia

Volume	2.1 mL
Abstinence	2 days
Concentration	1×10^6/mL
Progressive motility	25%
Non-progressive motility	25%
Immotile	50%
Normal forms	0%

Stimulation protocol	Agonist protocol (HMG)
Days of stimulation	9
Total dose	1450 IU
Estradiol at ovulation induction	739 ng/mL
Number of follicles ≥ 12 mm	10
Total number of COCs	7
Metaphase II	6
Injected/inseminated	6
Fertilization rate	83%
Cleavage rate	80%
Blastocyst rate	Day 4 vitrification
Culture medium	EmbryoAssist/BlastAssist

Fresh transfer

Quality of embryo(s)	No transfer because of suboptimal endometrium
Outcome	
Vitrification	2 compacting embryos, 2 morulae (all day 4)

Vitrified/warmed cycle: 2013

Stimulation	NC
Endometrium	11.0 mm
Quality before vitrification	Morula
Warming day	4
Survival	Yes
Assisted hatching	Yes
Transfer day	5
Quality	5ab
Duration of cryostorage	6 months
Time between warming and transfer	20h

Outcome: Live birth, healthy boy

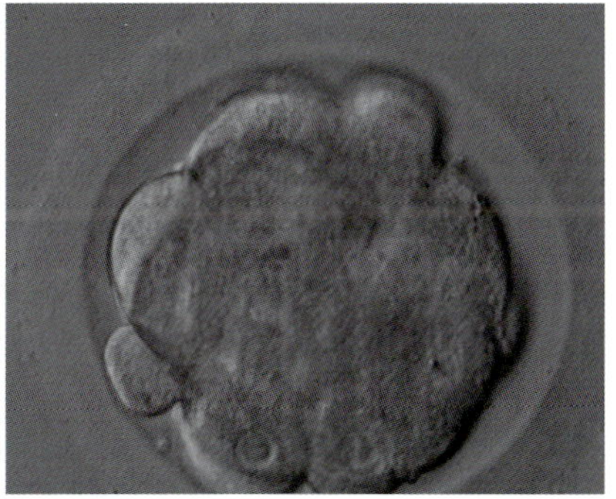

41-BV-1

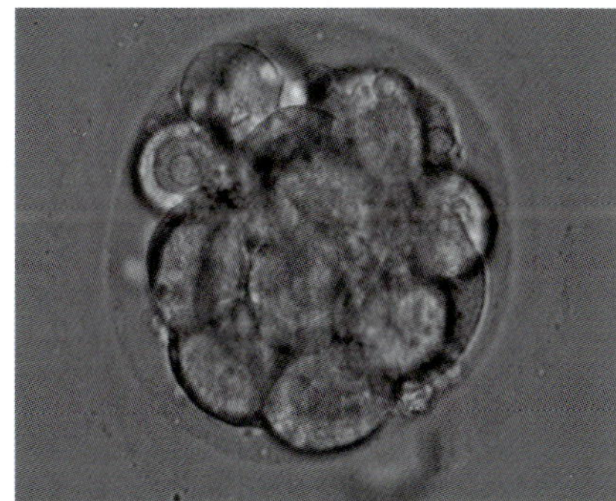

41-AW-1

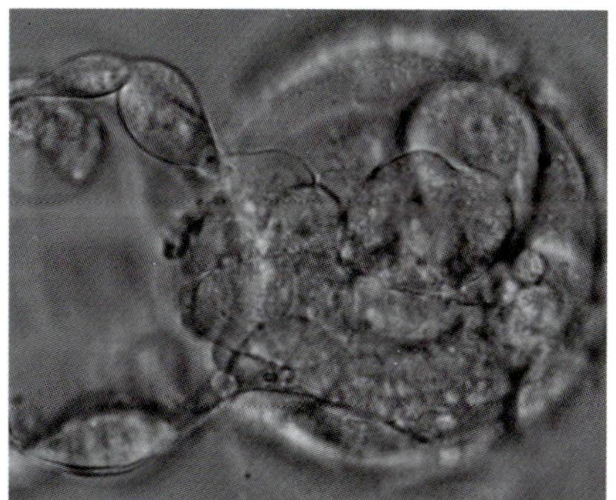

41-BT-1

41-BV-1   Morula with small vacuole (7 o'clock position)
41-AW-1   Same morula with vacuole at 10 o'clock position
41-BT-1   Hatching blastocyst with 2 blastomeres in blastocoel

Female partner

Age 26, hairdresser
Tubal status: unilateral patent
MH: dysmenorrhea
BMI: 23.4
Smoker, no alcohol
  consumption
Endometrioma on left ovary

Basal FSH: 8.1 IU/L
Basal LH: 2.7 IU/L
Basal estradiol: 33.7 pg/mL
Basal AMH: 4.19 ng/mL
Midluteal progesterone: 0.5 ng/mL
Midluteal prolactin: 15.5 ng/mL

Male partner

Age 28, electrician
History/examination: NAD
Smoker, no alcohol
  consumption

Previous treatments

2011 ICSI   Not pregnant

Fresh cycle: 2011 split IVF/ICSI
Semen assessment: normozoospermia

Volume	3 mL
Abstinence	4 days
Concentration	42×10^6/mL
Progressive motility	42%
Non-progressive motility	6%
Immotile	52%
Normal forms	15%

Stimulation protocol	Agonist protocol (HMG)
Days of stimulation	10
Total dose	2250 IU
Estradiol at ovulation induction	1150 ng/mL
Number of follicles $\geq$ 12 mm	12
Total number of COCs	7
Metaphase II	7
Injected/inseminated	4 (IVF), 3 (ICSI)
Fertilization rate	25% (IVF), 33% (ICSI)
Cleavage rate	100%, 100%
Blastocyst rate	100%, 100%
Culture medium	EmbryoAssist/BlastAssist

Fresh transfer

Quality of embryo(s)	4aa (IVF)
Outcome	Not pregnant
Vitrification	1 blastocyst (ICSI)

Vitrified/warmed cycle: 2012

Stimulation	HSP
Endometrium	11 mm
Quality before vitrification	4bb
Warming day	5
Survival	Yes
Assisted hatching	Yes
Transfer day	5
Quality	4bb
Duration of cryostorage	3 months
Time between warming and transfer	3h

Outcome: Live birth, healthy boy

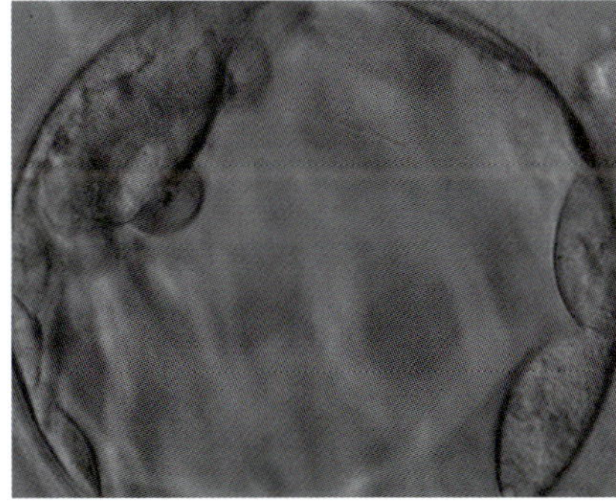 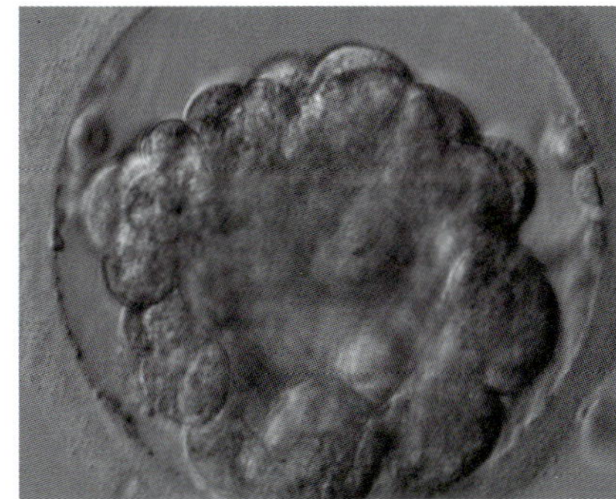 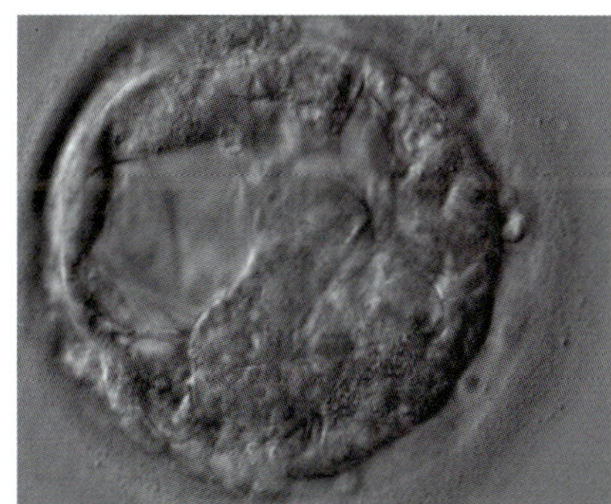

42-BV-1 42-AW-1 42-BT-1

42-BV-1 Expanded blastocyst showing non-homogeneous ZP
42-AW-1 Same blastocyst with granular cytoplasm
42-BT-1 Re-expanded blastocyst with non-homogeneous ZP

Female partner

Age 34, teacher
Tubal status: patent
MH: 4–5/31
BMI: 22.4
Non-smoker, no alcohol
    consumption
Normal female karyotype

Basal FSH: 8.0 IU/L
Basal LH: 7.5 IU/L
Basal estradiol: 45.8 pg/mL
Basal AMH: 8.25 ng/mL
Midluteal progesterone: 0.2 ng/mL
Midluteal prolactin: 5.1 ng/mL

Male partner

Age 35, social worker
History/examination: NAD
Non-smoker, no alcohol consumption
Normal male karyotype

Previous treatments

2009 TESE	Not pregnant
2010 vitrified/warmed cycle	Live birth, healthy boy

Fresh cycle: 2013 TESE
Semen assessment: azoospermia

Volume	2.9 mL
Abstinence	4 days
Concentration	0×10^6/mL
Progressive motility	0%
Non-progressive motility	0%
Immotile	0%
Normal forms	0%

Stimulation protocol	Agonist protocol (HMG)
Days of stimulation	17
Total dose	2813 IU
Estradiol at ovulation induction	4527 ng/mL
Number of follicles ≥ 12 mm	22
Total number of COCs	20
Metaphase II	17
Injected/inseminated	15
Fertilization rate	67%
Cleavage rate	70%
Blastocyst rate	Day 4 cryopreservation
Culture medium	EmbryoAssist/BlastAssist

Fresh transfer

Quality of embryo(s)	
Outcome	No fresh transfer because of OHSS
Vitrification	2 morulae (day 4), 2 blastocysts (day 5)

Vitrified/warmed cycle: 2013

Stimulation	HSP
Endometrium	9.5 mm
Quality before vitrification	3aa, 4ab
Warming day	5
Survival	Yes, Partial
Assisted hatching	Yes, No
Transfer day	5
Quality	2, no transfer
Duration of cryostorage	4 months
Time between warming and transfer	2h

Outcome: Missed abortion (no heart activity)

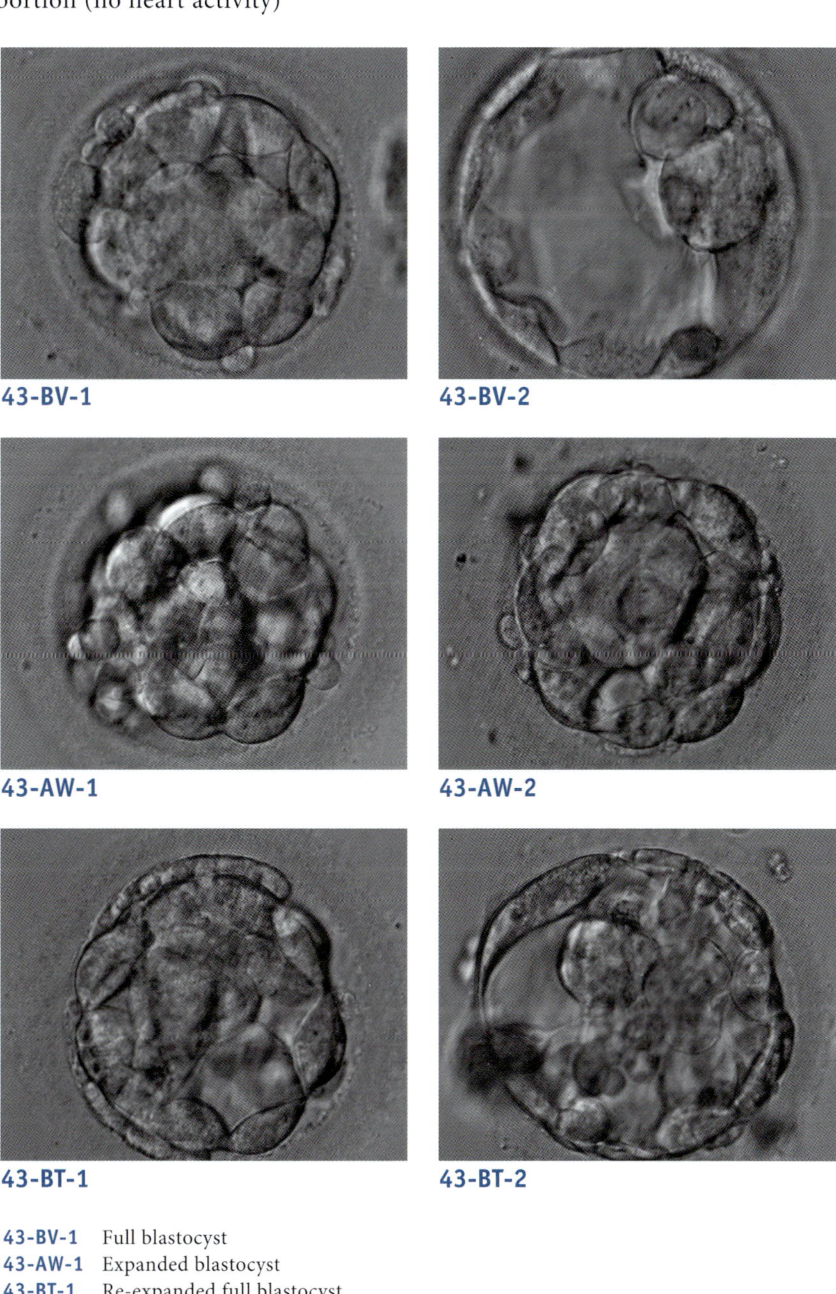

43-BV-1

43-BV-2

43-AW-1

43-AW-2

43-BT-1

43-BT-2

43-BV-1	Full blastocyst
43-AW-1	Expanded blastocyst
43-BT-1	Re-expanded full blastocyst
43-BV-2	Viable blastocyst with excluded fragments attached to the zona pellucida
43-AW-2	Non re-expanded blastocyst with extensive cytoplasmic granulation
43-BT-2	Partially re-expanded blastocyst with cytoplasmic granulation and necrotic foci (no transfer)

Female partner

Age 38, cook
Tubal status: patent
MH: 5/30–34
BMI: 28.3
Non-smoker, no alcohol
  consumption
Dysmenorrhea, hypertonia
Recurrent abortion

Basal FSH: 4.5 IU/L
Basal LH: 4.7 IU/L
Basal estradiol: 20.0 pg/mL
Basal AMH: 6.75 ng/mL
Midluteal progesterone: 8.46 ng/mL
Midluteal prolactin: 14.1 ng/mL

Male partner

Age 36, teacher
History/examination: NAD
Non-smoker, no alcohol consumption
Normal male karyotype

Previous treatments

2004 external insemination ×5	Not pregnant
2009 ICSI ×2	Not pregnant
2009 ICSI	Missed abortion
2010 vitrified/warmed cycle	Live birth, healthy girl
2012 vitrified/warmed cycle	Not pregnant
2012 ICSI ×2	Not pregnant

Fresh cycle: 2013 ICSI

Semen assessment: asthenozoospermia

Volume	1.8 mL
Abstinence	2 days
Concentration	32×10^6/mL
Progressive motility	21%
Non-progressive motility	9%
Immotile	70%
Normal forms	8%

Stimulation protocol	Agonist protocol (HMG, recombinant FSH)
Days of stimulation	13
Total dose	2775 IU
Estradiol at ovulation induction	7536 ng/mL
Number of follicles ≥ 12 mm	>30
Total number of COCs	30
Metaphase II	26
Injected/inseminated	26
Fertilization rate	92%
Cleavage rate	100%
Blastocyst rate	58%
Culture medium	EmbryoAssist/BlastAssist

Fresh transfer

Quality of embryo(s)	No transfer because of OHSS
Outcome	
Vitrification	4 compacted embryos, 2 morulae (all day 4); 6 blastocysts (day 5)

Vitrified/warmed cycle: 2013

TAB	HSP
Endometrium	11.0mm
Quality before vitrification	2 compacted embryos
Warming day	4
Survival	Yes
Assisted hatching	Yes
Transfer day	5
Quality	3ab, morula
Duration of cryostorage	2 months
Time between warming and transfer	21 hours

Outcome: Missed abortion (positive heart activity)

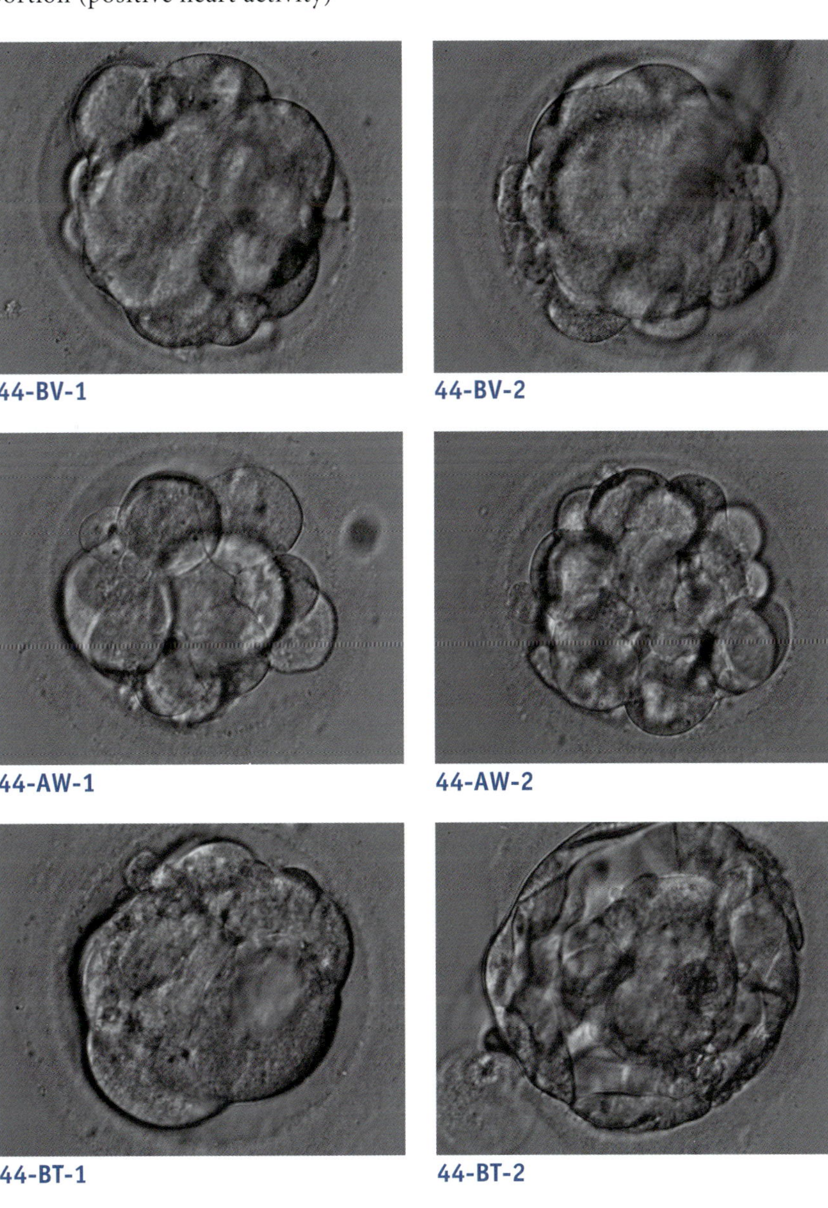

44-BV-1   44-BV-2

44-AW-1   44-AW-2

44-BT-1   44-BT-2

44-BV-1	Compacted embryo
44-AW-1	Embryo with disintegration of cells
44-BT-1	Morula
44-BV-2	Compacted embryo
44-AW-2	Embryo with disintegration of cells
44-BT-2	Full blastocyst with necrotic focus in inner cell mass

Case 45

10 years 2° infertility   Diagnosis: Male factor infertility

Female partner

Age 37, cleaner
Tubal status: patent
MH: 5/28
BMI: 29.1
Non-smoker, no alcohol
  consumption
Basal FSH: 6.0 IU/L
Basal LH: 4.1 IU/L
Basal estradiol: 37.8 pg/mL

Basal AMH: 7.10 ng/mL
Midluteal progesterone: 16.1 ng/mL
Midluteal prolactin: 30.0 ng/mL
TSH: 1.59 IU/L

Male partner

Age 38, painter
History/examination: NAD
Smoker, no alcohol consumption
Normal male karyotype

Previous treatments

2007 ICSI	Not pregnant
2007 vitrified/warmed cycle	Live birth, healthy girl

Fresh cycle: 2011 ICSI
Semen assessment: oligoasthenoteratozoospermia

Volume	5.0 mL
Abstinence	3 days
Concentration	1.3×10^6/mL
Progressive motility	20%
Non-progressive motility	20%
Immotile	60%
Normal forms	0%

Stimulation protocol	Agonist protocol (recombinant FSH)
Days of stimulation	9
Total dose	1775 IU
Estradiol at ovulation induction	1595 ng/mL
Number of follicles ≥ 12 mm	18
Total number of COCs	13
Metaphase II	11
Injected/inseminated	11
Fertilization rate	64%
Cleavage rate	100%
Blastocyst rate	57%
Culture medium	EmbryoAssist/BlastAssist

Fresh transfer

Quality of embryo(s)	4aa
Outcome	Not pregnant
Vitrification	2 blastocysts

Vitrified/warmed cycle: 2011

Stimulation	NC
Endometrium	7.0 mm
Quality before vitrification	5ab
Warming day	5
Survival	Yes
Assisted hatching	Yes
Transfer day	5
Quality	4ab
Duration of cryostorage	3 months
Time between warming and transfer	2h

Outcome: Missed abortion (positive heart activity)

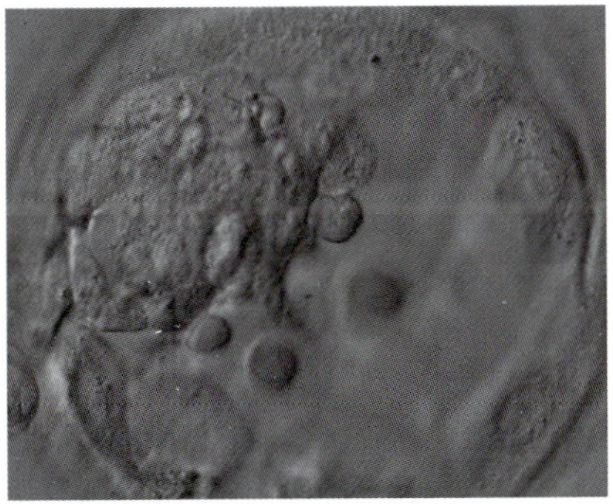

45-BV-1

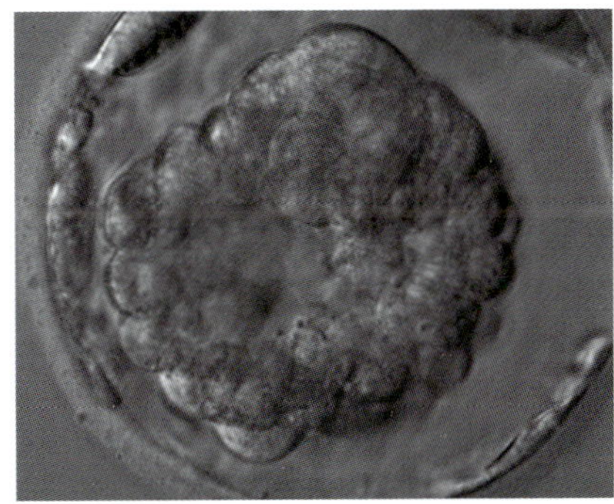

45-AW-1

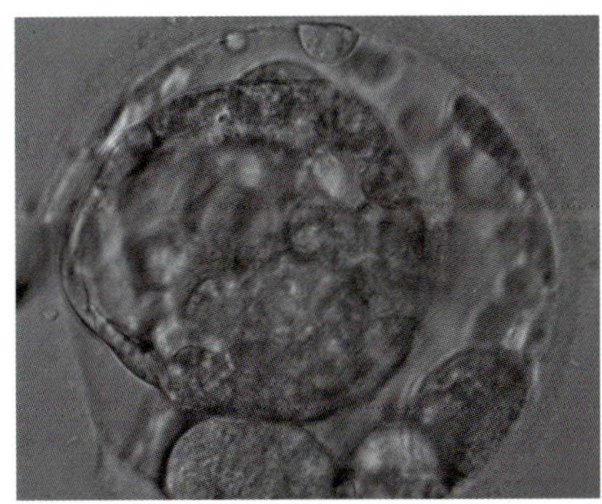

45-BT-1

45-BV-1 Hatching blastocyst with hatching site at 8 o'clock position
45-AW-1 Granulated blastocyst with no signs of re-expansion
45-BT-1 Blastocyst with excluded blastomeres in perivitelline space

Female partner

Age 26, hairdresser
Tubal status: bilateral blockage
MH: 5/32–46, dysmenorrhea
BMI: 20.8
Non-smoker, no alcohol
  consumption
Dyspareunia
PCO-like ovaries

Basal FSH: 6.0 IU/L
Basal LH: 3.2 IU/L
Basal estradiol: 30.3 pg/mL
Basal AMH: 3.53 ng/mL
Midluteal progesterone: 1.3 ng/mL
Midluteal prolactin: 6.5 ng/mL

Male partner

Age 27, bank employee
History/examination: NAD
Smoker, no alcohol consumption
Normal male karyotype

Previous treatments

None

Fresh cycle: 2012 IVF
Semen assessment: normozoospermia

Volume	3.0 mL
Abstinence	4 days
Concentration	42×10^6/mL
Progressive motility	52%
Non-progressive motility	10%
Immotile	38%
Normal forms	8%

Stimulation protocol	Agonist protocol (HMG)
Days of stimulation	11
Total dose	1650 IU
Estradiol at ovulation induction	3146 ng/mL
Number of follicles ≥ 12 mm	26
Total number of COCs	21
Metaphase II	20
Injected/inseminated	20
Fertilization rate	65%
Cleavage rate	100%
Blastocyst rate	54%
Culture medium	GM501

Fresh transfer

Quality of embryo(s)	No fresh transfer because of OHSS
Outcome	
Vitrification	6 blastocysts

Vitrified/warmed cycle: 2013

Stimulation	HSP
Endometrium	8.5 mm
Quality before vitrification	2
Warming day	5
Survival	Yes
Assisted hatching	Yes
Transfer day	5
Quality	3ab
Duration of cryostorage	2 months
Time between warming and transfer	2h

Outcome: Live birth, healthy girl

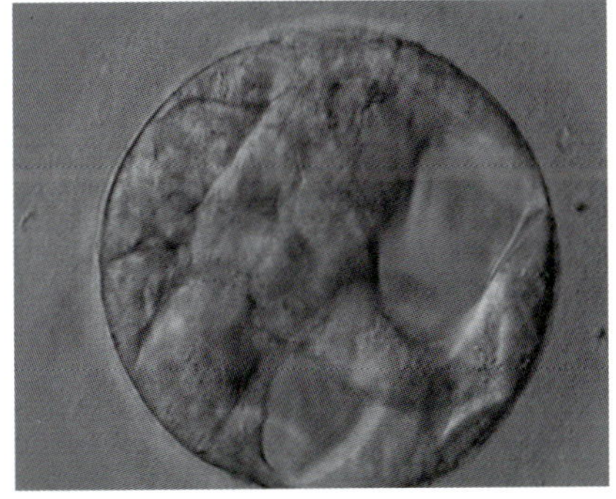

46-BV-1

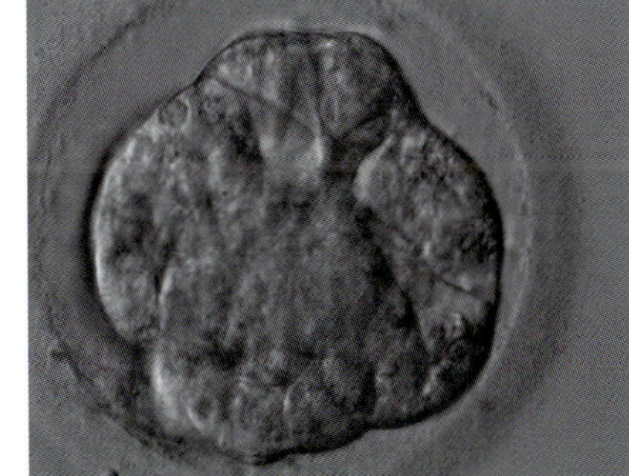

46-AW-1

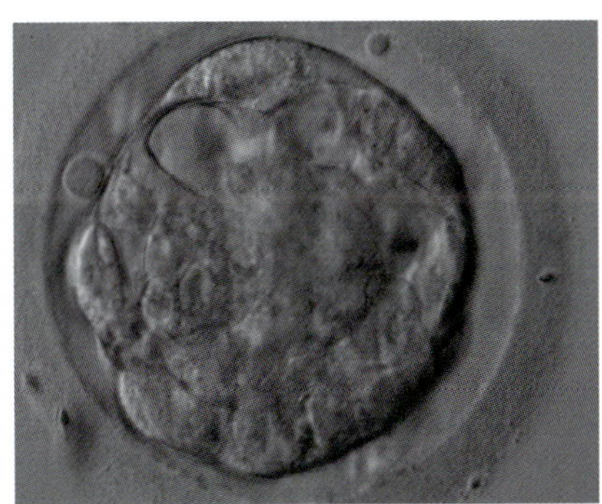

46-BT-1

46-BV-1 Early blastocyst
46-AW-1 Warmed blastocyst
46-BT-1 Full blastocyst

Female partner

Age 29, quality insurance
  representative
Tubal status: patent
MH: 5/28
BMI: 18.5
Smoker, no alcohol consumption
Basal FSH: 7.2 IU/L
Basal LH: 4.0 IU/L
Basal estradiol: 28.6 pg/mL

Basal AMH: 2.42 ng/mL
Midluteal progesterone: 18.0 ng/mL
Midluteal prolactin: 6.0 ng/mL

Male partner

Age 34, works council
History/examination: NAD
Non-smoker, no alcohol consumption

Previous treatments

None

Fresh cycle: 2011 ICSI with ionophore treatment
Semen assessment: cryptozoospermia

Volume	7.0 mL
Abstinence	10 days
Concentration	$<0.001 \times 10^6$/mL
Progressive motility	1%
Non-progressive motility	0%
Immotile	99%
Normal forms	0%

Stimulation protocol	Agonist protocol (recombinant FSH)
Days of stimulation	10
Total dose	1500 IU
Estradiol at ovulation induction	895 ng/mL
Number of follicles ≥ 12 mm	7
Total number of COCs	6
Metaphase II	6
Injected/inseminated	6
Fertilization rate	83%
Cleavage rate	100%
Blastocyst rate	80%
Culture medium	EmbryoAssist/BlastAssist

Fresh transfer

Quality of embryo(s)	5aa
Outcome	Not pregnant
Vitrification	2 blastocysts

Vitrified/warmed cycle: 2011

Stimulation	NC
Endometrium	7.5 mm
Quality before vitrification	4aa
Warming day	5
Survival	Yes
Assisted hatching	Yes
Transfer day	5
Quality	4aa
Duration of cryostorage	3 months
Time between warming and transfer	3h

Outcome: Biochemical pregnancy

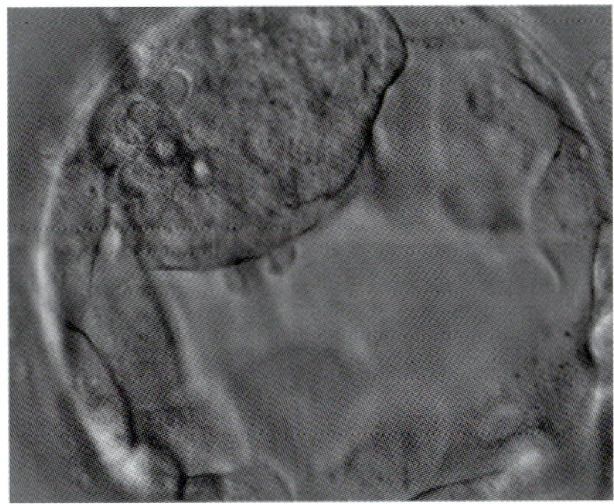

47-BV-1

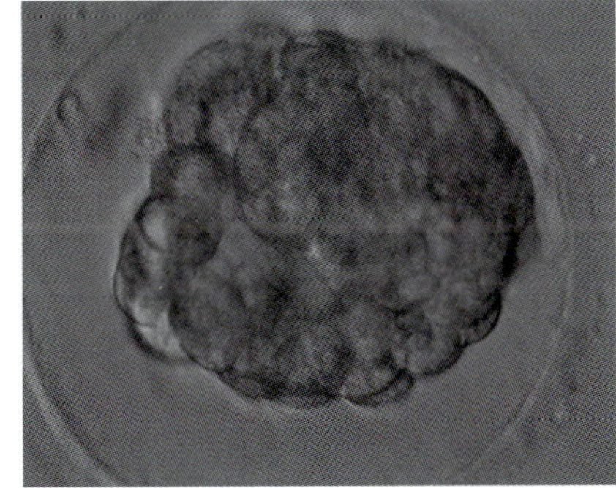

47-AW-1

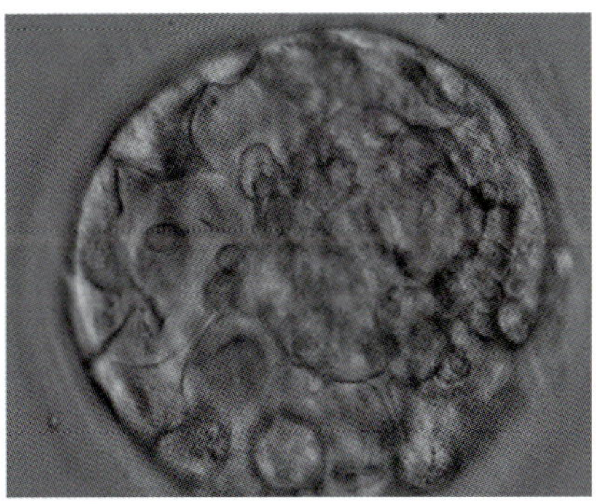

47-BT-1

47-BV-1 Expanded blastocyst with small vacuoles in inner cell mass
47-AW-1 Viable warmed blastocyst
47-BT-1 Expanded blastocyst with numerous cytoplasmic strings

Case 48

Female partner

Age 31, secretary
Tubal status: patent
MH: dysmenorrhea
BMI: 27.0
Non-smoker, no alcohol
  consumption

Basal FSH: 8.3 IU/L
Basal LH: 8.3 IU/L
Basal estradiol: 38.5 pg/mL
Basal AMH: 5.24 ng/mL

Male partner

Age 42, military man
History/examination: NAD
Non-smoker, no alcohol consumption

Previous treatments

2009 ICSI	Live birth, healthy boy
2011 vitrified/warmed cycle	Not pregnant
2011 vitrified/warmed cycle	Biochemical pregnancy

Fresh cycle: 2011 ICSI
Semen assessment: teratozoospermia

Volume	3.3 mL
Abstinence	5 days
Concentration	26×10^6/mL
Progressive motility	26%
Non-progressive motility	16%
Immotile	58%
Normal forms	1%

Stimulation protocol	Antagonist protocol (recombinant FSH)
Days of stimulation	8
Total dose	1275 IU
Estradiol at ovulation induction	701 ng/mL
Number of follicles ≥ 12 mm	4
Total number of COCs	3
Metaphase II	3
Injected/inseminated	3
Fertilization rate	100%
Cleavage rate	100%
Blastocyst rate	67%
Culture medium	GM501

Fresh transfer

Quality of embryo(s)	1
Outcome	Not pregnant
Vitrification	1 morula (day 5)

Vitrified/warmed cycle: 2012

Stimulation	HSP
Endometrium	7.5 mm
Quality before vitrification	Morula
Warming day	5
Survival	Yes
Assisted hatching	Yes
Transfer day	5
Quality	Morula
Duration of cryostorage	3 months
Time between warming and transfer	3h

Outcome: Live birth, healthy boy

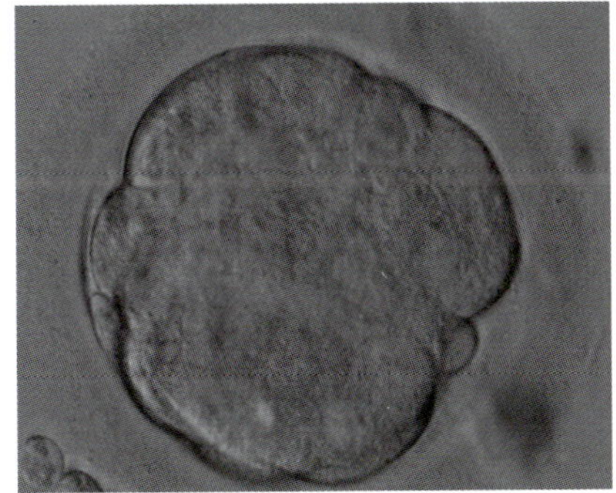

48-BV-1

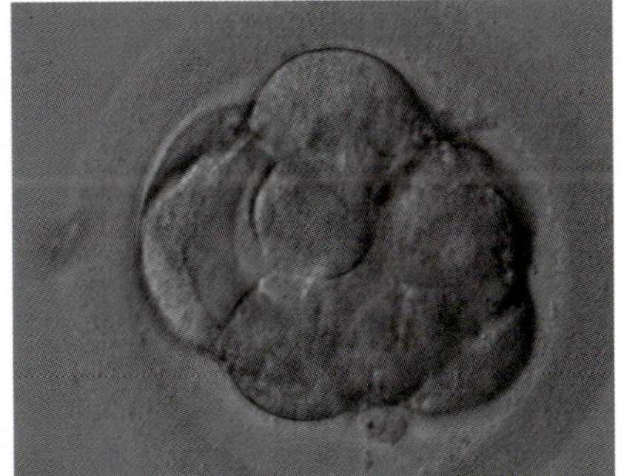

48-AW-1

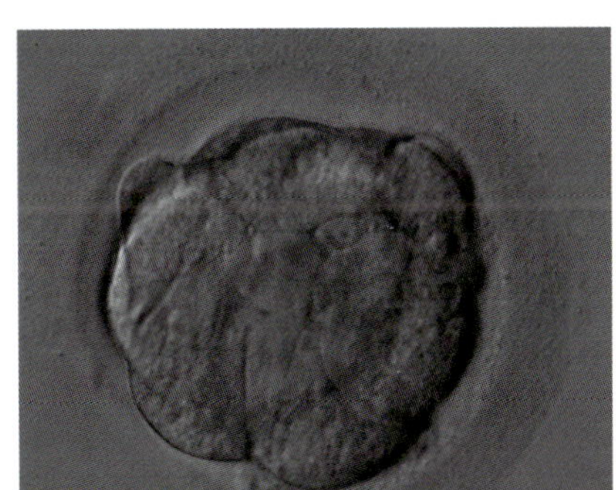

48-BT-1

48-BV-1 Morula
48-AW-1 Warmed morula
48-BT-1 Morula

Female partner

Age 29, employee
Tubal status: bilateral
   hydrosalpinx
MH: 4–5/28
BMI: 24.0
Non-smoker, no alcohol
   consumption
Bilateral removal of tubes
Normal female karyotype

Basal FSH: 4.5 IU/L
Basal LH: 3.0 IU/L
Basal estradiol: 20.2 pg/mL
Basal AMH: 4.2 ng/mL
Midluteal progesterone: 0.3 ng/mL
Midluteal prolactin: 5.9 ng/mL

Male partner

Age 46, author
History/examination: NAD
Non-smoker, no alcohol
   consumption
Normal male karyotype

Previous treatments

None

Fresh cycle: 2013 ICSI
Semen assessment: normoozoospermia

Volume	3.9 mL
Abstinence	2 days
Concentration	100×10^6/mL
Progressive motility	60%
Non-progressive motility	10%
Immotile	30%
Normal forms	13%

Stimulation protocol	Antagonist protocol (HMG)
Days of stimulation	11
Total dose	2175 IU
Estradiol at ovulation induction	4798 ng/mL
Number of follicles ≥ 12 mm	>25
Total number of COCs	30
Metaphase II	
Injected/inseminated	30
Fertilization rate	27%
Cleavage rate	100%
Blastocyst rate	63%
Culture medium	EmbryoAssist/BlastAssist

Fresh transfer

Quality of embryo(s)	No transfer because of OHSS
Outcome	
Vitrification	4 blastocysts

Vitrified/warmed cycle: 2013

Stimulation	HSP
Endometrium	7.5 mm
Quality before vitrification	4aa
Warming day	5
Survival	Partial
Assisted hatching	Yes
Transfer day	5
Quality	4ab
Duration of cryostorage	2 months
Time between warming and transfer	3h

Outcome: Ectopic pregnancy

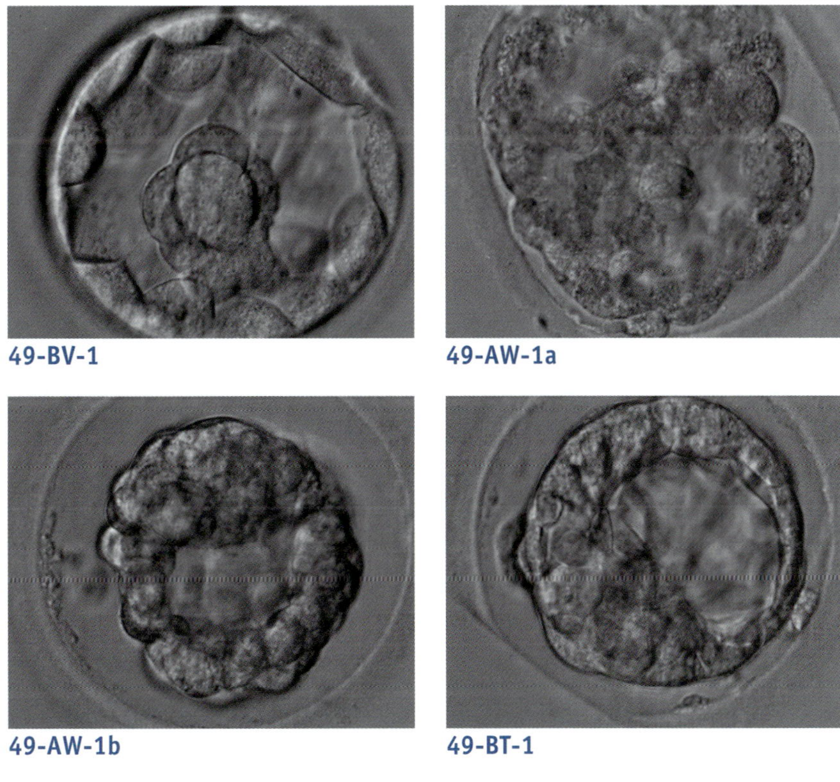

49-BV-1

49-AW-1a

49-AW-1b

49-BT-1

49-BV-1   Expanded blastocyst of good quality
49-AW-1a Warmed blastocyst with extensive granulation
49-AW-1b Recovery of the same blastocyst within 1h
49-BT-1   Blastocyst with lower quality trophectoderm

Case 50

4 years 2° infertility **Diagnosis: PCO, male factor infertility**

Female partner

Age 36, housewife
Tubal status: patent
MH: dysmenorrhea
BMI: 24.8
Non-smoker, no alcohol
  consumption
Basal FSH: 4.1 IU/L
Basal LH: 14.4 IU/L

Basal estradiol: 38.2 pg/mL
Basal AMH: 13.25 ng/mL
Midluteal progesterone: 0.7 ng/mL
Midluteal prolactin: 2.7 ng/mL
Androstenedione: 4.65 ng/mL
TSH: 0.96 IU/L

Male partner

Age 38, unskilled worker
History/examination: NAD
Non-smoker, no alcohol consumption

Previous treatments

2009 timed intercourse   Not pregnant
2011 IUI ×2   Not pregnant

Fresh cycle: 2011 ICSI
Semen assessment: asthenoteratozoospermia

Volume	4.0 mL
Abstinence	2 days
Concentration	26×10^6/mL
Progressive motility	12%
Non-progressive motility	0%
Immotile	88%
Normal forms	2%

Stimulation protocol	Antagonist protocol (recombinant FSH)
Days of stimulation	9
Total dose	1150 IU
Estradiol at ovulation induction	5902 ng/mL
Number of follicles ≥ 12 mm	>30
Total number of COCs	31
Metaphase II	28
Injected/inseminated	28
Fertilization rate	71%
Cleavage rate	100%
Blastocyst rate	20%
Culture medium	EmbryoAssist/BlastAssist

Fresh transfer

Quality of embryo(s)	No transfer because of OHSS
Outcome	
Vitrification	1 compacting embryo, 2 morulae, 4 blastocysts (all day 5)

Vitrified/warmed cycle: 2012

Stimulation	HSP
Endometrium	15.0 mm
Quality before vitrification	1, 2
Warming day	5
Survival	Yes, No
Assisted hatching	Yes, No
Transfer day	5
Quality	3bb
Duration of cryostorage	11 months
Time between warming and transfer	3h

Outcome: Biochemical pregnancy

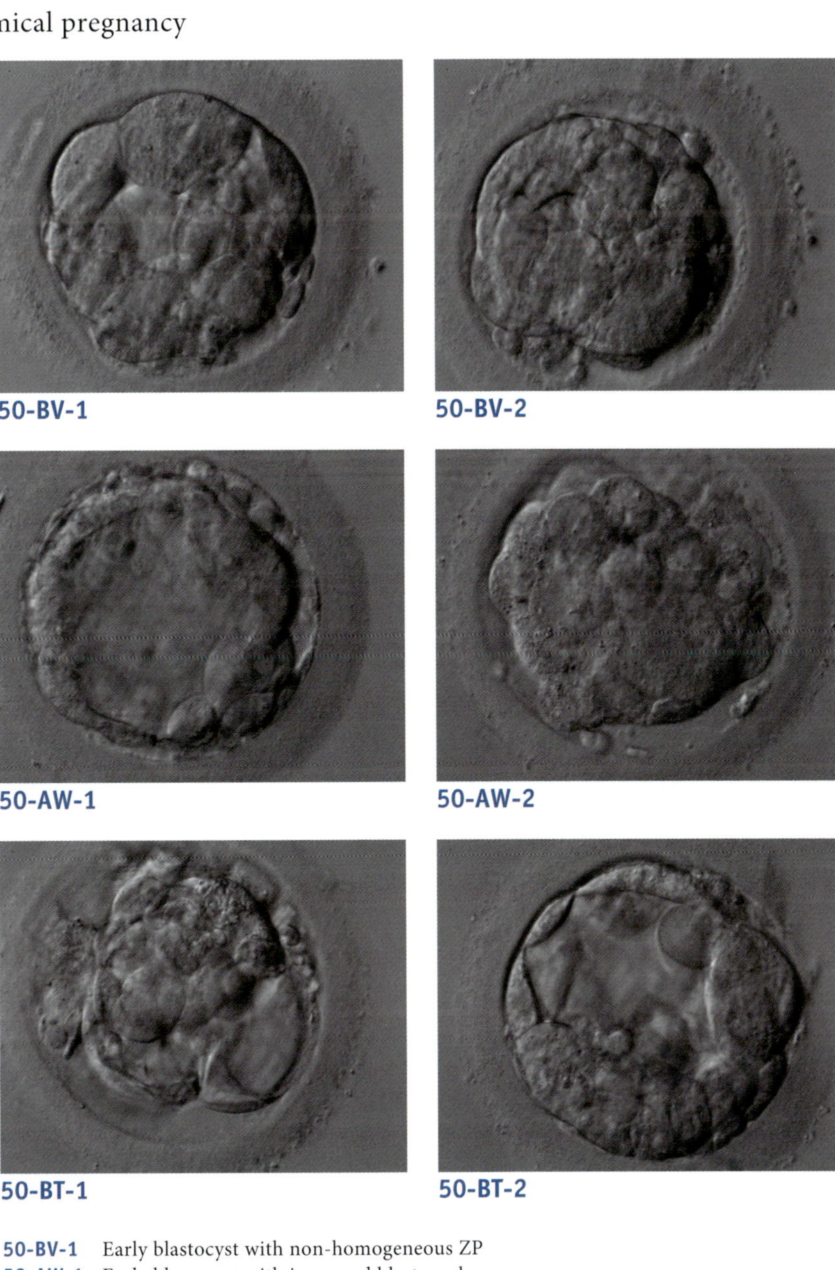

50-BV-1   50-BV-2

50-AW-1   50-AW-2

50-BT-1   50-BT-2

50-BV-1	Early blastocyst with non-homogeneous ZP
50-AW-1	Early blastocyst with increased blastocoel
50-BV-2	Early blastocyst
50-AW-2	Early blastocyst with signs of degeneration
50-BT-1	Worst quality early blastocyst with excluded cells (no transfer)
50-BT-2	Poor quality early blastocyst

Female partner

Age 31, medical engineer
Tubal status: patent
MH: 6/28
BMI: 22.8
Smoker, no alcohol
   consumption
Adhesiolysis
Urethra dilatation

Basal FSH: 7.4 IU/L
Basal LH: 8.2 IU/L
Basal estradiol: 62.2 pg/mL
Basal AMH: 4.88 ng/mL
Midluteal progesterone: 14.4 ng/mL
Midluteal prolactin: 9.0 ng/mL

Male partner

Age 29, engineer
History/examination: NAD
Smoker, no alcohol consumption

Previous treatments

2011 timed intercourse   Not pregnant

Fresh cycle: 2011 ICSI (patient wish)
Semen assessment: normozoospermia

Volume	3.6 mL
Abstinence	4 days
Concentration	210×10^6/mL
Progressive motility	50%
Non-progressive motility	1%
Immotile	49%
Normal forms	7%

Stimulation protocol	Antagonist protocol (recombinant FSH)
Days of stimulation	9
Total dose	1450 IU
Estradiol at ovulation induction	3937 ng/mL
Number of follicles ≥ 12 mm	12
Total number of COCs	10
Metaphase II	8
Injected/inseminated	8
Fertilization rate	63%
Cleavage rate	100%
Blastocyst rate	40%
Culture medium	EmbryoAssist/BlastAssist

Fresh transfer

Quality of embryo(s)	
Outcome	No fresh transfer because of OHSS
Vitrification	1 compacting embryo (day 4), 1 early blastocyst (day 5)

Vitrified/warmed cycle: 2012

Stimulation	HSP
Endometrium	6.5 mm
Quality before vitrification	1
Warming day	5
Survival	Yes
Assisted hatching	Yes
Transfer day	5
Quality	3ab
Duration of cryostorage	2 months
Time between warming and transfer	3h

Outcome: Live birth, healthy boy

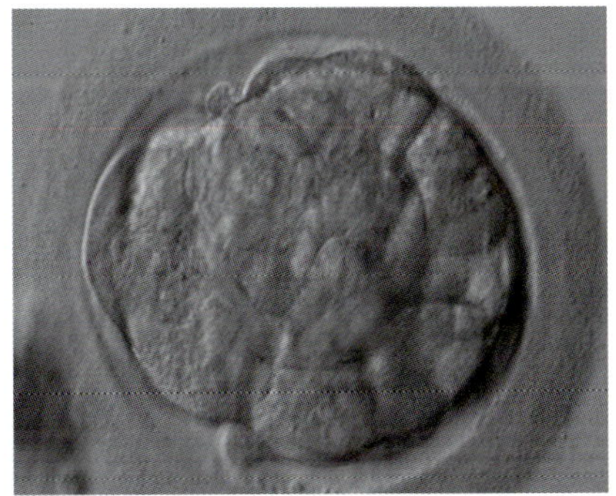

51-BV-1

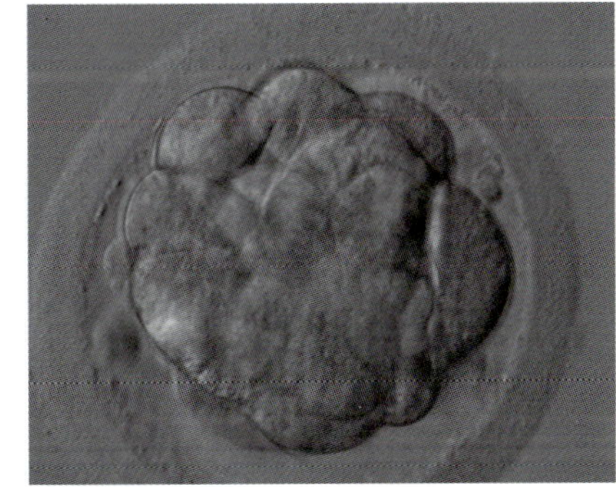

51-AW-1

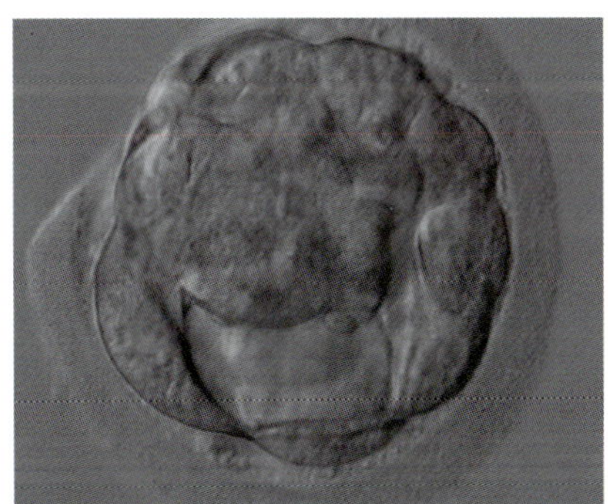

51-BT-1

51-BV-1 Early blastocyst
51-AW-1 Almost re-expanded early blastocyst
51-BT-1 Full blastocyst

Female partner

Age 26, employee
Tubal status: patent
MH: 5/28–30
BMI: 22.5
Non-smoker, no alcohol
  consumption
Basal FSH: 7.5 IU/L
Basal LH: 9.2 IU/L

Basal estradiol: 31.1 pg/mL
Basal AMH: 5.56 ng/mL
Midluteal progesterone: 0.2 ng/mL
Midluteal prolactin: 18.5 ng/mL

Male partner

Age 48, teacher
History/examination: NAD
Smoker, no alcohol consumption
Child with other partner

Previous treatments

2010 ICSI	Not pregnant
2010 vitrified/warmed cycle	Not pregnant

Fresh cycle: 2010 ICSI
Semen assessment: oligoasthenoteratozoospermia

Volume	3.5 mL
Abstinence	5 days
Concentration	8×10^6/mL
Progressive motility	15%
Non-progressive motility	4%
Immotile	81%
Normal forms	1%

Stimulation protocol	Antagonist protocol (recombinant FSH)
Days of stimulation	9
Total dose	1275 IU
Estradiol at ovulation induction	1989 ng/mL
Number of follicles ≥ 12 mm	17
Total number of COCs	17
Metaphase II	16
Injected/inseminated	16
Fertilization rate	94%
Cleavage rate	100%
Blastocyst rate	773%
Culture medium	GM501

Fresh transfer

Quality of embryo(s)	5aa
Outcome	Not pregnant
Vitrification	4 compacting embryos (day 4), 7 blastocysts (day 5)

Vitrified/warmed cycle: 2011

Stimulation	HSP
Endometrium	7.5 mm
Quality before vitrification	Compacting embryo (day 4)
Warming day	4
Survival	Yes
Assisted hatching	Yes
Transfer day	5
Quality	5aa
Duration of cryostorage	1 year
Time between warming and transfer	18h

Outcome: Live birth, healthy boy

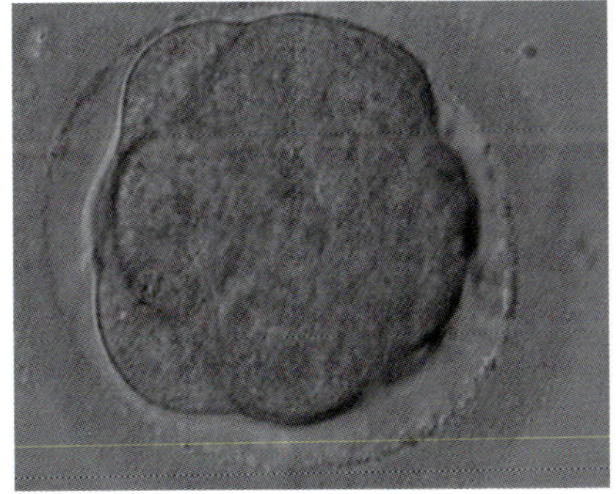

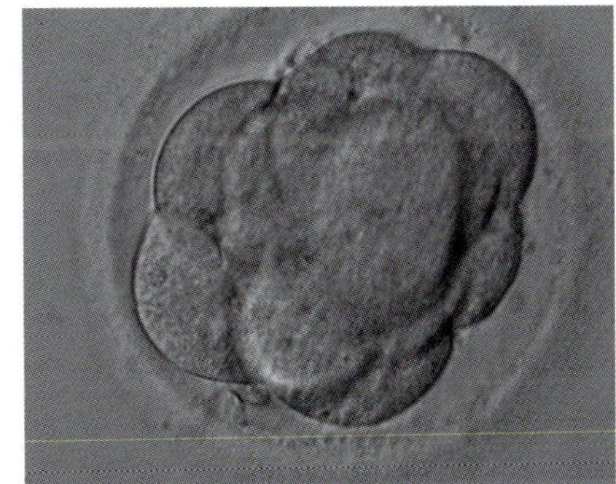

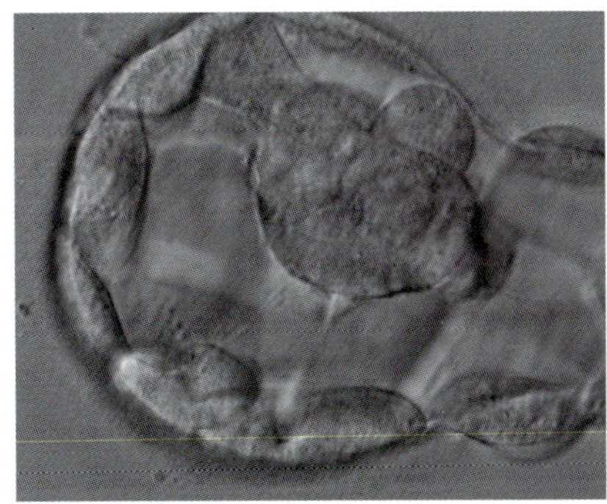

52-BV-1   **52-AW-1**   **52-BT-1**

52-BV-1 Fully compacted embryo
52-AW-1 Fully compacted embryo after warming
52-BT-1 Hatching blastocyst showing cytoplasmic strings in the blastocoel

Female partner

Age 42, cook

Tubal status: patent

MH: 4/28–30

BMI: 28.2

Smoker, no alcohol
  consumption

Normal female karyotype

Basal FSH: 5.2 IU/L

Basal LH: 7.9 IU/L

Basal estradiol: 22.1 pg/mL

Basal AMH: 5.60 ng/mL

Midluteal progesterone: 11.2 ng/mL

Midluteal prolactin: 16.9 ng/mL

Male partner

Age 67, retiree

History/examination: NAD

Smoker, no alcohol consumption

Normal male karyotype

Previous treatments

2004 ICSI	Not pregnant
2004 ICSI	Missed abortion
2005 ICSI × 2	Not pregnant
2006 ICSI	Missed abortion
2010 ICSI	Extrauterine gravidity
2010 vitrified/warmed cycle	Not pregnant

Fresh cycle: 2012 ICSI with ionophore treatment

Semen assessment: severe oligoasthenoteratozoospermia

Volume	1.6 mL
Abstinence	2 days
Concentration	1×10^6/mL
Progressive motility	0%
Non-progressive motility	2%
Immotile	98%
Normal forms	0%

Stimulation protocol	Antagonist protocol (recombinant FSH)
Days of stimulation	10
Total dose	1050 IU
Estradiol at ovulation induction	3180 ng/mL
Number of follicles ≥ 12 mm	16
Total number of COCs	16
Metaphase II	14
Injected/inseminated	14
Fertilization rate	36%
Cleavage rate	100%
Blastocyst rate	60%
Culture medium	GM501

Fresh transfer

Quality of embryo(s)	4aa, 5aa
Outcome	Live birth, healthy girl
Vitrification	2 blastocysts, 1 morula (all day 5)

Vitrified/warmed cycle: 2014

Stimulation	HSP
Endometrium	9.0 mm
Quality before vitrification	4ab
Warming day	5
Survival	Yes
Assisted hatching	Yes
Transfer day	5
Quality	5ab
Duration of cryostorage	22 months
Time between warming and transfer	6h

Outcome: Not pregnant

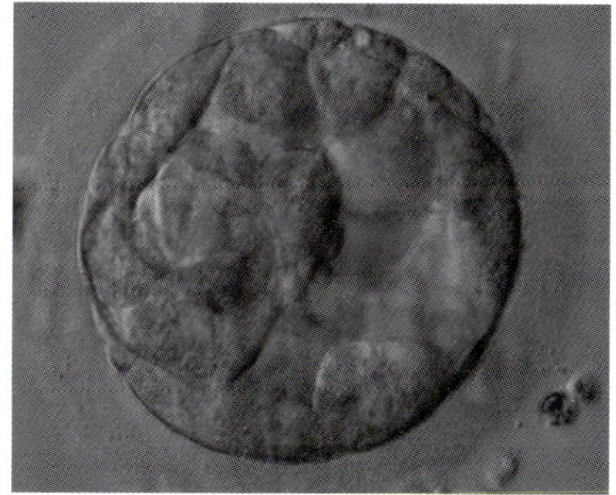

53-BV-1

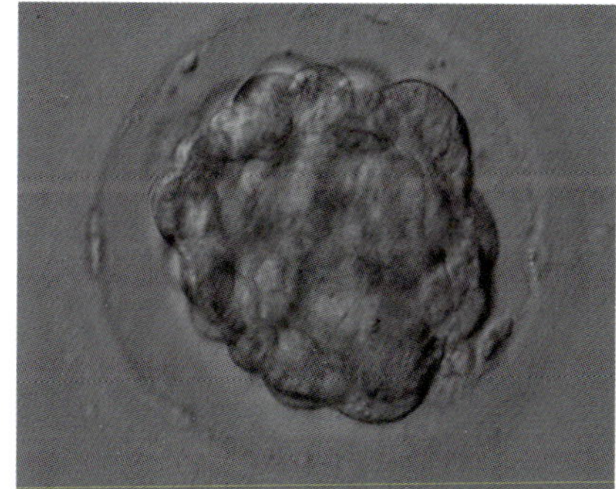

53-AW-1

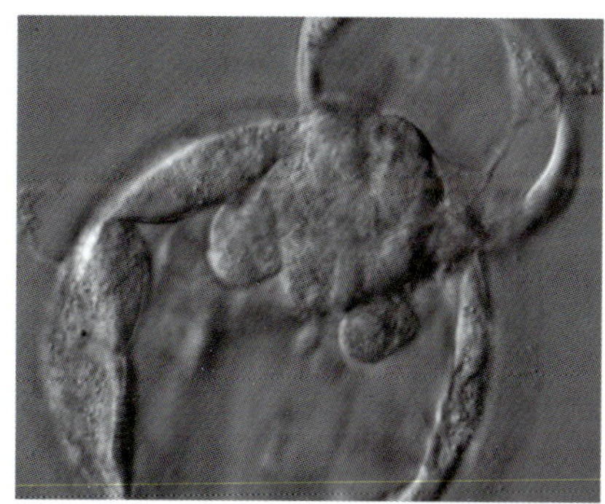

53-BT-1

53-BV-1 Full blastocyst
53-AW-1 Viable blastocyst with minor fragments excluded
53-BT-1 Hatching blastocyst with cytoplasmic string

Case 54

7 years 2° infertility   **Diagnosis: Unexplained infertility**

Female partner

Age 38, civil servant
Tubal status: patent
MH: 3–4/28–41
BMI: 16.5
Non-smoker, no alcohol
  consumption
Uterine polyp
Anovulation

Basal FSH: 4.2 IU/L
Basal LH: 1.9 IU/L
Basal estradiol: 39.5 pg/mL
Basal AMH: 9.95 ng/mL
Midluteal progesterone: 4.3 ng/mL
Midluteal prolactin: 5.9 ng/mL

Male partner

Age 38, civil servant
History/examination: NAD
Smoker, no alcohol consumption

Previous treatments

2006 timed intercourse × 4	Not pregnant
2007 insemination × 2	Not pregnant
2008 IVF	Not pregnant
2008 vitrified/warmed cycle	Not pregnant
2008 vitrified/warmed cycle	Live birth, healthy boy

Fresh cycle: 2010 IVF
Semen assessment: normozoospermia

Volume	2.0 mL
Abstinence	4 days
Concentration	46×10^6/mL
Progressive motility	35%
Non-progressive motility	9%
Immotile	56%
Normal forms	15%

Stimulation protocol	Antagonist protocol (recombinant FSH, HMG)
Days of stimulation	8
Total dose	1275 IU
Estradiol at ovulation induction	1881 ng/mL
Number of follicles ≥ 12 mm	14
Total number of COCs	14
Metaphase II	
Injected/inseminated	14
Fertilization rate	57%
Cleavage rate	88%
Blastocyst rate	86%
Culture medium	EmbryoAssist/BlastAssist

Fresh transfer

Quality of embryo(s)	5aa
Outcome	Missed abortion
Vitrification	5 blastocysts

Previous vitrified warmed cycle

Quality of embryo(s)	4aa
Outcome	Not pregnant

Vitrified/warmed cycle: 2012

Stimulation	HSP
Endometrium	7.0 mm
Quality before vitrification	4ab
Warming day	5
Survival	Yes
Assisted hatching	Yes
Transfer day	5
Quality	4ab
Duration of cryostorage	2 years
Time between warming and transfer	3h

Outcome: Biochemical pregnancy

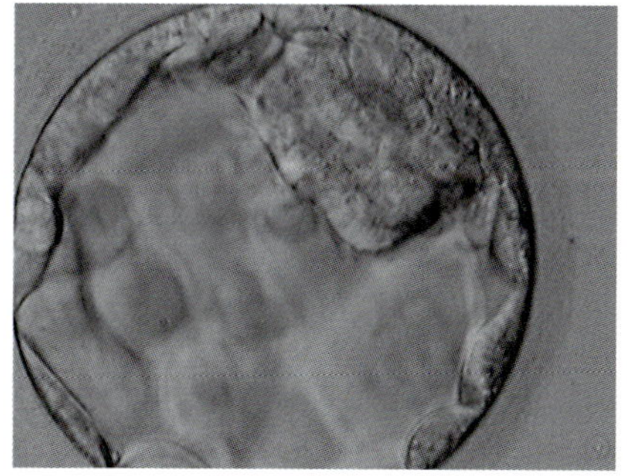

54-BV-1

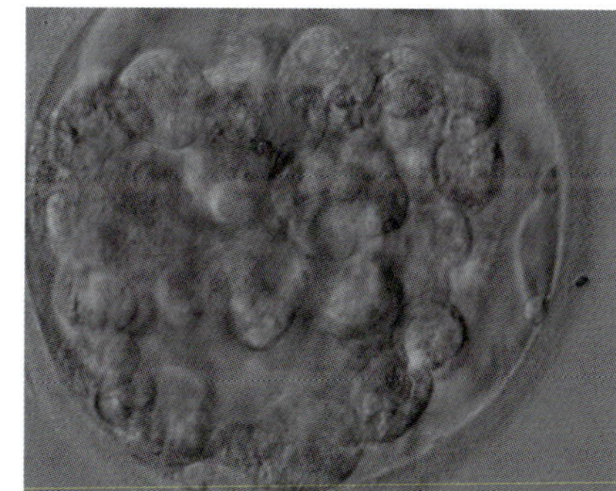

54-AW-1

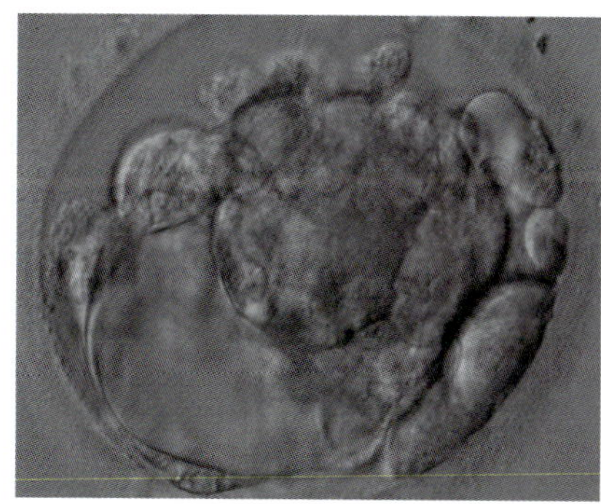

54-BT-1

54-BV-1 Expanded blastocyst
54-AW-1 Blastocyst with granulated cytoplasm
54-BT-1 Partly re-expanded blastocyst with excluded fragments/blastomeres

Female partner

Age 36, civil servant
Tubal status: patent
MH: 5/28
BMI: 28.2
Smoker, no alcohol
  consumption
Normal female karyotype
History of thrombosis

Basal FSH: 10.3 IU/L
Basal LH: 6.0 IU/L
Basal estradiol: 39.1 pg/mL
Basal AMH: 0.97 ng/mL

Male partner

Age 46, civil servant
History/examination: NAD
Non-smoker, no alcohol
  consumption
Normal male karyotype

Previous treatments

2006 spontaneous

Termination of pregnancy

Fresh cycle: 2011 ICSI
Semen assessment: asthenoteratozoospermia

Volume	4.2 mL
Abstinence	4 days
Concentration	18×10^6/mL
Progressive motility	7%
Non-progressive motility	16%
Immotile	77%
Normal forms	2%

Stimulation protocol	Antagonist protocol (HMG)
Days of stimulation	13
Total dose	3600 IU
Estradiol at ovulation induction	752 ng/mL
Number of follicles $\geq$ 12 mm	3
Total number of COCs	3
Metaphase II	3
Injected/inseminated	3
Fertilization rate	100%
Cleavage rate	100%
Blastocyst rate	100%
Culture medium	GM501

Fresh transfer

Quality of embryo(s)	5ab
Outcome	Not pregnant
Vitrification	2 blastocysts

Vitrified/warmed cycle: 2011

Stimulation	HSP
Endometrium	8.5 mm
Quality before vitrification	3ab
Warming day	5
Survival	Yes
Assisted hatching	Yes
Transfer day	5
Quality	3ab
Duration of cryostorage	1
Time between warming and transfer	5h

Outcome: Live birth, healthy boy

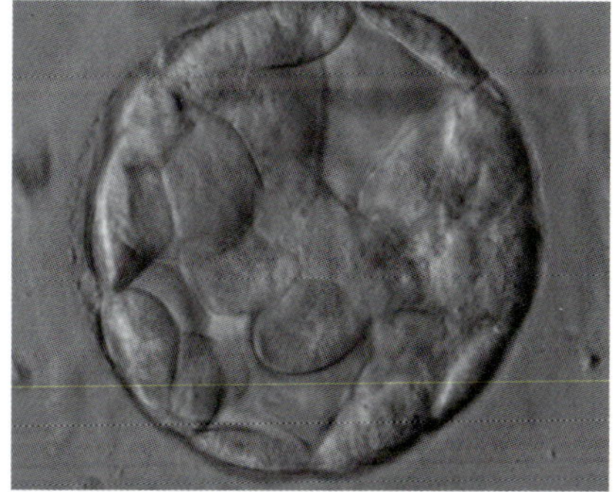

55-BV-1

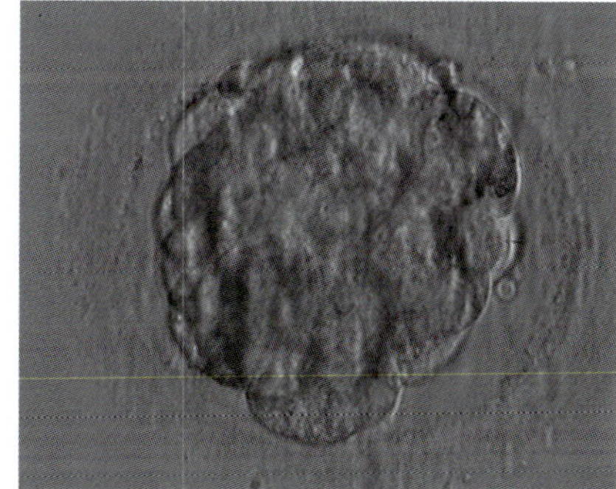

55-AW-1

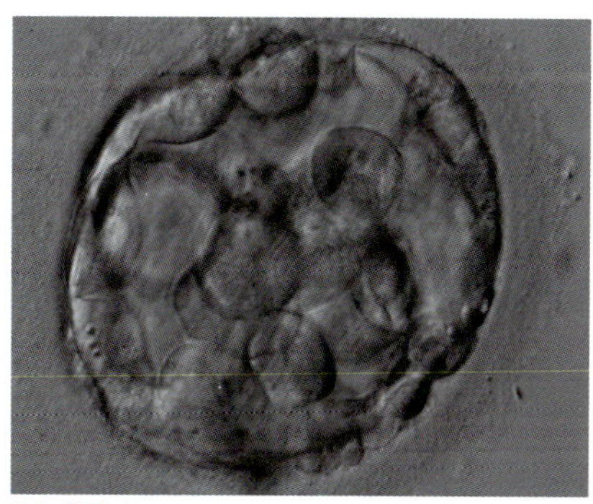

55-BT-1

55-BV-1 Full blastocyst (inner cell mass composed of few cells)
55-AW-1 Same blastocyst with extensive granulation after warming
55-BT-1 Re‑expanded blastocyst

Case 56

Female partner

Age 31, teacher
Tubal status: patent
MH: dysmenorrhea
BMI: 22.2
Smoker, no alcohol
  consumption
Anovulation

Basal FSH: 4.4 IU/L
Basal LH: 0.6 IU/L
Basal estradiol: 18 pg/mL
Basal AMH: 4.32 ng/mL

Male partner

Age 28, teacher
History/examination: history
  of cryptorchism
Non-smoker, no alcohol consumption

Previous treatments

2009 ICSI × 3   Not pregnant
2009 vitrified/warmed cycle   Extrauterine gravity
2010 ICSI   Not pregnant

Fresh cycle: 2011 ICSI
Semen assessment: severe oligoasthenoteratozoospermia

Volume	3.3 mL
Abstinence	5 days
Concentration	1.3×10^6/mL
Progressive motility	10%
Non-progressive motility	10%
Immotile	80%
Normal forms	1%

Stimulation protocol	Agonist protocol (HMG)
Days of stimulation	13
Total dose	1800 IU
Estradiol at ovulation induction	5139 ng/mL
Number of follicles $\geq$ 12 mm	12
Total number of COCs	10
Metaphase II	10
Injected/inseminated	10
Fertilization rate	80%
Cleavage rate	100%
Blastocyst rate	38%
Culture medium	GM501

Fresh transfer

Quality of embryo(s)	3ab
Outcome	Not pregnant
Vitrification	1 embryo with beginning compaction, 1 morula (day 5)

Vitrified/warmed cycle: 2011

Stimulation	HSP
Endometrium	9.0 mm
Quality before vitrification	Embryo with beginning compaction, morula
Warming day	5
Survival	Yes, Yes
Assisted hatching	Yes, Yes
Transfer day	5
Quality	Compacting embryo, morula
Duration of cryostorage	1
Time between warming and transfer	2h

Outcome: Live birth, healthy boy

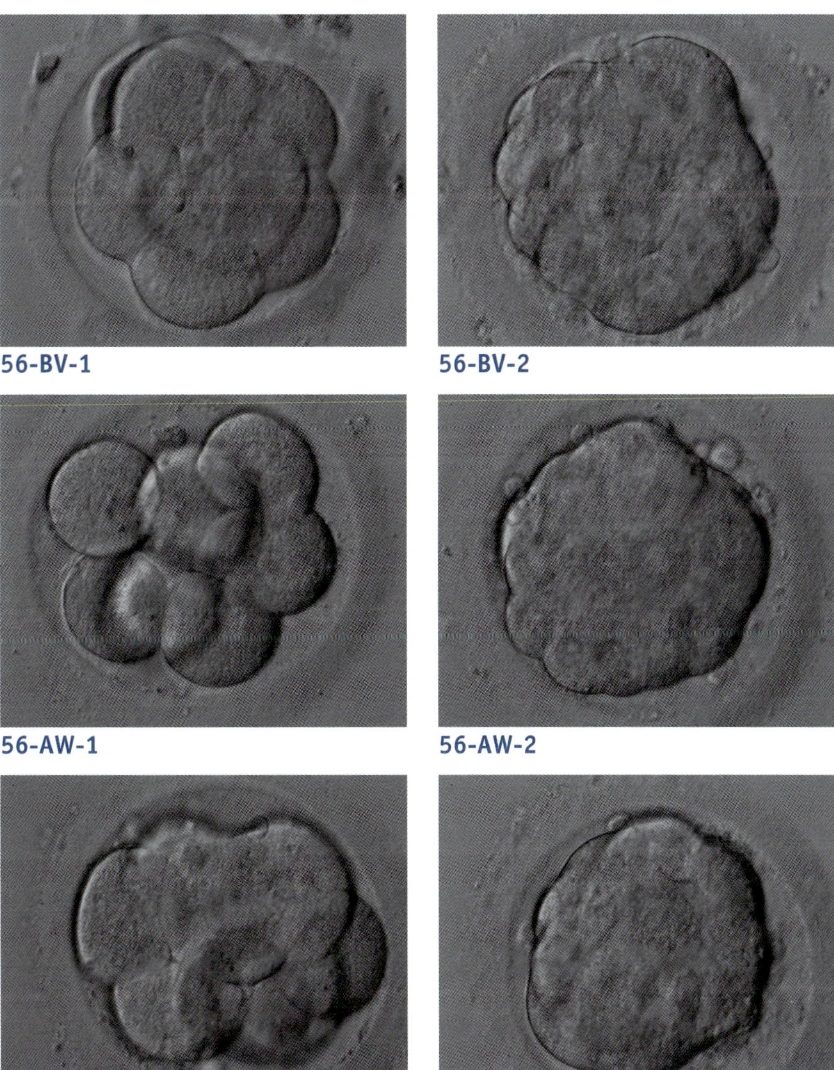

56-BV-1

56-BV-2

56-AW-1

56-AW-2

56-BT-1

56-BT-2

56-BV-1 10-cell embryo of good quality showing signs of compaction. Remark: Regression of cell–cell contacts should be noted in embryo #1

56-AW-1 10-cell embryo

56-BT-1 Compacting embryo

56-BV-2 Morula of optimal quality

56-AW-2 Viable morula (not fully re-expanded)

56-BT-2 Viable morula (not fully re-expanded)

Female partner

Age 36, employee
Tubal status: patent
MH: 5/28
BMI: 21.7
Non-smoker, no alcohol
  consumption
Hypoferremia

Basal FSH: 7.1 IU/L
Basal LH: 5.7 IU/L
Basal estradiol: 36.6 pg/mL
Basal AMH: 6.06 ng/mL
Midluteal progesterone: 12.9 ng/mL
Midluteal prolactin: 16.1 ng/mL

Male partner

Age 44, employee
History/examination: NAD
Non-smoker, no alcohol
  consumption
Hepatitis B

Previous treatments

None

Fresh cycle: 2011 ICSI

Semen assessment: severe oligoasthenoteratozoospermia

Volume	4.4 mL
Abstinence	3 days
Concentration	0.5×10^6/mL
Progressive motility	25%
Non-progressive motility	25%
Immotile	50%
Normal forms	0%

Stimulation protocol	Antagonist protocol (HMG, recombinant FSH)
Days of stimulation	11
Total dose	1450 IU
Estradiol at ovulation induction	1685 ng/mL
Number of follicles ≥ 12 mm	13
Total number of COCs	6 (from one ovary only)
Metaphase II	6
Injected/inseminated	6
Fertilization rate	83%
Cleavage rate	100%
Blastocyst rate	60%
Culture medium	EmbryoAssist/BlastAssist

Fresh transfer

Quality of embryo(s)	5aa
Outcome	Missed abortion (no heart activity)
Vitrification	2 blastocysts

Vitrified/warmed cycle: 2013

Stimulation	NC
Endometrium	10.0 mm
Quality before vitrification	4aa
Warming day	5
Survival	Yes
Assisted hatching	Yes
Transfer day	5
Quality	4aa
Duration of cryostorage	2.5 years
Time between warming and transfer	2h

Outcome: Live birth, healthy girl

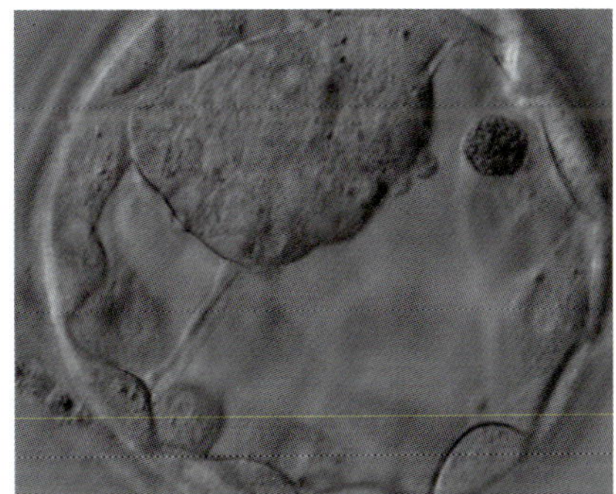

57-BV-1

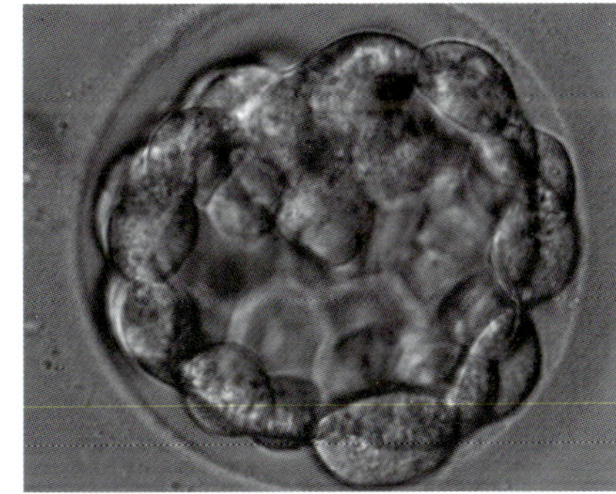

57-AW-1

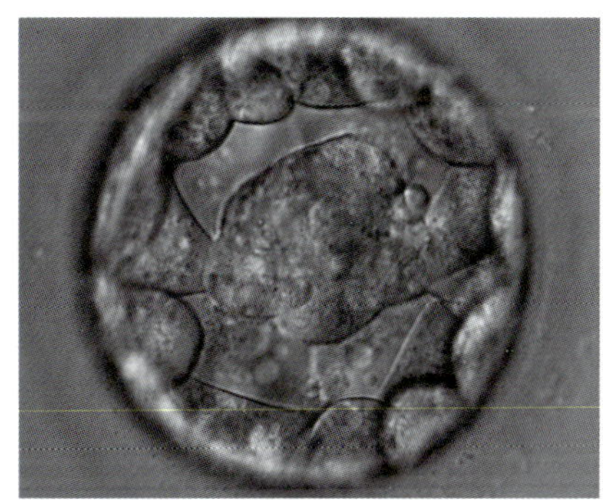

57-BT-1

57-BV-1 Expanded blastocyst with necrotic cell in blastocoel
57-AW-1 Partly re-expanded blastocyst
57-BT-1 Fully re-expanded blastocyst of optimal quality

Female partner

Age 25, saleswoman
Tubal status: patent
MH: 3–4/28
BMI: 18.8
Non-smoker, no alcohol
  consumption
Dysmenorrhea

Basal FSH: 8.2 IU/L
Basal LH: 6.0 IU/L
Basal estradiol: 31.4 pg/mL
Basal AMH: 4.12 ng/mL
Midluteal progesterone: 5.6 ng/mL
Midluteal prolactin: 10.5 ng/mL

Male partner

Age 25, salesman
History/examination: NAD
Smoker, no alcohol
  consumption

Fresh cycle: 2013 ICSI
Semen assessment: teratozoospermia

Volume	3 mL
Abstinence	4 days
Concentration	26×10^6/mL
Progressive motility	61%
Non-progressive motility	8%
Immotile	31%
Normal forms	2%

Stimulation protocol	Agonist protocol (HMG)
Days of stimulation	13
Total dose	1500 IU
Estradiol at ovulation induction	3022 ng/mL
Number of follicles $\geq$ 12 mm	16
Total number of COCs	16
Metaphase II	14
Injected/inseminated	14
Fertilization rate	86%
Cleavage rate	100%
Blastocyst rate	75%
Culture medium	EmbryoAssist/BlastAssist

Fresh transfer

Quality of embryo(s)	5aa
Outcome	Not pregnant
Vitrification	7 blastocysts

Previous vitrified/warmed cycles

2013 ×2   Not pregnant

Vitrified/warmed cycle: 2013

Stimulation	HSP
Endometrium	10.0 mm
Quality before vitrification	4aa
Warming day	5
Survival	Yes
Assisted hatching	Yes
Transfer day	5
Quality	4aa
Duration of cryostorage	6 months
Time between warming and transfer	2h

Outcome: Live birth, healthy girl

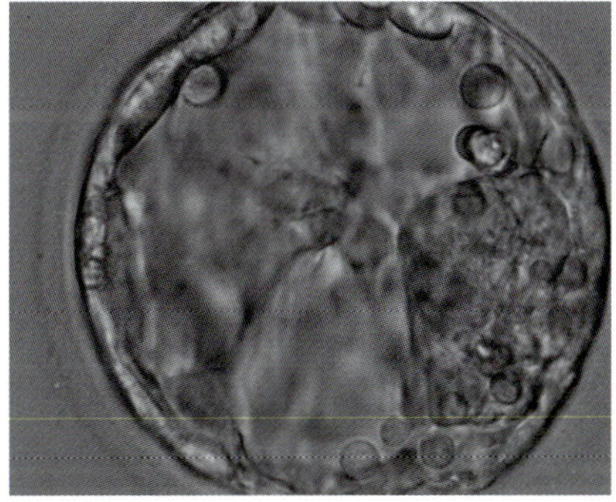
58-BV-1

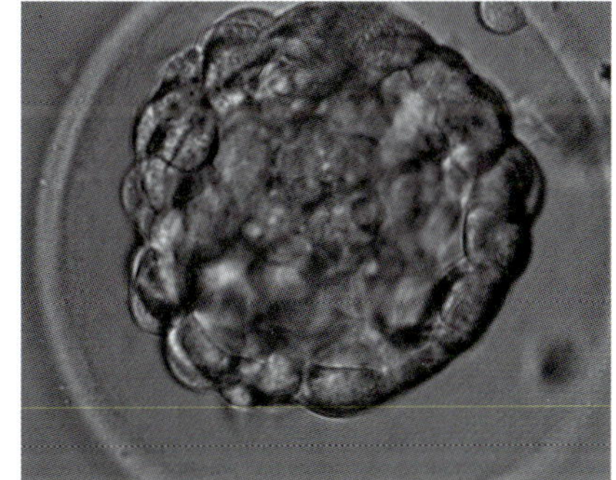
58-AW-1

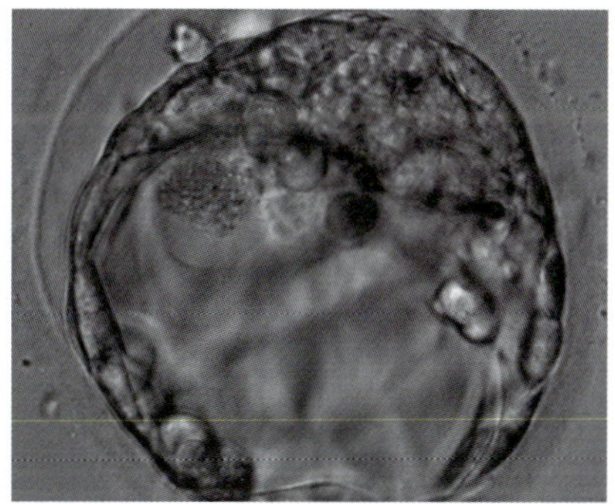
58-BT-1

58-BV-1 Expanded blastocyst
58-AW-1 Blastocyst not fully re-expanded
58-BT-1 Re-expanded blastocyst with necrotic cell in blastocoel

Female partner

Age 39, social worker
Tubal status: patent
MH: 3–4/30–35
BMI: 24.5
Non-smoker, no alcohol
  consumption
Anovulation

Basal FSH: 5.2 IU/L
Basal LH: 7.8 IU/L
Basal estradiol: 78.2 pg/mL
Basal AMH: 10.03 ng/mL
Midluteal progesterone: 0.2 ng/mL
Midluteal prolactin: 8.4 ng/mL

Male partner

Age 50, civil servant
History/examination: NAD
Non-smoker, no alcohol
  consumption
Psoriasis, ankylosing spondylitis

Previous treatments

None

Fresh cycle: 2012 ICSI
Semen assessment: oligoasthenoteratozoospermia

Volume	0.6 mL
Abstinence	5 days
Concentration	28×10^6/mL
Progressive motility	18%
Non-progressive motility	10%
Immotile	72%
Normal forms	1%

Stimulation protocol	Antagonist protocol (recombinant FSH)
Days of stimulation	8
Total dose	1086 IU
Estradiol at ovulation induction	3300 ng/mL
Number of follicles ≥ 12 mm	20
Total number of COCs	13
Metaphase II	11
Injected/inseminated	10
Fertilization rate	70%
Cleavage rate	100%
Blastocyst rate	71%
Culture medium	EmbryoAssist/BlastAssist

Fresh transfer

Quality of embryo(s)	4aa
Outcome	Live birth, healthy boy
Vitrification	4 blastocysts

Vitrified/warmed cycle: 2013

Stimulation	HSP
Endometrium	10.0 mm
Quality before vitrification	4ab
Warming day	5
Survival	Yes
Assisted hatching	Yes
Transfer day	5
Quality	4ab
Duration of cryostorage	2 years
Time between warming and transfer	3h

Outcome: Not pregnant

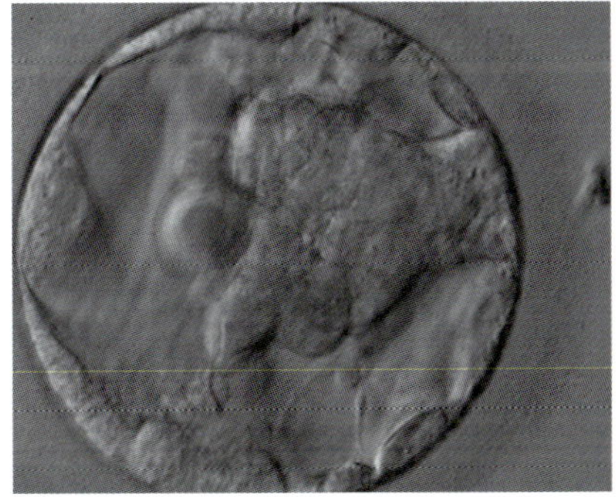
59-BV-1

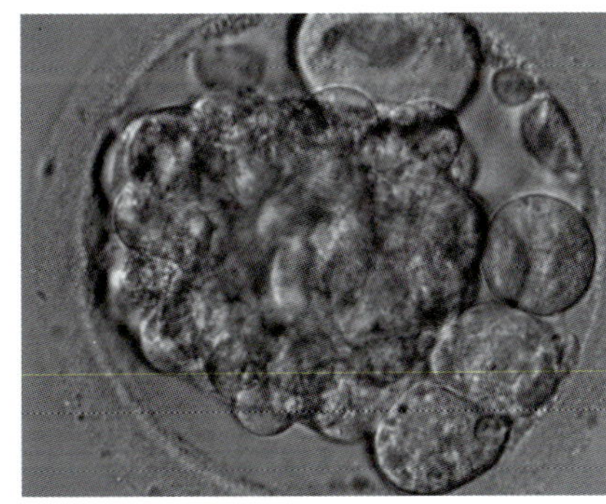
59-AW-1

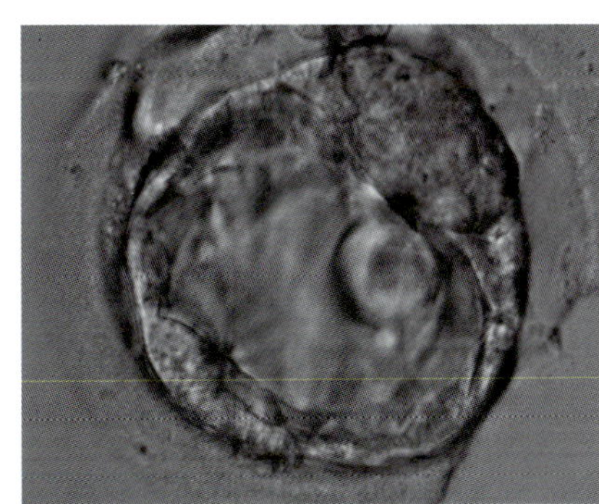
59-BT-1

59-BV-1 Expanded blastocyst with moderate trophectoderm
59-AW-1 Warmed blastocyst with cytoplasmic granulation and 4 excluded blastomeres in perivitelline space
59-BT-1 Same blastocyst as 59-AW-1 after removal of excluded blastomeres

Case 60

2 years 2° infertility   Diagnosis: Male factor infertility

Female partner

Age 24, waitress
Tubal status: patent
MH: dysmenorrhea
BMI: 15.6
Smoker, no alcohol
  consumption
Anovulation

Basal FSH: 9.6 IU/L
Basal LH: 3.5 IU/L
Basal estradiol: 50.0 pg/mL
Basal AMH: 3.61 ng/mL
Midluteal progesterone: 4.4 ng/mL
Midluteal prolactin: 3.2 ng/mL

Male partner

Age 41, carpenter
History/examination: NAD
Non-smoker, no alcohol
  consumption
Normal male karyotype

Previous treatments

None

Fresh cycle: 2011 ICSI
Semen assessment: asthenoteratozoospermia

Volume	4.8 mL
Abstinence	3 days
Concentration	16×10^6/mL
Progressive motility	27%
Non-progressive motility	6%
Immotile	67%
Normal forms	3%

Stimulation protocol	Antagonist protocol (recombinant FSH)
Days of stimulation	9
Total dose	950 IU
Estradiol at ovulation induction	3538 ng/mL
Number of follicles ≥ 12 mm	25
Total number of COCs	22
Metaphase II	16
Injected/inseminated	16
Fertilization rate	50%
Cleavage rate	100%
Blastocyst rate	50%
Culture medium	GM501

Fresh transfer

Quality of embryo(s)	No fresh transfer because of OHSS
Outcome	
Vitrification	One compacting embryo, 2 early blastocysts (day 4), 2 blastocysts (day 5)

Vitrified/warmed cycle: 2012

Stimulation	NC
Endometrium	10.0 mm
Quality before vitrification	3ab
Warming day	5
Survival	Yes
Assisted hatching	Yes
Transfer day	5
Quality	4ab
Duration of cryostorage	2 months
Time between warming and transfer	4h

Outcome: Live birth, healthy girl

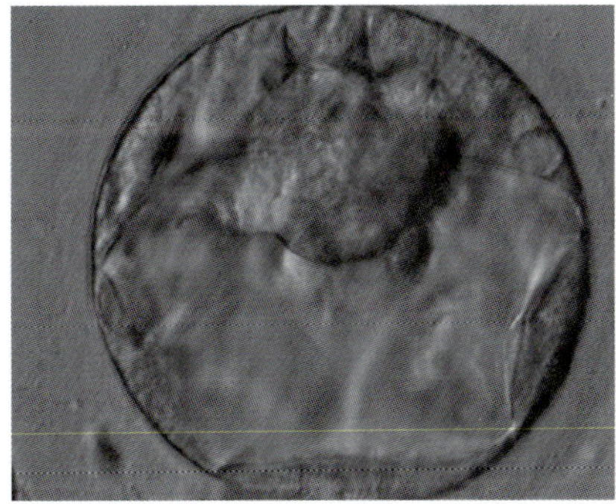

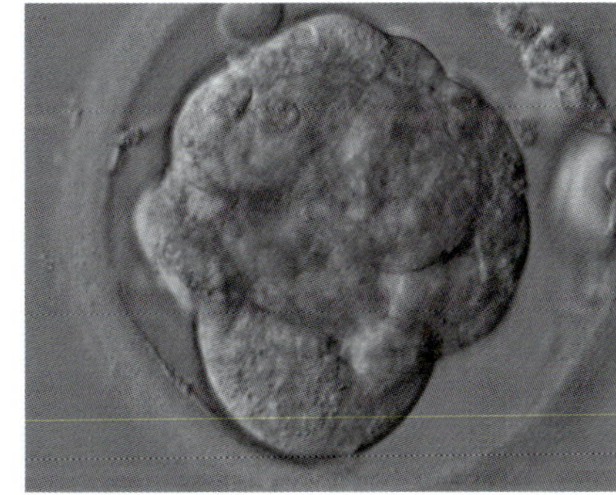

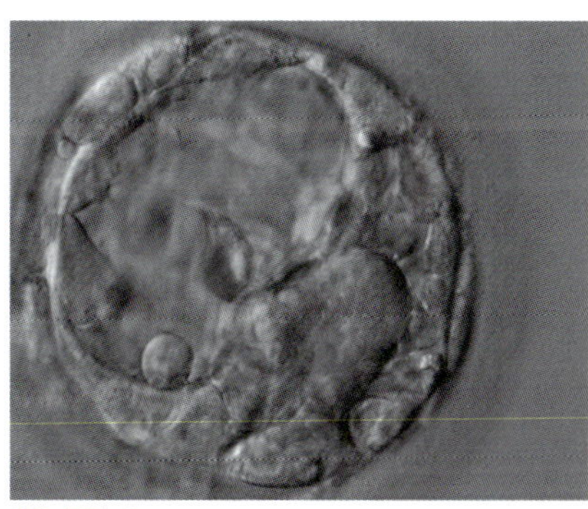

60-BV-1   **60-AW-1**   **60-BT-1**

60-BV-1   Full blastocyst with necrotic focus at 5 o'clock position of inner cell mass
60-AW-1   Non re-expanded blastocyst with minor fragmentation in perivitelline space
60-BT-1   Re-expanded blastocyst with excluded fragments in the top left quadrant

Case 61

7 years 2° infertility   Diagnosis: Tubal infertility

Female partner

Age 35, cleaning woman
Tubal status: bilateral
  blockage
MH: 5/28
BMI: 21.3
Smoker, no alcohol
  consumption
Massive adhesions
Basal FSH: 8.6 IU/L

Basal LH: 3.2 IU/L
Basal estradiol: 36.8 pg/mL
Basal AMH: 2.28 ng/mL
Midluteal progesterone: 11.3 ng/mL
Midluteal prolactin: 25.2 ng/mL
TSH: 2.99 IU/L

Male partner

Age 41, lorry driver
History/examination: NAD
Smoker, no alcohol
  consumption

Previous treatments

None

Fresh cycle: 2008 IVF

Semen assessment: normozoospermia

Volume	3.6 mL
Abstinence	4 days
Concentration	72×10^6/mL
Progressive motility	61%
Non-progressive motility	8%
Immotile	31%
Normal forms	12%

Stimulation protocol	Agonist protocol (recombinant FSH)
Days of stimulation	9
Total dose	1450 IU
Estradiol at ovulation induction	2227 ng/mL
Number of follicles ≥ 12 mm	17
Total number of COCs	16
Metaphase II	
Injected/inseminated	16
Fertilization rate	38%
Cleavage rate	100%
Blastocyst rate	50%
Culture medium	EmbryoAssist/BlastAssist

Fresh transfer

Quality of embryo(s)	3aa
Outcome	Live birth, healthy boy
Vitrification	2 blastocysts

Vitrified/warmed cycle: 2013

Stimulation	NC
Endometrium	7.5 mm
Quality before vitrification	3ab
Warming day	5
Survival	Yes
Assisted hatching	Yes
Transfer day	5
Quality	3ab
Duration of cryostorage	5 years
Time between warming and transfer	3h

Outcome: Live birth, healthy girl

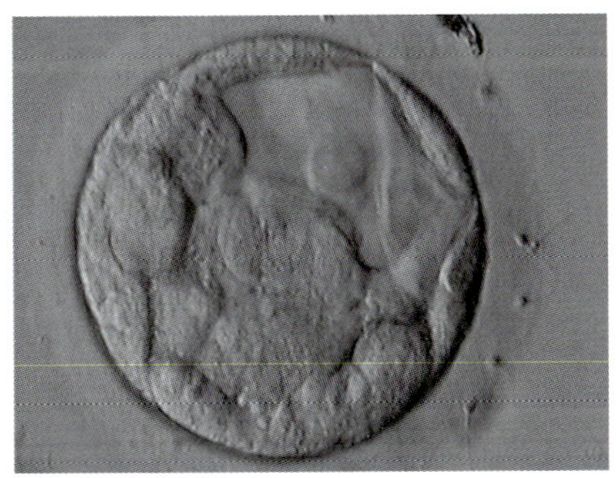

61-BV-1

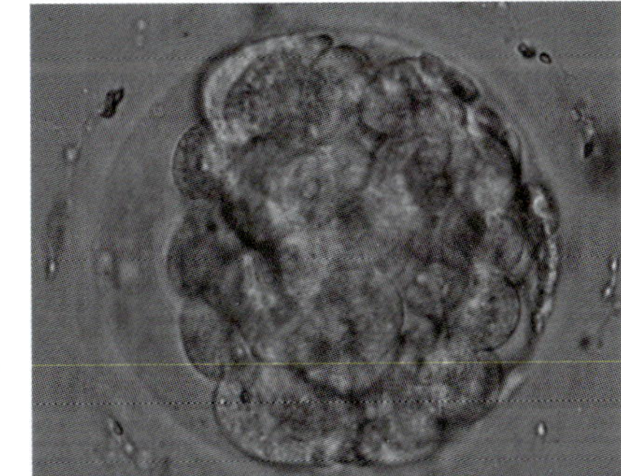

61-AW-1

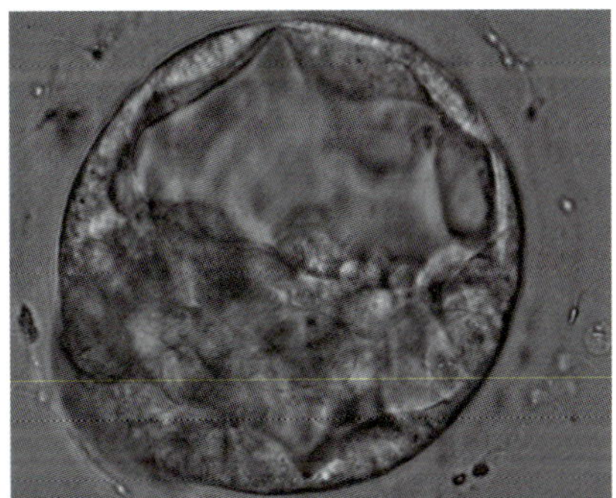

61-BT-1

61-BV-1 Full blastocyst
61-AW-1 Warmed blastocyst with minor cytoplasmic granulation
61-BT-1 Re-expanded full blastocyst

Female partner

Age 36, worker

Tubal status: bilateral sactosalpinx

MH: 1–2/21–28

BMI: 23.3

Smoker, no alcohol consumption

Dyspareunia

Penicillin allergy, neurodermatitis

Basal FSH: 7.5 IU/L

Basal LH: 6.5 IU/L

Basal estradiol: 38.5 pg/mL

Basal AMH: 2.19 ng/mL

Midluteal progesterone: 5.0 ng/mL

Midluteal prolactin: 21.1 ng/mL

Male partner

Age 33, fork-lift driver

History/examination: leucospermia

Smoker, no alcohol consumption

Adipositas

BMI: 39.0

Previous treatments

2011 timed intercourse	Not pregnant
2012 insemination	Not pregnant

Fresh cycle: 2012 ICSI

Semen assessment: oligoasthenoteratozoospermia

Volume	2.4 mL
Abstinence	2 days
Concentration	5×10^6/mL
Progressive motility	24%
Non-progressive motility	6%
Immotile	70%
Normal forms	3%

Stimulation protocol	Antagonist protocol (recombinant FSH)
Days of stimulation	8
Total dose	1250 IU
Estradiol at ovulation induction	752 ng/mL
Number of follicles $\geq$ 12 mm	9
Total number of COCs	4
Metaphase II	4
Injected/inseminated	4
Fertilization rate	75%
Cleavage rate	100%
Blastocyst rate	100%
Culture medium	EmbryoAssist/BlastAssist

Fresh transfer

Quality of embryo(s)	5aa
Outcome	Not pregnant
Vitrification	2 blastocysts

Vitrified/warmed cycle: 2012

Stimulation	HSP
Endometrium	9 mm
Quality before vitrification	4aa
Warming day	5
Survival	Yes
Assisted hatching	Yes
Transfer day	5
Quality	4ab
Duration of cryostorage	2 months
Time between warming and transfer	2h

Outcome: Pregnant, missed abortion (no heart activity)

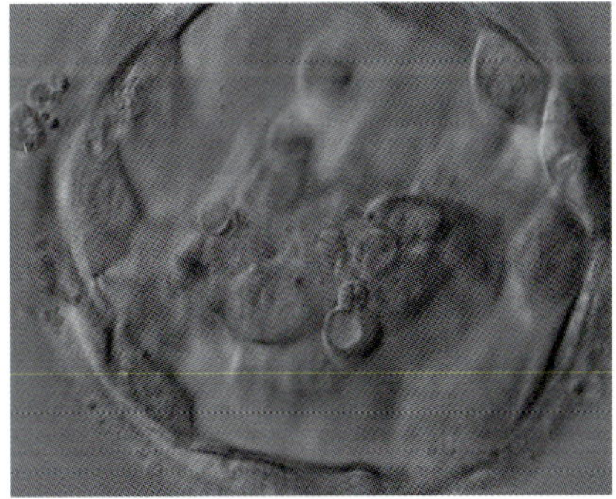
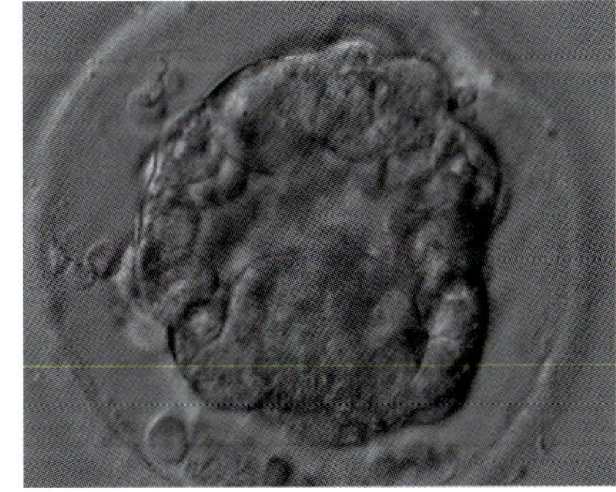
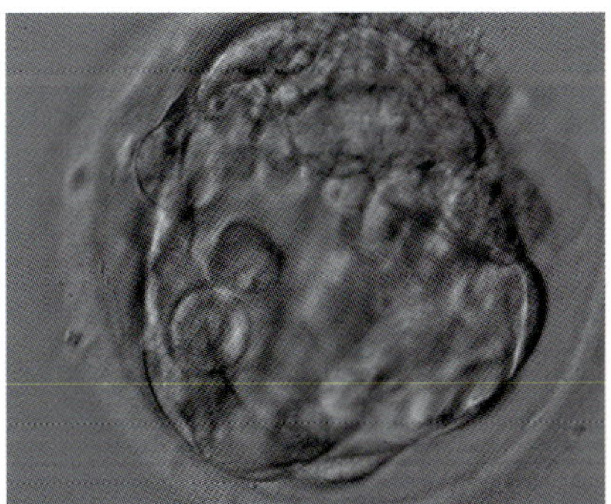

62-BV-1

62-AW-1

62-BT-1

62-BV-1 Expanded blastocyst with reduced trophectoderm
62-AW-1 Expanded blastocyst with no signs of re-expansion
62-BT-1 Partly re-expanded blastocyst with fragments in the blastocoel (8 o'clock position)

Female partner

Age 38, farmer
Tubal status: patent
MH: 3–4/28
BMI: 33.5
Non-smoker, no alcohol
  consumption
Adipositas, struma
Autoimmune disease
  (M. Hashimoto)

Basal FSH: 7.2 IU/L
Basal LH: 2.8 IU/L
Basal estradiol: 44.4 pg/mL
Basal AMH: 3.91 ng/mL
Midluteal progesterone: 7.8 ng/mL
Midluteal prolactin: 20.9 ng/mL

Male partner

Age 41, farmer
History/examination: NAD
Non-smoker, no alcohol
  consumption

Previous treatments

2011 ICSI	Not pregnant
2011 ICSI	Stillbirth
2012 vitrified/warmed cycle	Not pregnant

Fresh cycle: 2012 ICSI
Semen assessment: oligoteratozoospermia

Volume	2.1 mL
Abstinence	4 days
Concentration	12×10^6/mL
Progressive motility	35%
Non-progressive motility	0%
Immotile	65%
Normal forms	1%

Stimulation protocol	Agonist protocol (HMG)
Days of stimulation	11
Total dose	2700 IU
Estradiol at ovulation induction	3073 ng/mL
Number of follicles ≥ 12 mm	21

Total number of COCs	14
Metaphase II	9
Injected/inseminated	9
Fertilization rate	89%
Cleavage rate	100%
Blastocyst rate	25%
Culture medium	EmbryoAssist/BlastAssist

Fresh transfer

Quality of embryo(s)	Morula (day 5)
Outcome	Biochemical pregnancy
Vitrification	1 morula (day 5)

Vitrified/warmed cycle: 2013

Stimulation	HSP
Endometrium	10.0 mm
Quality before vitrification	Morula (day 5)
Warming day	5
Survival	Yes
Assisted hatching	Yes
Transfer day	5
Quality	2
Duration of cryostorage	8 months
Time between warming and transfer	3h

Outcome: Live birth, healthy girl

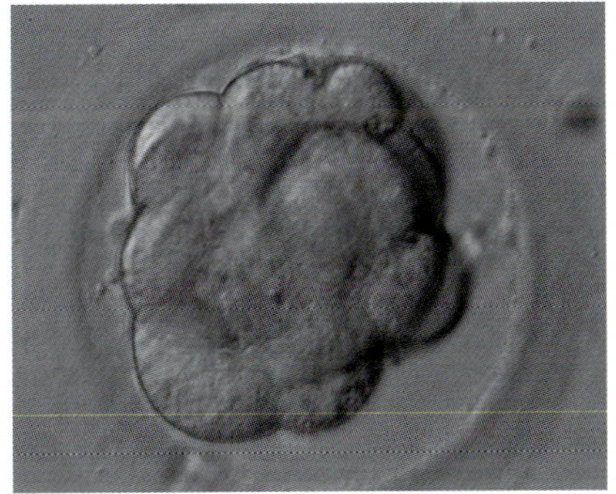

63-BV-1

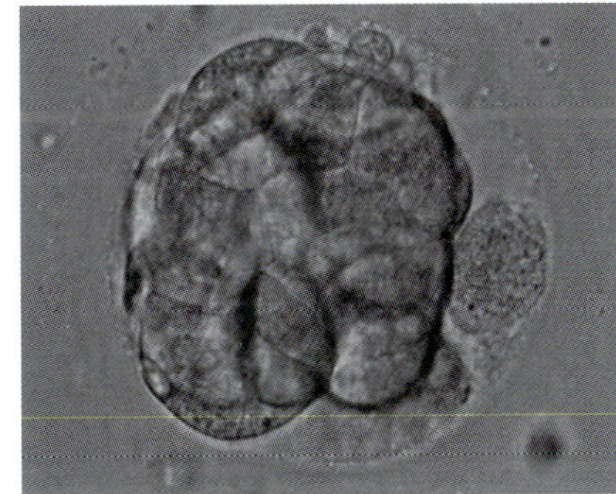

63-AW-1

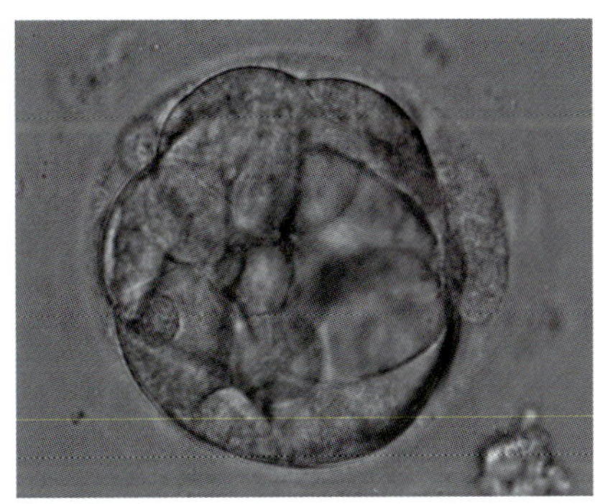

63-BT-1

63-BV-1 Morula
63-AW-1 Morula with beginning cavitation
63-BT-1 Early blastocyst with necrotic focus at 9 o'clock position

Female partner

Age 36, cook
Tubal status: patent
MH: 5/28
BMI: 24.2
Non-smoker, no alcohol
  consumption

Basal FSH: 7.7 IU/L
Basal LH: 5.1 IU/L
Basal estradiol: 56.9 pg/mL
Basal AMH: 6.7 ng/mL

Male partner

Age 42, farmer
History/examination: NAD
Non-smoker, no alcohol
  consumption
Normal male karyotype

Previous treatments

None

Fresh cycle: 2011 ICSI
Semen assessment: oligoasthenoteratozoospermia

Volume	2.0 mL
Abstinence	4 days
Concentration	6×10^6/mL
Progressive motility	22%
Non-progressive motility	3%
Immotile	75%
Normal forms	2%

Stimulation protocol	Agonist protocol (HMG)
Days of stimulation	9
Total dose	IU
Estradiol at ovulation induction	2571 ng/mL
Number of follicles ≥ 12 mm	15
Total number of COCs	15
Metaphase II	14
Injected/inseminated	14
Fertilization rate	86%
Cleavage rate	92%
Blastocyst rate	42%
Culture medium	EmbryoAssist/BlastAssist

Fresh transfer

Quality of embryo(s)	One compacting embryo, one early blastocyst (day 5)
Outcome	Not pregnant
Vitrification	3 early blastocysts

Previous vitrified/warmed cycles

2011   Not pregnant

Vitrified/warmed cycle: 2011

Stimulation	HSP
Endometrium	8.5 mm
Quality before vitrification	1 (day 5)
Warming day	5
Survival	Yes
Assisted hatching	Yes
Transfer day	5
Quality	2
Duration of cryostorage	9 months
Time between warming and transfer	2h

Outcome: Live birth, healthy boy

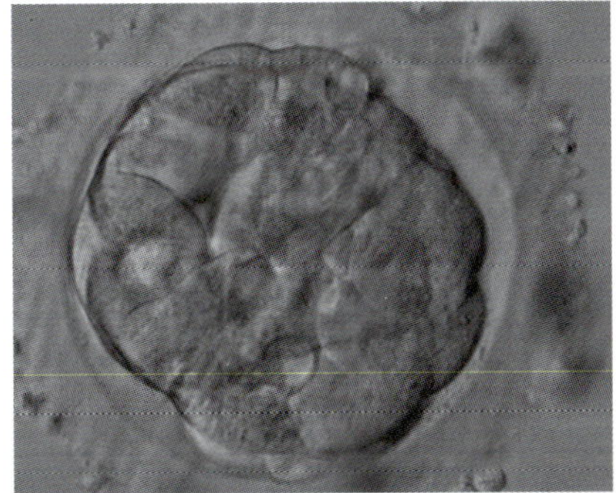

64-BV-1

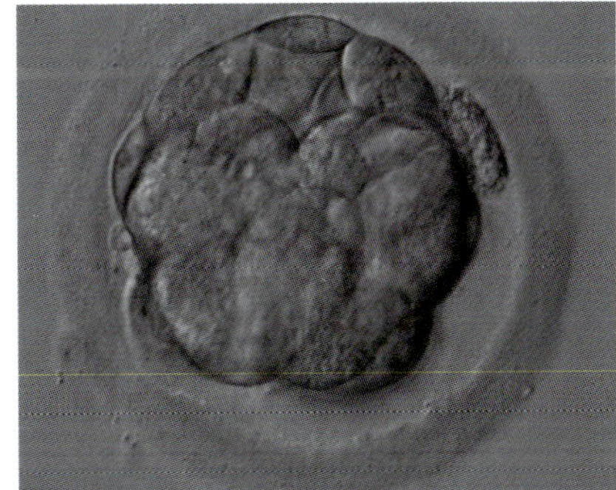

64-AW-1

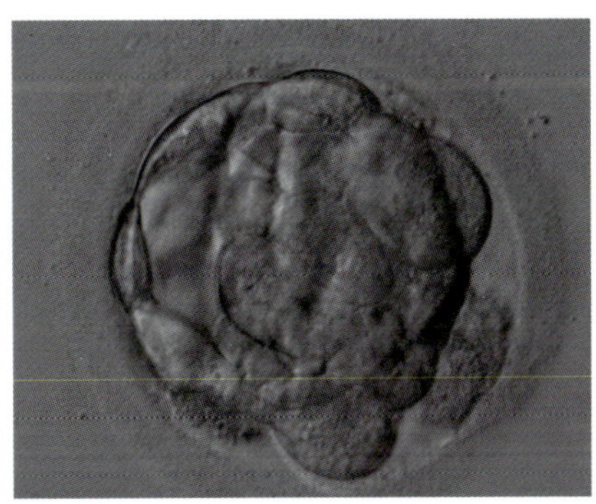

64-BT-1

64-BV-1 Early blastocyst with 2 vacuoles (1 and 6 o'clock position)
64-AW-1 Immediate survival (necrotic polar body should be noted)
64-BT-1 Early blastocyst with necrotic polar body

Female partner

Age 40, teacher
Tubal status: patent
MH: dysmenorrhea
BMI: 26.1
Non-smoker, no alcohol
  consumption
Acne

Basal FSH: 6.0 IU/L
Basal LH: 2.0 IU/L
Basal estradiol: 72.2 pg/mL
Basal AMH: 3.33 ng/mL

Male partner

Age 40, biologist
History/examination:
  cryptorchism
Non-smoker, no alcohol
  consumption
Normal male karyotype

Previous treatments

2003 TESE	Not pregnant
2005 TESE	Biochemical pregnancy
2007 TESE	Extrauterine pregnancy

Fresh cycle: 2009 TESE
Semen assessment: azoospermia

Volume	3.1 mL
Abstinence	5 days
Concentration	0×10^6/mL
Progressive motility	0%
Non-progressive motility	0%
Immotile	0%
Normal forms	0%

Stimulation protocol	Antagonist protocol (recombinant FSH)
Days of stimulation	11
Total dose	1375 IU
Estradiol at ovulation induction	2302 ng/mL
Number of follicles ≥ 12 mm	20
Total number of COCs	17
Metaphase II	15
Injected/inseminated	15
Fertilization rate	93%
Cleavage rate	93%
Blastocyst rate	43%
Culture medium	EmbryoAssist/BlastAssist

Fresh transfer

Quality of embryo(s)	5aa, 3ab
Outcome	Live birth, healthy boy
Vitrification	4 blastocysts

Vitrified/warmed cycle: 2012

Stimulation	HSP
Endometrium	9.0 mm
Quality before vitrification	4aa, 4bb
Warming day	5
Survival	Partly, Yes
Assisted hatching	Yes, Yes
Transfer day	5
Quality	4ab, 4bb
Duration of cryostorage	3.5 years
Time between warming and transfer	3h

Outcome: Missed abortions (2 positive heart activities)

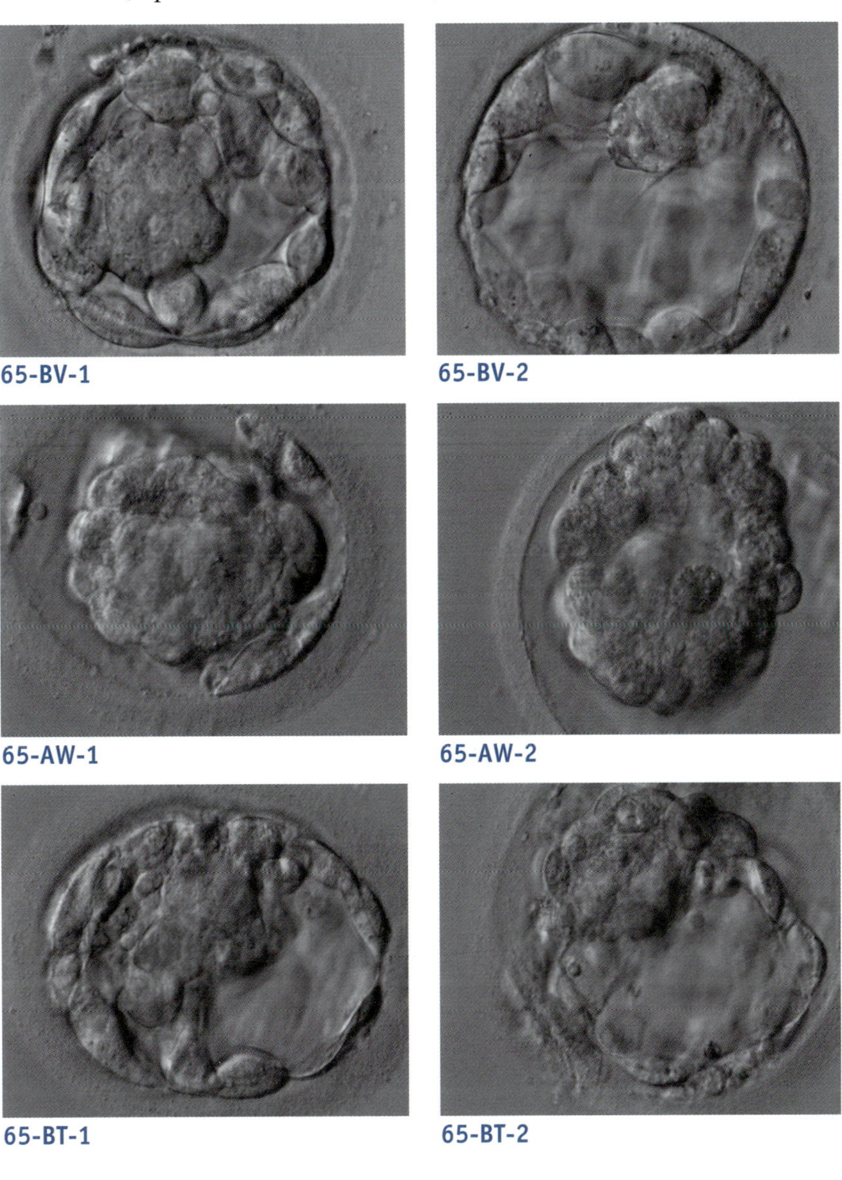

65-BV-1

65-BV-2

65-AW-1

65-AW-2

65-BT-1

65-BT-2

65-BV-1	Expanded blastocyst
65-AW-1	Blastocyst with necrotic area at 10 o'clock position
65-BT-1	Re-expanded blastocyst with excluded fragments at 9 o'clock position
65-BV-2	Expanded blastocyst
65-AW-2	Heavily granulated blastocyst
65-BT-2	Poor quality blastocyst

Case 66

2 years 2° infertility **Diagnosis: Tubal infertility, male factor infertility**

Female partner

Age 28, nurse
Tubal status: unilateral
 blockage
MH: 5–7/28–31
BMI: 20.6
Smoker, no alcohol
 consumption
Basal FSH: 4.8 IU/L
Basal LH: 3.8 IU/L

Basal estradiol: 45.3 pg/mL
Basal AMH: 5.74 ng/mL
Midluteal progesterone: 10.0 ng/mL
Midluteal prolactin: 10.8 ng/mL

Male partner

Age 28, mechanic
History/examination: NAD
Smoker, no alcohol consumption

Previous treatments

None

Fresh cycle: 2010 ICSI
Semen assessment: teratozoospermia

Volume	3.6 mL
Abstinence	4 days
Concentration	167×10^6/mL
Progressive motility	28%
Non-progressive motility	6%
Immotile	66%
Normal forms	1%

Stimulation protocol	Agonist protocol (recombinant FSH)
Days of stimulation	11
Total dose	1460 IU
Estradiol at ovulation induction	3328 ng/mL
Number of follicles ≥ 12 mm	18
Total number of COCs	11
Metaphase II	11
Injected/inseminated	11
Fertilization rate	64%
Cleavage rate	100%
Blastocyst rate	71%
Culture medium	EmbryoAssist/BlastAssist

Fresh transfer

Quality of embryo(s)	4aa
Outcome	Live birth, healthy girl
Vitrification	3 morulae (day 5)

Previous vitrified/warmed cycle

Quality of embryo(s)	1
Outcome	Not pregnant

Vitrified/warmed cycle: 2012

Stimulation	NC
Endometrium	10.0 mm
Quality before vitrification	1
Warming day	5
Survival	Yes
Assisted hatching	Yes
Transfer day	5
Quality	1
Duration of cryostorage	2 years
Time between warming and transfer	2h

Outcome: Missed abortion (positive heart activity)

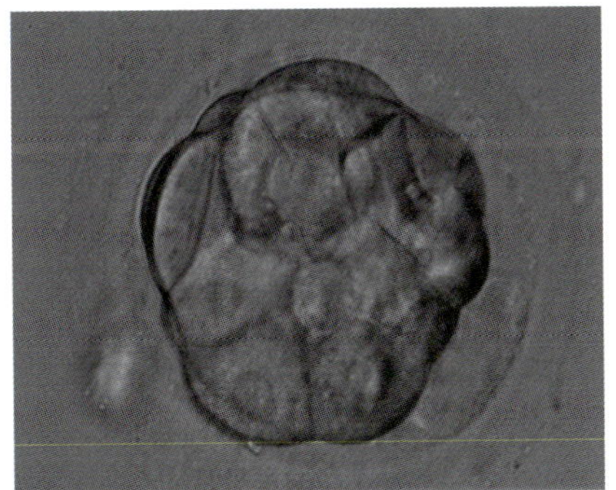

66-BV-1

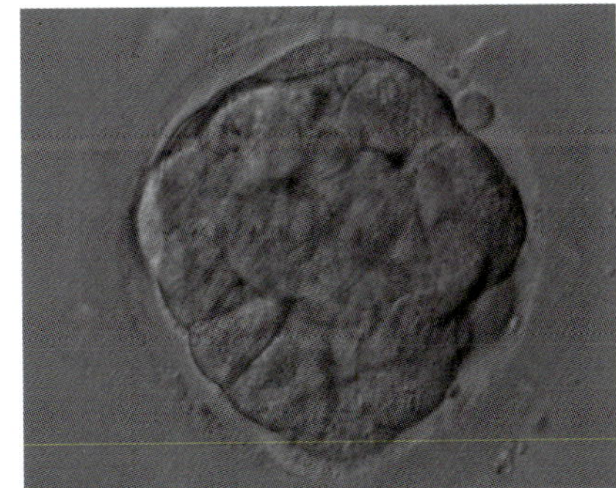

66-AW-1

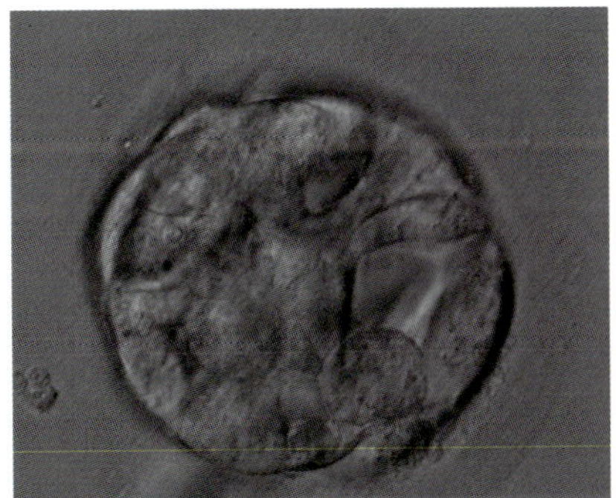

66-BT-1

66-BV-1   Early blastocyst
66-AW-1   Early blastocyst with artificial hatching at 1 o'clock position
66-BT-1   Early blastocyst

Female partner

Age 34, secretary
Tubal status: patent
MH: 5/28
BMI: 23.2
Smoker, no alcohol
   consumption

Basal FSH: 9 IU/L
Basal LH: 8.8 IU/L
Basal estradiol: 41.7 pg/mL
Basal AMH: 3.03 ng/mL

Male partner

Age 35, teacher
History/examination:
   vasectomy
Non-smoker, no alcohol
   consumption
Normal male karyotype

Previous treatments

2009 TESE　　Live birth, healthy boy

Fresh cycle: 2011 TESE
Semen assessment: azoospermia

Volume	4.5 mL
Abstinence	4 days
Concentration	0×10^6/mL
Progressive motility	0%
Non-progressive motility	0%
Immotile	0%
Normal forms	0%

Stimulation protocol	Agonist protocol (HMG)
Days of stimulation	10
Total dose	1500 IU
Estradiol at ovulation induction	2993 ng/mL
Number of follicles ≥ 12 mm	12

Total number of COCs	11
Metaphase II	9
Injected/inseminated	8
Fertilization rate	100%
Cleavage rate	88%
Blastocyst rate	100%
Culture medium	EmbryoAssist/BlastAssist

Fresh transfer

Quality of embryo(s)	5aa
Outcome	Not pregnant
Vitrification	6 blastocysts

Previous vitrified/warmed cycle

2011　Not pregnant

Vitrified/warmed cycle: 2012

Stimulation	HSP
Endometrium	8.0 mm (2 layers only)
Quality before vitrification	5ab
Warming day	5
Survival	Yes
Assisted hatching	No
Transfer day	5
Quality	5ab
Duration of cryostorage	5 months
Time between warming and transfer	3h

Outcome: Live birth, healthy girl

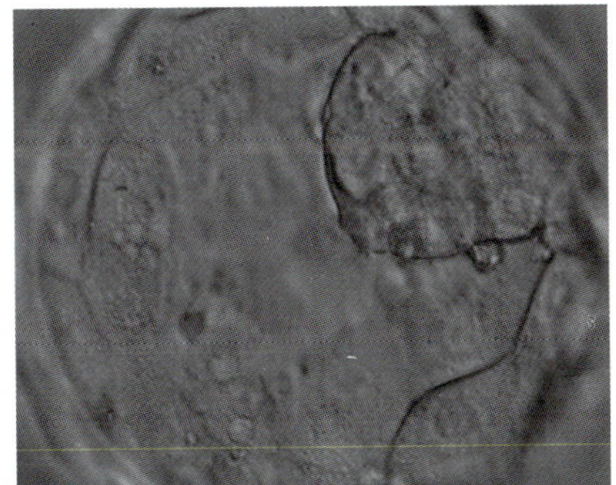

67-BV-1

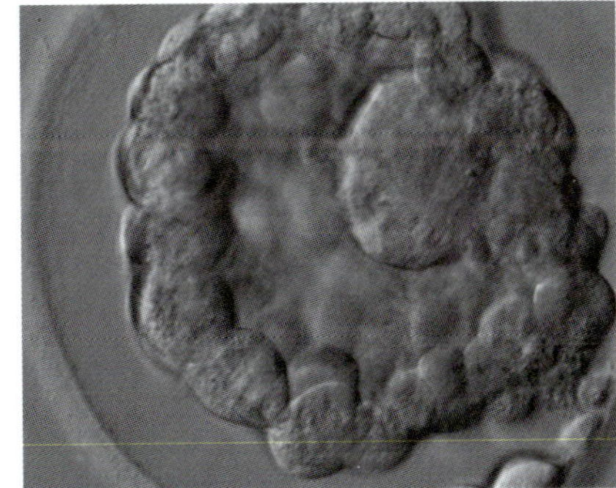

67-AW-1

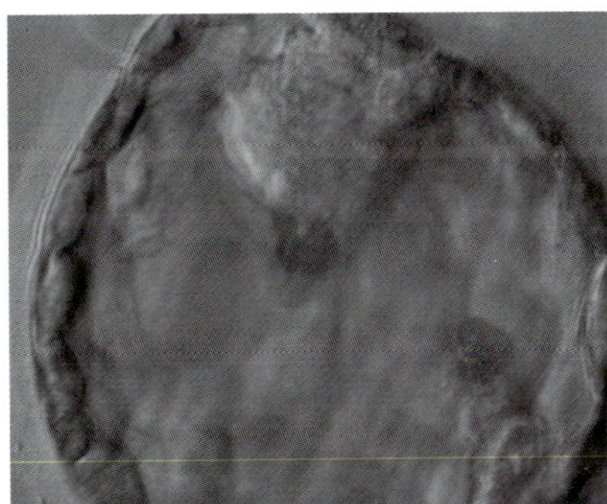

67-BT-1

67-BV-1 Hatching blastocyst with hatching site out of focus (4 o'clock position)
67-AW-1 Blastocyst with beginning re-expansion (previous site of hatching at 5 o'clock position)
67-BT-1 Hatching blastocyst

Female partner

Age 31, kindergartener
Tubal status: patent
MH: 6/30–35
BMI: 23.3
Non-smoker, no alcohol
 consumption
History of pituitary
 adenoma
History of chlamydia
 infection

Basal FSH: 7.1 IU/L
Basal LH: 3.1 IU/L
Basal estradiol: 33.4 pg/mL
Basal AMH: 8.04 ng/mL
Midluteal progesterone: 9.0 ng/mL
Midluteal prolactin: 25.8 ng/mL

Male partner

Age 29, lawyer
History/examination: NAD
Non-smoker, no alcohol
 consumption

Previous treatments

2011 timed intercourse × 3	Not pregnant
2011 insemination × 2	Not pregnant

Fresh cycle: 2012 IVF
Semen assessment: normozoospermia

Volume	2.0 mL
Abstinence	3 days
Concentration	100×10^6/mL
Progressive motility	50%
Non-progressive motility	10%
Immotile	40%
Normal forms	11%

Stimulation protocol	Antagonist protocol (recombinant FSH)
Days of stimulation	9
Total dose	1050 IU
Estradiol at ovulation induction	2556 ng/mL
Number of follicles ≥ 12 mm	34
Total number of COCs	29
Metaphase II	26
Injected/inseminated	26
Fertilization rate	58%
Cleavage rate	100%
Blastocyst rate	47
Culture medium	EmbryoAssist/BlastAssist

Fresh transfer

Quality of embryo(s)	No fresh transfer because of OHSS
Outcome	
Vitrification	

Vitrified/warmed cycle: 2013

Stimulation	HSP
Endometrium	8 mm
Quality before vitrification	1
Warming day	5
Survival	Yes
Assisted hatching	Yes
Transfer day	5
Quality	2
Duration of cryostorage	2 months
Time between warming and transfer	3 hours

Outcome: Live birth, healthy boy

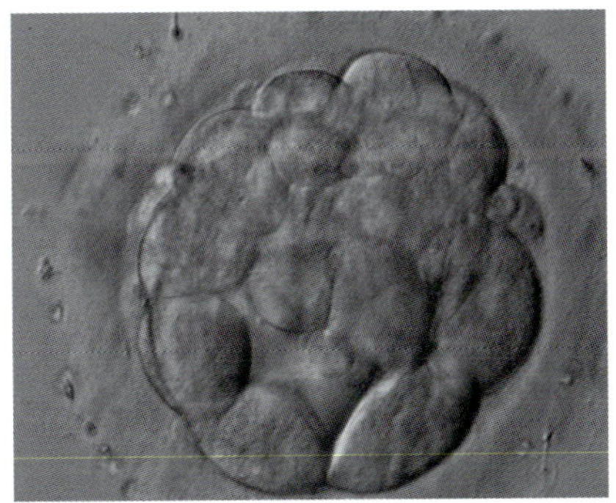

68-BV-1

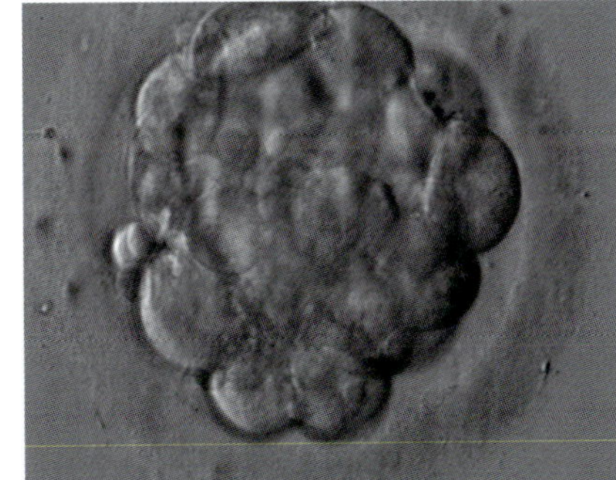

68-AW-1

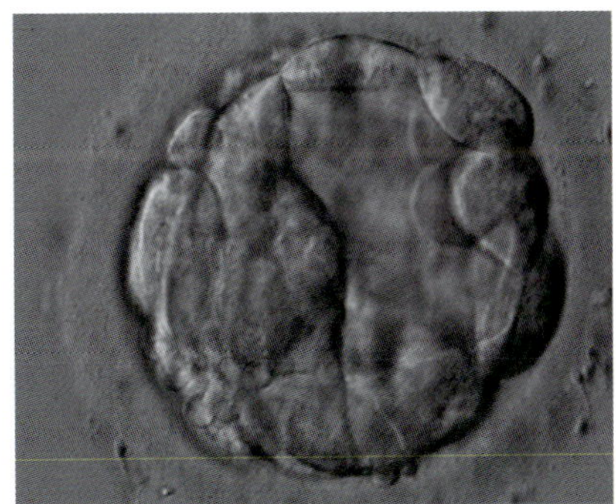

68-BT-1

68-BV-1   Early blastocyst
68-AW-1   Early blastocyst after warming
68-BT-1   Viable early blastocyst with excluded fragments

Case 69

1.5 years 1° infertility

Diagnosis: Male factor infertility, hypothalamic pituitary failure

Female partner

Age 33, technician
Tubal status: patent
MH: secondary
  amenorrhea
BMI: 28.2
Non-smoker, no alcohol
  consumption

Basal FSH: 0.4 IU/L
Basal LH: 0.1 IU/L
Basal estradiol: 53.0 pg/mL
Basal AMH: 0.88 ng/mL

Male partner

Age 46, civil servant
History/examination: NAD
Non-smoker, no alcohol
  consumption

Previous treatments

2011 ICSI	Not pregnant
2011 vitrified/warmed cycle	Not pregnant

Fresh cycle: 2011 ICSI
Semen assessment: teratozoospermia

Volume	2.8 mL
Abstinence	2 days
Concentration	27×10^6/mL
Progressive motility	36%
Non-progressive motility	12%
Immotile	42%
Normal forms	2%

Stimulation protocol	Antagonist protocol (HMG)
Days of stimulation	15
Total dose	1500 IU
Estradiol at ovulation induction	2409 ng/mL
Number of follicles ≥ 12 mm	8
Total number of COCs	8
Metaphase II	8
Injected/inseminated	8
Fertilization rate	50%
Cleavage rate	75%
Blastocyst rate	100%
Culture medium	EmbryoAssist/BlastAssist

Fresh transfer

Quality of embryo(s)	4aa
Outcome	Not pregnant
Vitrification	3 blastocysts

Vitrified/warmed cycle: 2011

Stimulation	HSP
Endometrium	11.0 mm
Quality before vitrification	3ab
Warming day	5
Survival	Yes
Assisted hatching	Yes
Transfer day	5
Quality	3ab
Duration of cryostorage	7 months
Time between warming and transfer	3h

Outcome: Live birth, healthy girl

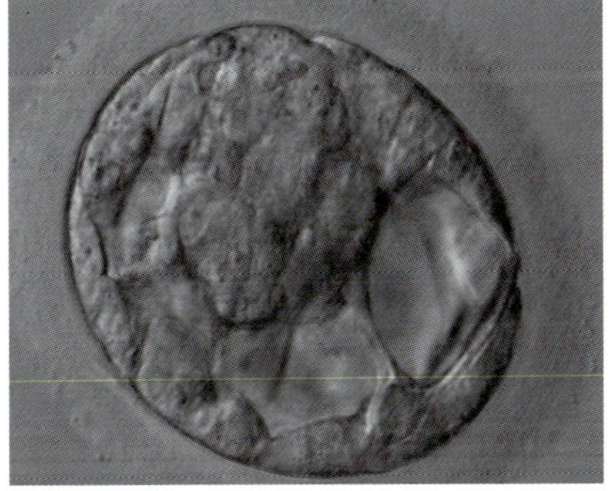

69-BV-1

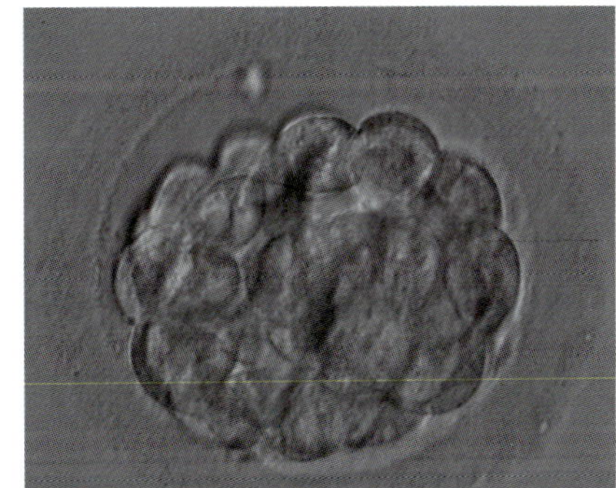

69-AW-1

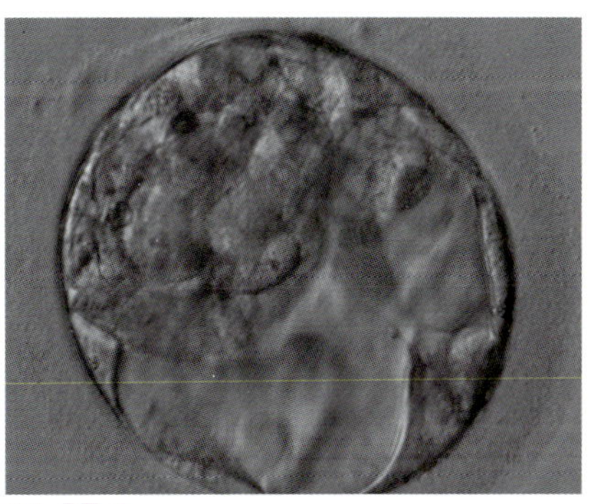

69-BT-1

69-BV-1 Slightly ovoid full blastocyst
69-AW-1 Full blastocyst with starting re-expansion
69-BT-1 Fully re-expanded blastocyst with suboptimal trophectoderm

Case 70

1.5 years 1° infertility   Diagnosis: Endometriosis

Female partner

Age 31, pastry cook
Tubal status: patent
MH: 5/28
BMI: 20.6
Non-smoker, no alcohol
    consumption
Basal FSH: 3.4 IU/L
Basal LH: 4.7 IU/L

Basal estradiol: 128 pg/mL
Basal AMH: 8.09 ng/mL
Midluteal progesterone: 2.3 ng/mL
Midluteal prolactin: 12.6 ng/mL
TSH: 2.71 IU/L

Male partner

Age 35, civil servant
History/examination: NAD
Non-smoker, no alcohol
    consumption

Previous treatments

2009 timed intercourse	Not pregnant
2009 ICSI	Not pregnant

Fresh cycle: 2010 ICSI
Semen assessment: teratozoospermia

Volume	2.2 mL
Abstinence	2 days
Concentration	90×10^6/mL
Progressive motility	75%
Non-progressive motility	7%
Immotile	18%
Normal forms	3%

Stimulation protocol	Agonist protocol (recombinant FSH)
Days of stimulation	11
Total dose	1250 IU
Estradiol at ovulation induction	4131 ng/mL
Number of follicles ≥ 12 mm	19
Total number of COCs	18
Metaphase II	13
Injected/inseminated	13
Fertilization rate	85%
Cleavage rate	100%
Blastocyst rate	31%
Culture medium	EmbryoAssist/BlastAssist, GM501

Fresh transfer

Quality of embryo(s)	Fully compacting embryo (day 4)
Outcome	Not pregnant
Vitrification	3 blastocysts (day 5)

Vitrified/warmed cycle: 2011

Stimulation	HSP
Endometrium	7.5 mm
Quality before vitrification	5ab (GM501)
Warming day	5
Survival	Yes
Assisted hatching	Yes
Transfer day	5
Quality	4ab
Duration of cryostorage	8 months
Time between warming and transfer	3h

Outcome: Live birth, healthy girl

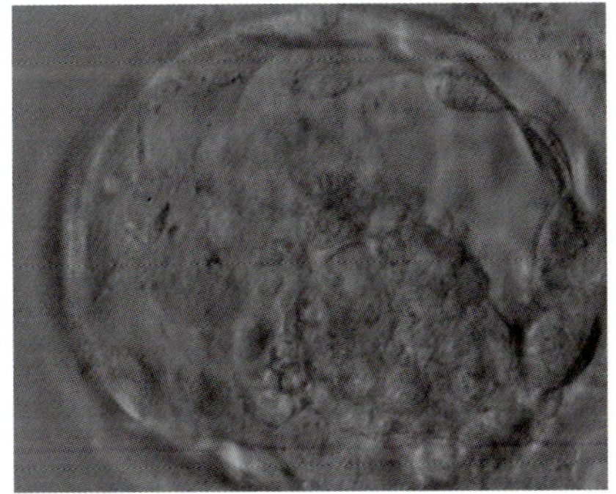

70-BV-1

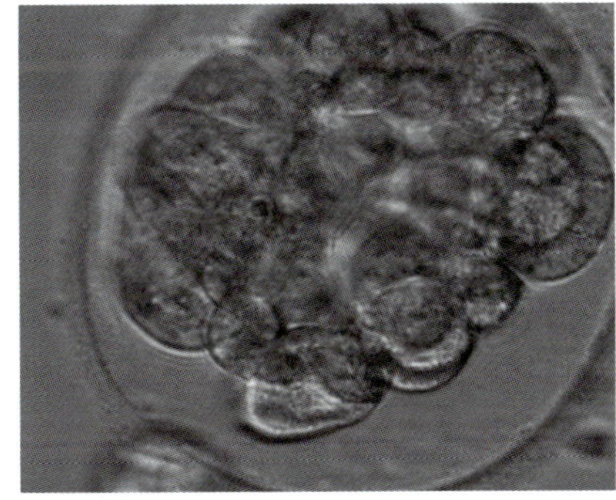

70-AW-1

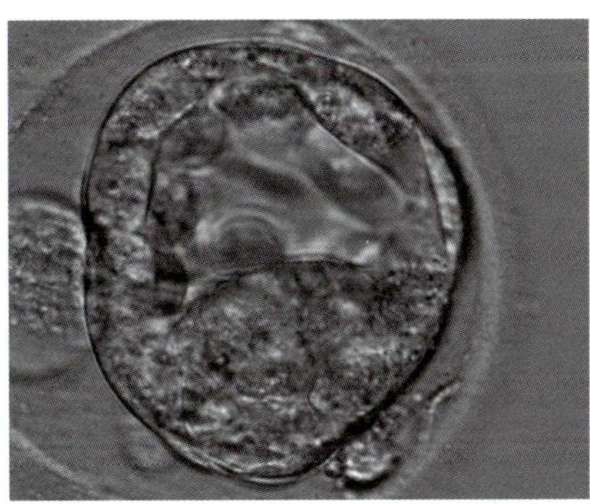

70-BT-1

70-BV-1 Hatching blastocyst with hatching site close to the ICM
70-AW-1 Warmed blastocyst showing strangulation of already hatched cells (7 o'clock position)
70-BT-1 Expanded blastocyst (previously hatched cells degenerated)

Part B

Closed Vitrification Method

Female partner

Age 27, shop assistant
Tubal status: patent
MH: 28–32
BMI: 23.9
Non-smoker, no alcohol
  consumption
TSH: 0.61 µU/mL

Basal FSH: 5.7 IU/L
Basal LH: 4.1 IU/L
Basal estradiol: 168 pg/mL
Prolactin: 103 ng/mL

Male partner

Age 36, machinist
History/examination: NAD
BMI: 24.3
Oligoasthenoteratozoospermia
Smoker, moderate alcohol consumption

Previous treatments

| 2010 | ICSI cycle (external) | Not pregnant |
| 2010–2011 | Frozen/thawed cycles (×4) | Not pregnant |

Fresh cycle: 2013 IMSI
Semen assessment: oligoasthenoteratozoospermia

Volume	1.4 mL
Abstinence	1 day
Concentration	8×10^6/mL
Total sperm number	11.2×10^6/mL
Progressive motility	25%
Non-progressive motility	0%
Immotile	75%
Normal forms	0%
IMSI-Classification Class I/II/III	0%/37%/63%

Stimulation protocol and outcome

Stimulation protocol	Long protocol
Days of stimulation	11
Total dose	1500 IU
Number of follicles ≥ 12 mm	38
Total number of COCs	33
Metaphase II	31
Fertilization rate	77%
Cleavage rate	100%
Blastocyst rate	50%

Fresh transfer

Quality of embryo(s)	No transfer due to OHSS
Vitrification	10 blastocysts (day 5)
	2 blastocysts (day 6)

Vitrified/warmed cycle: 2013

Stimulation	Hormonal substitution protocol
Endometrium	13.3 mm
Quality before vitrification	Blastocyst 4ba, blastocyst 4ca
Warming day	5
Survival	Yes/Yes
Assisted hatching	Yes/Yes
Transfer day	5
Quality	Blastocyst 4ba hatching, blastocyst 4cc hatching
Duration of cryostorage	3 months
Time between warming and transfer	3.5 hours

Outcome: Live birth, 2 healthy twin boys

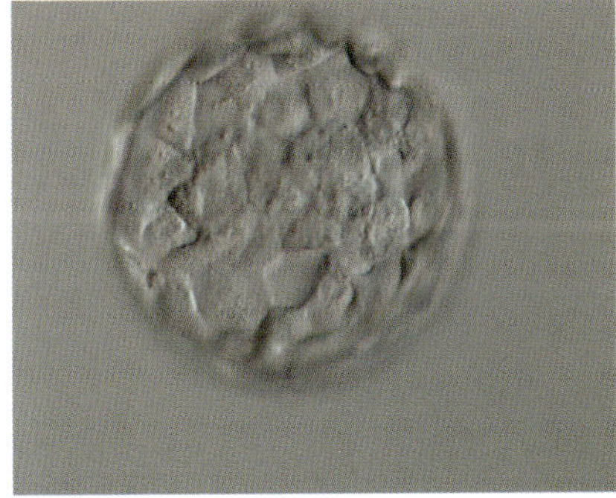

71-BV-1

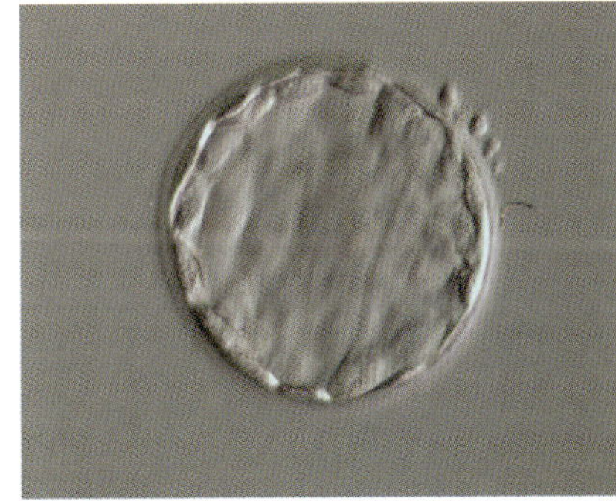

71-BV-2

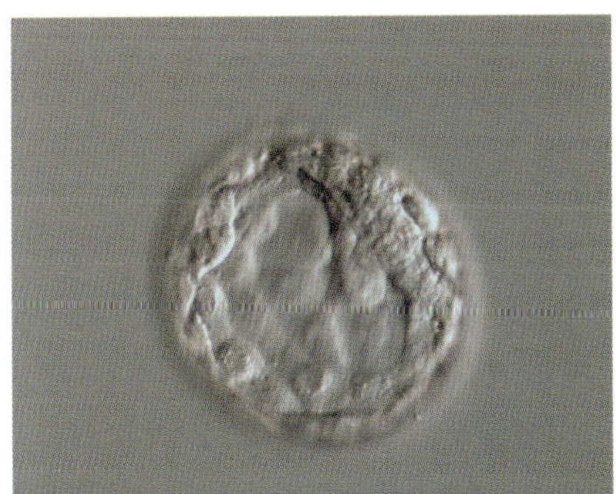

71-AW-1

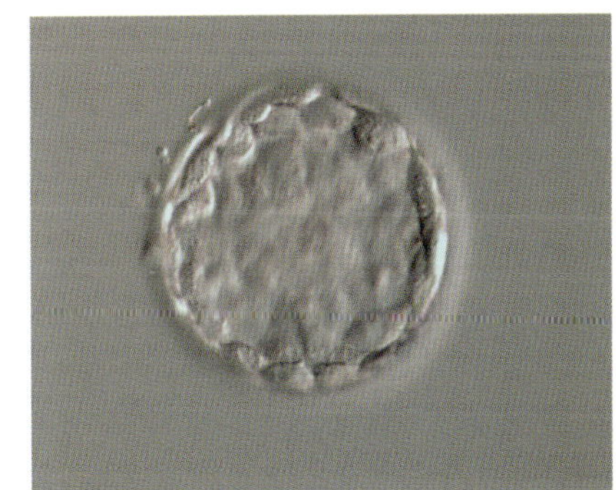

71-AW-2

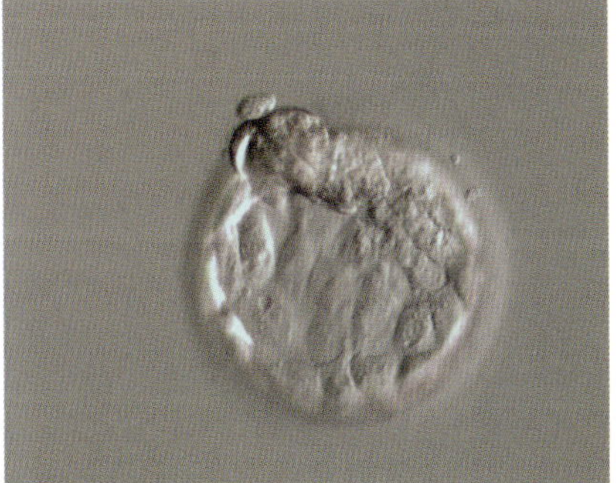

71-BT-1

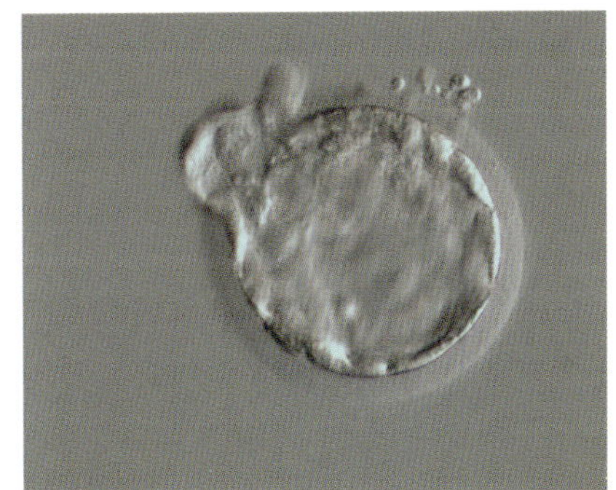

71-BT-2

71-BV-1	Blastocyst 4ba with flat, poorly defined inner cell mass before vitrification
71-BV-2	Blastocyst 4ca with nice cohesive trophectoderm and thinned zona pellucida
71-AW-1	Fully expanded blastocyst after warming
71-AW-2	Fully expanded blastocyst after warming, clear trophectoderm cells
71-BT-1	Expanded and hatching blastocyst with intact cells before transfer
71-BT-2	Trophectoderm poor and granular with necrotic cells at 12 o'clock, blastocyst vital, fully re-expanded and hatching

Female partner

Age 35, employee
Tubal status: patent
MH: 26
BMI: 19.5
PAI 1 homozygote, MTHFR
  heterozygote
Previous surgeries: hysteroscopy
  and cervical dilation due to
  stenosis
Non-smoker, no alcohol
  consumption
Basal FSH: 7.4 IU/L

Basal LH: 2 IU/L
Basal estradiol: 79 pg/mL
Midluteal progesterone: 1.2 ng/mL
Prolactin: 269 mIU/L

Male partner

Age 38, economist
History/examination: NAD
BMI: 22.9
Teratozoospermia

Previous treatments

2010	Intrauterine insemination ×4 (external)	Not pregnant
2010	IVF (external)	Not pregnant
2010	Frozen/thawed cycle (external)	Not pregnant
2011	IVF cycle (external)	Not pregnant
2011	IVF cycle (external)	Abortion gestation week 11 (1 positive heart activity)
2011	ICSI cycle (external)	Not pregnant
2012	ICSI cycle (external)	Not pregnant
2012	Frozen/thawed cycle (external)	Not pregnant
2013	IMSI	Not pregnant

Fresh cycle: 2013 IMSI

Semen assessment: teratozoospermia

Volume	2 mL
Abstinence	1 day
Concentration	38×10^6/mL
Total sperm number	76×10^6/mL
Progressive motility	48%
Non-progressive motility	24%
Immotile	28%
Normal forms	0%
IMSI-Classification	0%/53%/47%
Class I/II/III	

Stimulation protocol and outcome

Stimulation protocol	Long protocol
Days of stimulation	12
Total dose	2625 IU
Number of follicles ≥ 12 mm	24
Total number of COCs	21
Metaphase II	20

Fertilization rate	100%
Cleavage rate	100%
Blastocyst rate	75%

Fresh transfer

Quality of embryo(s)	Blastocyst 5bb, blastocyst 4ab
Outcome	Pregnant, 1 heart activity, abortion gestation week 8
Vitrification	11 blastocysts (day 5)

Vitrified/warmed cycle: 2013

Stimulation	Hormonal substitution protocol
Endometrium	14 mm
Quality before vitrification	Blastocyst 4ba, blastocyst 4ac
Warming day	5
Survival	Yes/Yes
Assisted hatching	No/Yes
Transfer day	5
Quality	Blastocyst 4bb, blastocyst 3bc
Duration of cryostorage	7 months
Time between warming and transfer	3.5 hours

Outcome: Clinical pregnancy, abortion gestation week 7

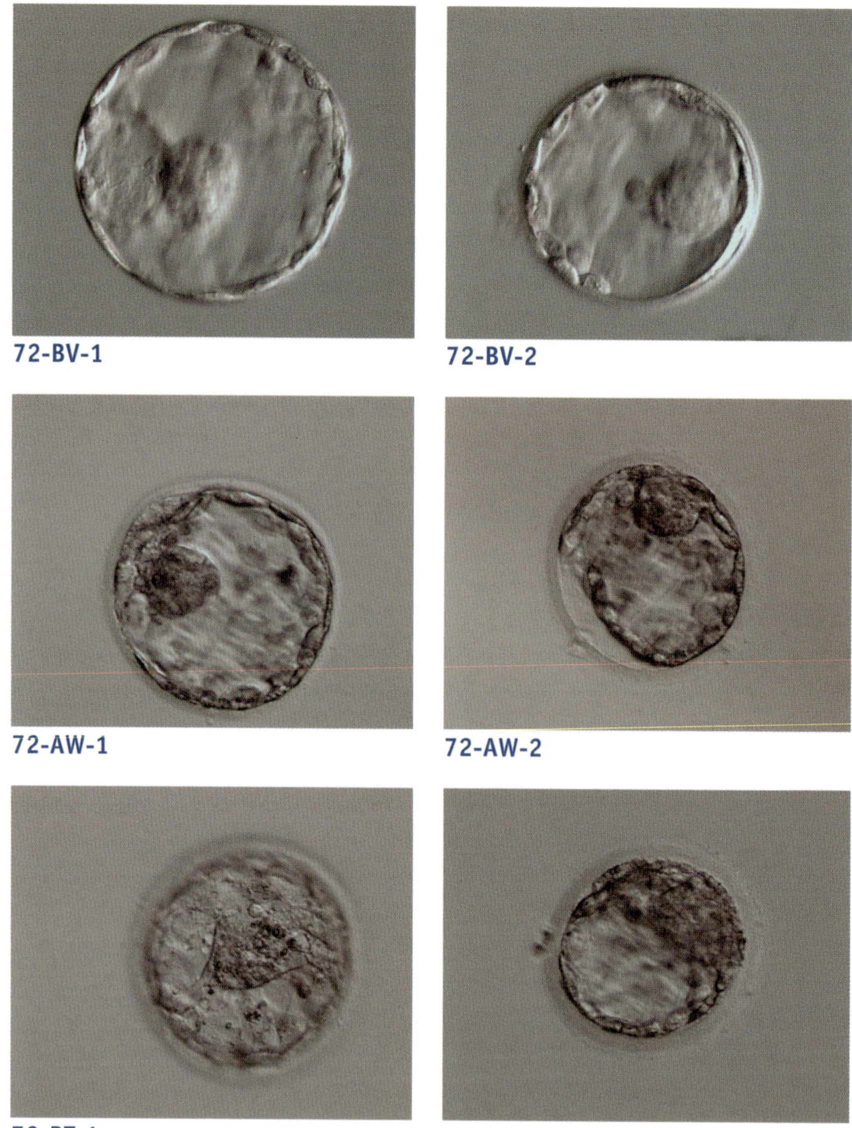

72-BV-1

72-BV-2

72-AW-1

72-AW-2

72-BT-1

72-BT-2

72-BV-1 Fully expanded blastocyst with nice cohesive trophectoderm and a compact inner cell mass in the background, on the left a large vacuole formed by TE cells

72-BV-2 Expanded blastocyst grade 4ab, inner cell mass compact at 3 o'clock, one excluded fragment attached to ICM, trophectoderm consists of few elongated cells

72-AW-1 No signs of contraction directly after warming

72-AW-2 Minor contraction after warming on the left side of the blastocyst

72-BT-1 Blastocyst fully re-expanded, focus on inner cell mass which appears flattened and covered with small dark fragments

72-BT-2 Blastocyst re-expanded but without thinning of the zona pellucida, cells dark granular, inner cell mass compact

Female partner

Age 31, teacher
Tubal status: patent
MH: oligomenorrhea
   (5–9 weeks)
BMI: 22.8
Non-smoker, no alcohol abuse
Basal FSH: 6.1 IU/L

Basal LH: 13.7 IU/L
Basal estradiol: 82 pg/mL
Prolactin: 22.7 ng/mL
Midluteal progesterone: 1.2 ng/mL

Male partner

Age 37, butcher
History/examination: NAD
BMI: 26.3
Normozoospermia
Smoker, no alcohol abuse

Previous treatments

2012   Timed intercourse with clomiphene treatment ×4   Not pregnant

Fresh cycle: 2013 IMSI
Semen assessment: normozoospermia

Volume	4 mL
Abstinence	1 day
Concentration	127×10^6/mL
Total sperm number	508×10^6/mL
Progressive motility	81%
Non-progressive motility	3%
Immotile	16%
Normal forms	4%
IMSI-Classification	4%/41%/55%
Class I/II/III	

Stimulation protocol and outcome

Stimulation protocol	Long protocol
Days of stimulation	11
Total dose	2025 IU
Number of follicles ≥ 12 mm	11
Total number of COCs	11
Metaphase II	9
Fertilization rate	100%
Cleavage rate	100%
Blastocyst rate	100%

Fresh transfer

Quality of embryo(s)	Blastocyst 5ba
Outcome	Not pregnant
Vitrification	8 blastocysts day 5

Vitrified/warmed cycle: 2013

Stimulation	Hormonal substitution protocol
Endometrium	5.8 mm
Quality before vitrification	Blastocyst 5ba
Warming day	5
Survival	Yes
Assisted hatching	No
Transfer day	5
Quality	Blastocyst 5ba
Duration of cryostorage	2 months
Time between warming and transfer	2.5 hours

Outcome: Live birth, healthy boy

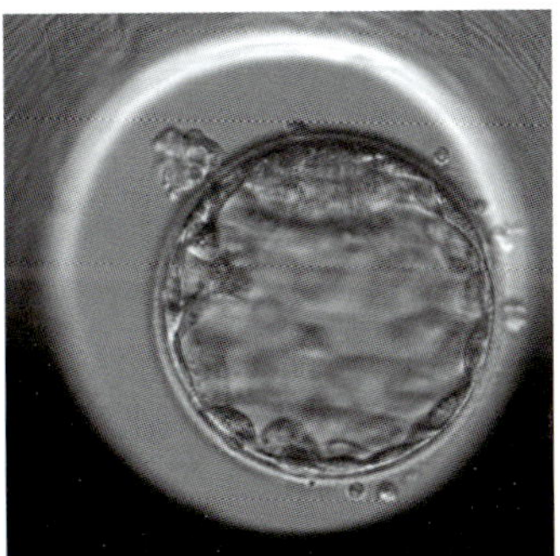

73-BV-1

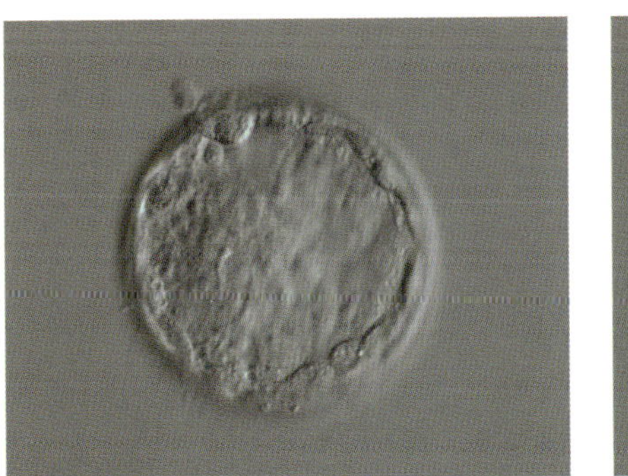

73-AW-1a

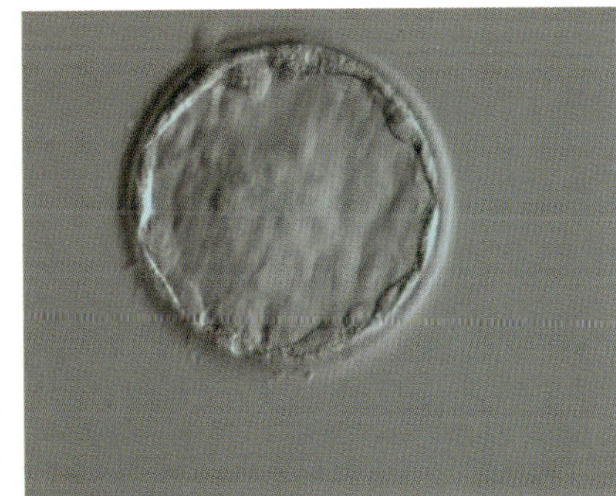

73-AW-1b

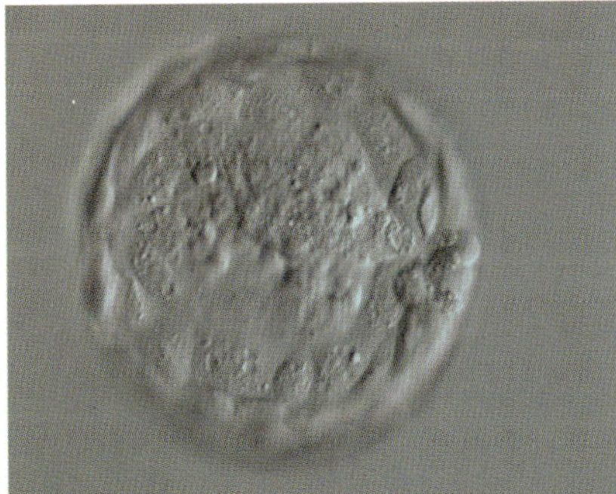

73-BT-1a

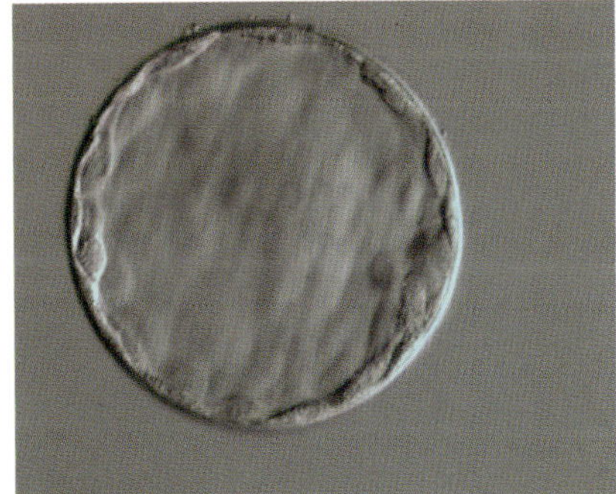

73-BT-1b

73-BV-1   Before vitrification blastocyst hatching at 11 o'clock with flat inner cell mass
73-AW-1a   Blastocyst fully re-expanded during the exposure to the sucrose solutions
73-AW-1b   Trophectoderm cells granular, some with microvacuoles, flat inner cell mass
73-BT-1a   Blastocyst fully re-expanded, hatching at 3 o'clock position, large flat but visible inner cell mass
73-BT-1b   Trophectoderm cells appear less granular and vital before embryo transfer

2 years 2° infertility **Diagnosis: Endometriosis, male factor infertility**

Female partner

Age 40, businesswoman
Tubal status: patent
MH: 30
BMI: 19.9
Previous surgeries: laparoscopic chromo-perturbation
Thin endometrial layer after abrasio uteri
Non-smoker, no alcohol abuse
Basal FSH: 8.9 IU/L
Basal LH: 5.5 IU/L
Basal estradiol: 27.3 pg/mL
Midluteal progesterone: 0.23 ng/mL

Male partner

Age 46, engineer
History/examination: undescended testes
BMI: 23.9
Teratozoospermia
Non-smoker, no alcohol abuse

Previous treatments

2009	ICSI cycle	Live birth, healthy boy
2012	Vitrified/warmed transfer	Clinical pregnancy, abortion gestation week 8
2012	IMSI cycle	Not pregnant
2012	Vitrified/warmed transfer	Not pregnant

Fresh cycle: 2013 IMSI

Semen assessment: teratozoospermia

Volume	1.6 mL
Abstinence	7 days
Concentration	18×10^6/mL
Total sperm number	28.8×10^6/mL
Progressive motility	27%
Non-progressive motility	22%
Immotile	51%
Normal forms	0%
IMSI-Classification Class I/II/III	0%/5%/95%

Stimulation protocol and outcome

Stimulation protocol	Long protocol
Days of stimulation	11
Total dose	2925 IU
Number of follicles ≥ 12 mm	6
Total number of COCs	3
Metaphase II	3
Fertilization rate	100%
Cleavage rate	100%
Blastocyst rate	100%

Fresh transfer

Quality of embryo(s)	No fresh transfer because of poor endometrium build-up
Vitrification	3 blastocysts day 5

Vitrified/warmed cycle: 2013

Stimulation	Hormonal substitution protocol
Endometrium	8.0 mm
Quality before vitrification	Blastocyst 4aa contracted
Warming day	5
Survival	Yes
Assisted hatching	No
Transfer day	5
Quality	Blastocyst 4ba
Duration of cryostorage	2 months
Time between warming and transfer	3 hours

Outcome: Not pregnant

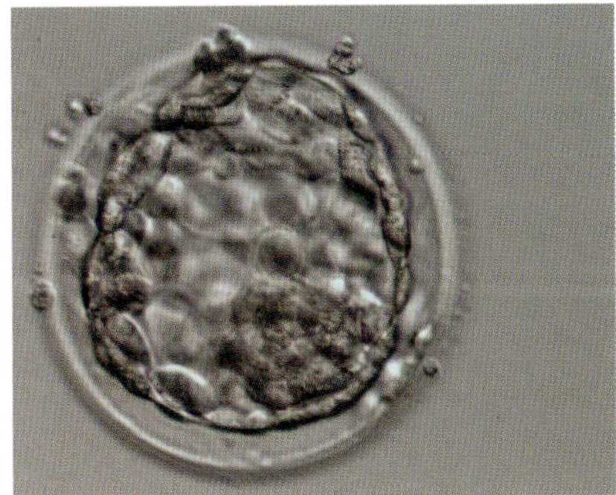

74-BV-1a

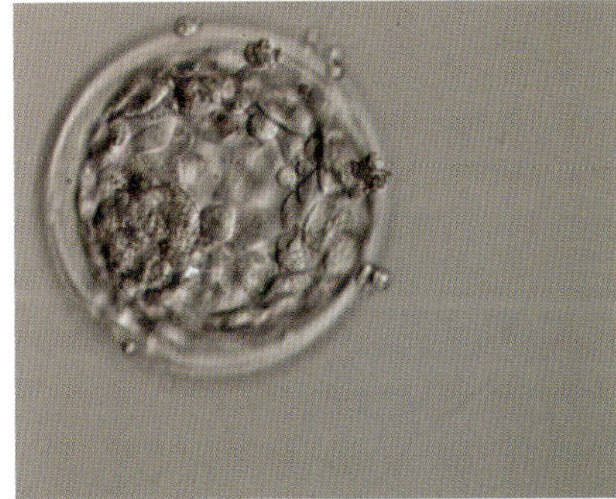

74-BV-1b

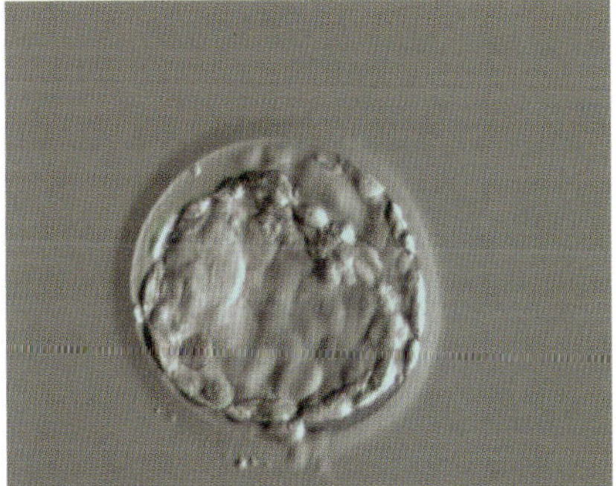

74-AW-1a

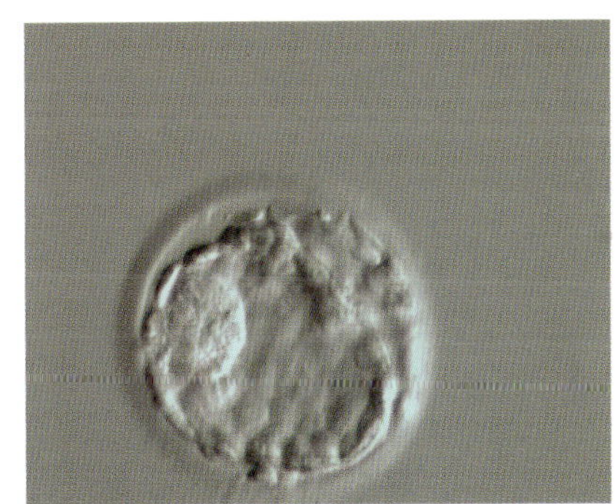

74-AW-1b

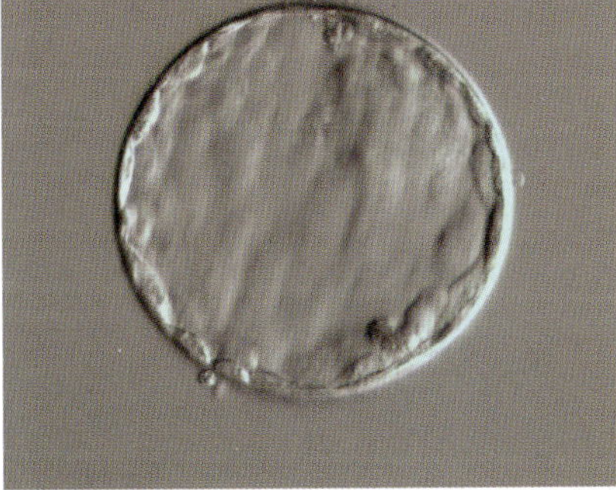

74-BT-1a

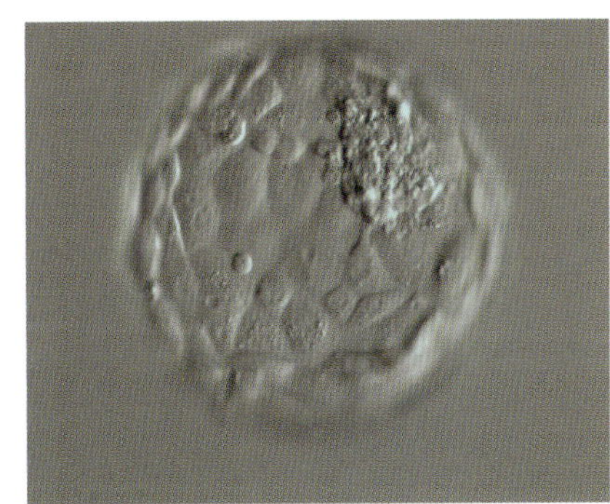

74-BT-1b

74-BV-1a	Slightly contracting blastocyst, nice trophectoderm
74-BV-1b	Large, compact inner cell mass
74-AW-1a	After warming same appearance as before vitrification
74-AW-1b	Focus on inner cell mass, blastocyst slightly contracted as before vitrification, some excluded fragments attached to the ZP
74-BT-1a	Blastocyst fully re-expanded, clear cohesive trophectoderm cells, very thin ZP
74-BT-1b	Focus on inner cell mass, cells slightly granular

Case 75

6 years 1° infertility   Diagnosis: PCOS, male factor infertility

Female partner

Age 26, employee
Tubal status: patent
MH: >30
BMI: 22.6
Non-smoker, no alcohol abuse
Basal FSH: 4 IU/L
Basal LH: 3.4 IU/L
Basal estradiol: 125 pg/mL
Prolactin: 14.8 ng/mL
Midluteal progesterone: 9.2 ng/mL

Male partner

Age 31, electrician
History/examination: NAD
BMI: 31.0
Oligoasthenoteratozoospermia
Non-smoker, no alcohol abuse

Previous treatments

2008	ICSI-cycle (external)	Not pregnant
2011	ICSI-cycle (external)	Not pregnant
2009, 2010, 2011	Frozen/thawed cycles ×6 (external)	Not pregnant

Fresh cycle: 2013 ICSI
Semen assessment: oligoasthenoteratozoospermia

Volume	4 mL
Abstinence	3 days
Concentration	0.02×10^6/mL
Total sperm number	0.08×10^6/mL
Progressive motility	10%
Non-progressive motility	10%
Immotile	80%
Normal forms	2%

Stimulation protocol and outcome

Stimulation protocol	Long protocol
Days of stimulation	11
Total dose	1050 IU
Number of follicles ≥ 12 mm	25
Total number of COCs	25
Metaphase II	23
Fertilization rate	96%
Cleavage rate	100%
Blastocyst rate	59%

Fresh transfer

Quality of embryo(s)	No fresh transfer because of OHSS
Outcome	
Vitrification	12 blastocysts day 5

Vitrified/warmed cycle: 2013

Stimulation	Hormonal substitution protocol
Endometrium	10 mm
Quality before vitrification	Blastocyst 4aa, blastocyst 4bc
Warming day	5
Survival	Yes/Yes
Assisted hatching	No/No
Transfer day	5
Quality	Blastocyst 4bb, blastocyst 5cb
Duration of cryostorage	3 months
Time between warming and transfer	3 hours

Outcome: Live birth twins, 2 healthy boys

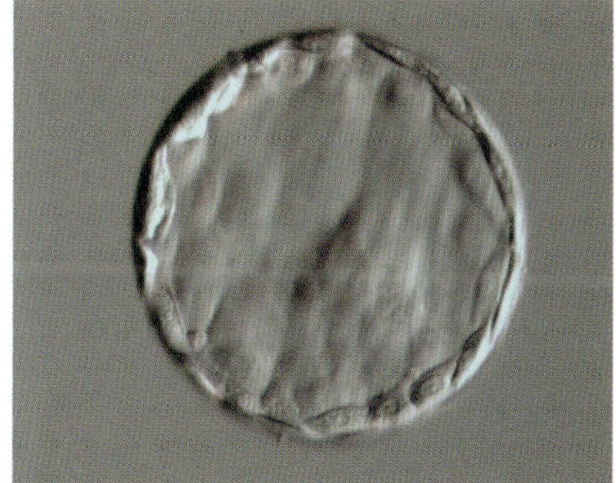

75-BV-1

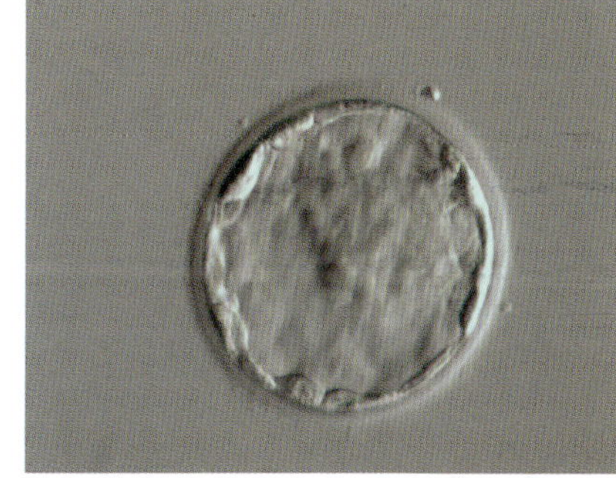

75-BV-2

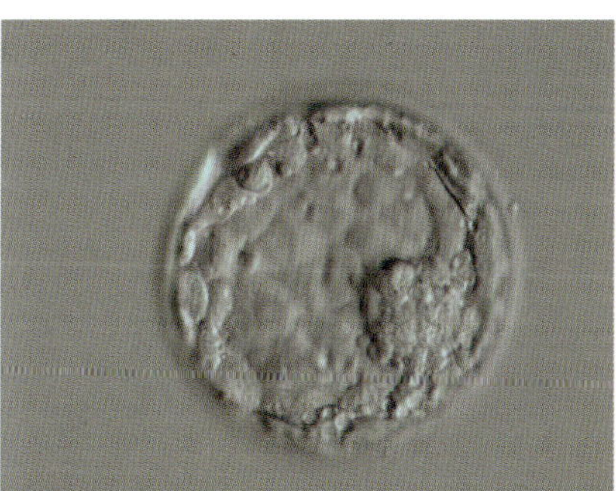

75-AW-1

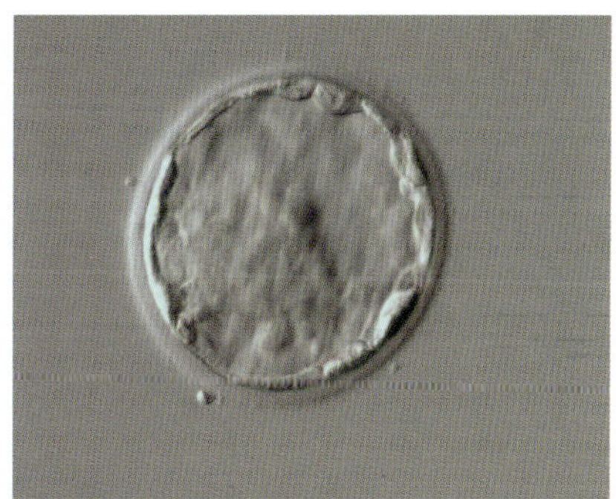

75-AW-2

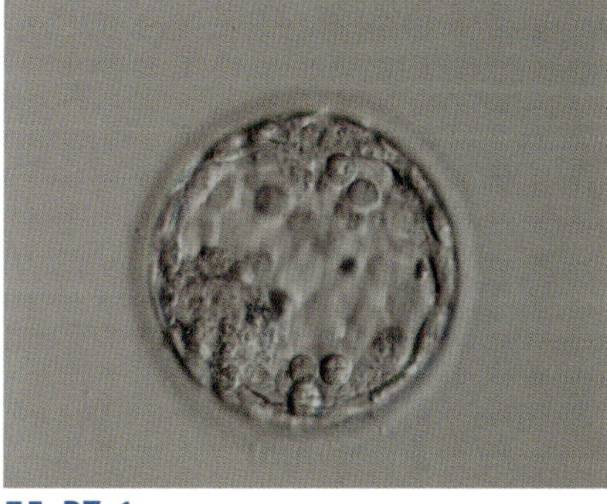

75-BT-1

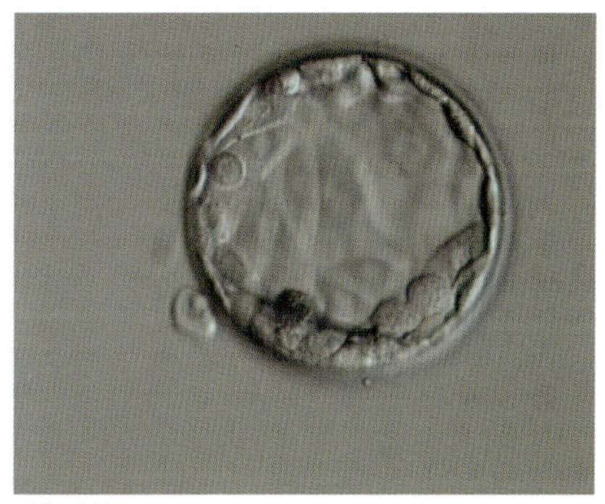

75-BT-2

75-BV-1 Blastocyst 4aa before vitrification, nice cohesive trophectoderm, inner cell mass compact, slightly visible in the background at 5 o'clock

75-BV-2 Blastocyst 4bc before vitrification, zona pellucida not fully thinned

75-AW-1 After warming granular cells with microvacuoles, only slightly contracted blastocyst

75-AW-2 Intact blastocyst after warming

75-BT-1 Blastocyst fully re-expanded, granular cells, loose fragments in blastocoel, some necrotic cells

75-BT-2 Fully re-expanded blastocyst, one necrotic cell at 7 o'clock position, starting to hatch at 8 o'clock position, flat inner cell mass

Case 76

4 years 2° infertility   Diagnosis: PCOS

Female partner

Age: 38, worker

Tubal status: patent

MH: 28

Previous surgeries: hysteroscopy due to endometrial polyp in 2009

Abortion/Deliveries: spontaneous abortion in 2009

Smoker, no alcohol abuse

BMI: 23.1

Basal FSH: 4.3 IU/L

Basal LH: 8.9 IU/L

Basal estradiol: 112 pg/mL

Prolactin: 7 ng/mL

Midluteal progesterone: 0.1 ng/mL

Male partner

Age 34, mechanic

BMI: 28.4

History/examination: NAD

Smoker, no alcohol abuse

One child after natural conception with another partner

Previous treatments

2011	ICSI cycle ×1 (external)	Not pregnant
2011	Vitrified/warmed cycle ×1 (external)	Not pregnant

Fresh cycle: 2013 IMSI

Semen assessment: normozoospermia

Volume	1.6 mL
Abstinence	1 day
Concentration	56×10^6/mL
Total sperm number	89.6×10^6/mL
Progressive motility	34%
Non-progressive motility	14%
Immotile	52%
Normal forms	7%
IMSI-Classification	7%/56%/37%
Class I/II/III	

Stimulation protocol and outcome

Stimulation protocol	Long protocol
Days of stimulation	10
Total dose	1425 IU
Number of follicles ≥ 12 mm	24
Total number of COCs	19
Metaphase II	18
Fertilization rate	89%
Cleavage rate	100%
Blastocyst rate	50%

Fresh transfer

Quality of embryo(s)	Blastocyst 3bb, early blastocyst
Outcome	Not pregnant
Vitrification	5 blastocysts (day 5)

Vitrified/warmed cycle: 2013

Stimulation	Hormonal substitution protocol
Endometrium	10.0 mm
Quality before vitrification	Blastocyst 2bb, bastocyst 3cc
Warming day	5
Survival	Yes
Assisted hatching	Yes
Transfer day	5
Quality	Blastocyst 2bc, blastocyst 3cc
Duration of cryostorage	5 months
Time between warming and transfer	3 hours

Outcome: Stillbirth after premature labor and loss of amniotic fluid in gestation week 24

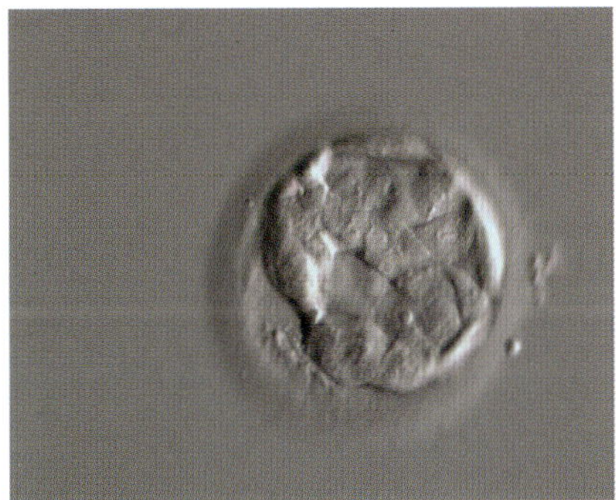

76-BV-1

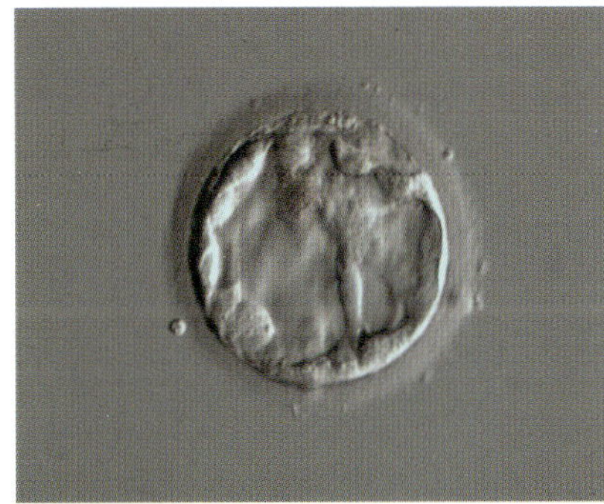

76-BV-2

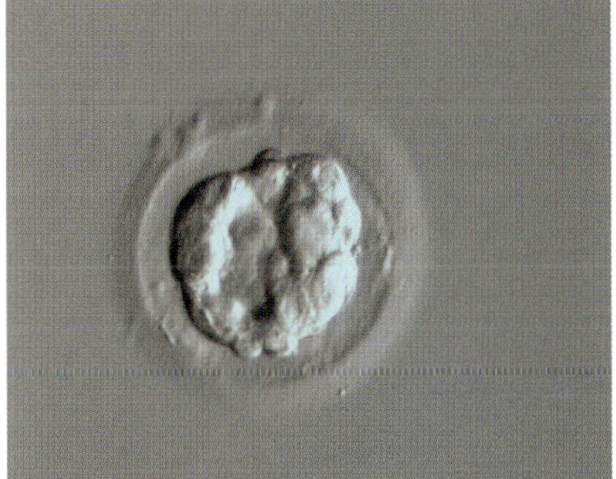

76-AW-1

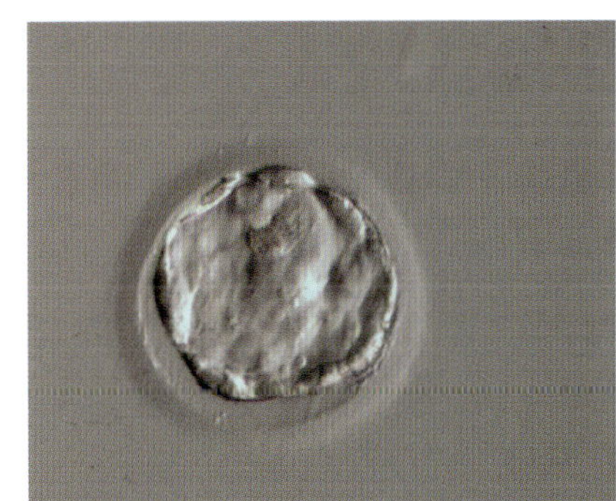

76-AW-2

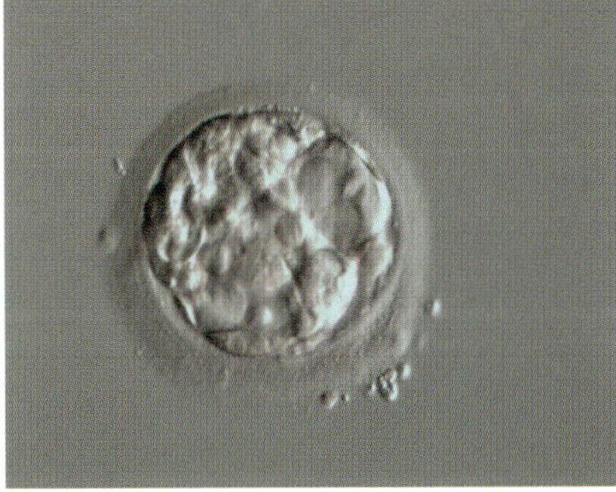

76-BT-1

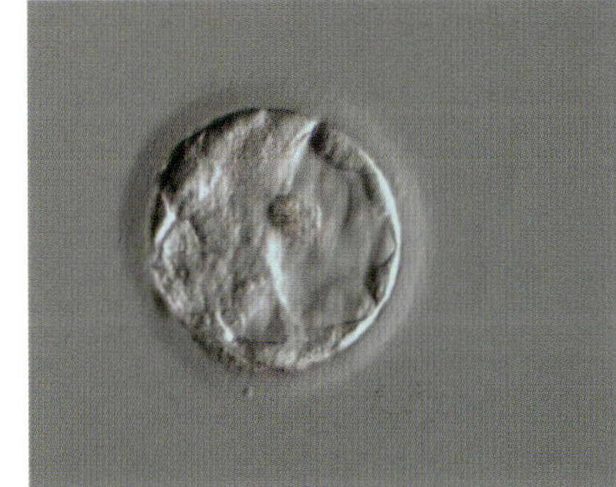

76-BT-2

76-BV-1 Blastocyst 2bb in contraction phase before vitrification
76-BV-2 Bl 3cc before vitrification, poor trophectoderm, one necrotic cell at 12 o'clock position, thick zona pellucida
76-AW-1 Collapsed blastocyst after warming
76-AW-2 Blastocyst slightly contracted after exposure to sucrose solutions
76-BT-1 No full re-expansions, adhesions within the blastocyst
76-BT-2 Fully re-expanded blastocyst, granular cells, presence of necrotic cells

Female partner

Age: 31, housewife

Tubal status: patent

MH: oligomenorrhea

BMI: 19.0

Abortion/Deliveries: spontaneous pregnancy, birth of a healthy boy in 2010, same partner

Non-smoker, no alcohol abuse

Basal FSH: 6.1 IU/L

Basal LH: 8.1 IU/L

Basal estradiol: 33 pg/mL

Prolactin: 16.2 ng/mL

Midluteal progesterone: 0.99 ng/mL

Male partner

Age 32, employee

BMI: 22.1

History/examination: NAD

Non-smoker, no alcohol abuse

Teratozoospermia

Previous treatments

None

Fresh cycle: 2013 IMSI

Semen assessment: teratozoospermia

Volume	5 mL
Abstinence	1 day
Concentration	41×10^6/mL
Total sperm number	205×10^6/mL
Progressive motility	68%
Non-progressive motility	27%
Immotile	5%
Normal forms	2%
IMSI-Classification Class I/II/III	2%/41%/57%

Stimulation protocol and outcome

Stimulation protocol	Long protocol
Days of stimulation	11
Total dose	1557 IU
Number of follicles ≥ 12 mm	15
Total number of COCs	14
Metaphase II	12
Fertilization rate	92%
Cleavage rate	100%
Blastocyst rate	100%

Fresh transfer

Quality of embryo(s)	Blastocyst 4aa
Outcome	Not pregnant
Vitrification	11 blastocysts day 5

Vitrified/warmed cycle: August 2013

Stimulation	Hormonal substitution protocol
Endometrium	6.7 mm
Quality before vitrification	Blastocyst 4aa
Warming day	5
Survival	Yes
Assisted hatching	No
Transfer day	5
Quality	Blastocyst 4aa
Duration of cryostorage	2 months
Time between warming and transfer	3.5 hours

Outcome: Not pregnant

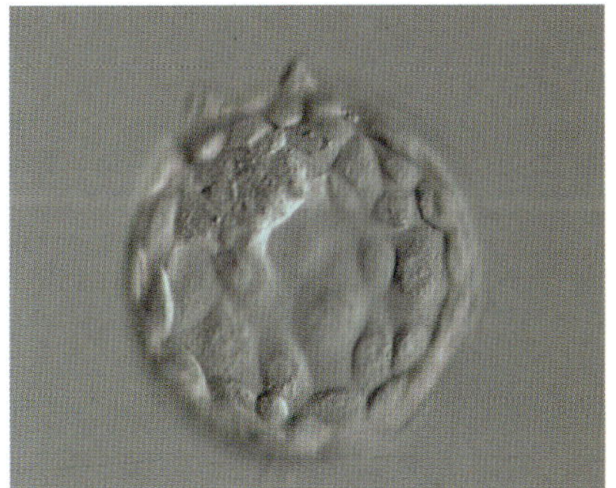
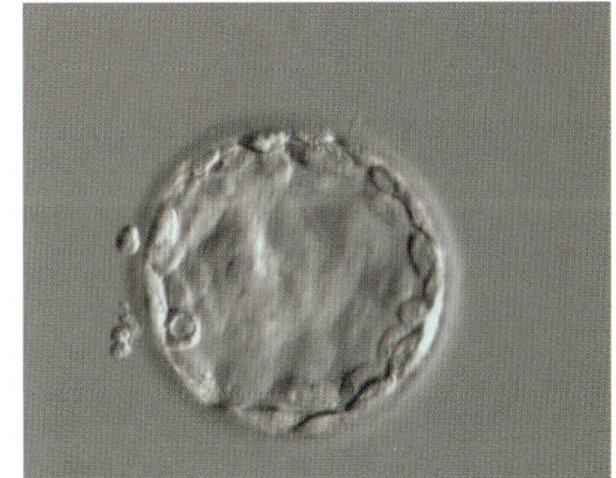
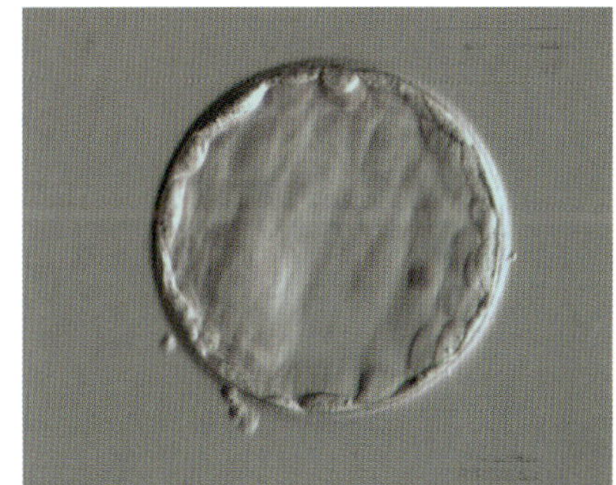

77-BV-1   **77-AW-1**   **77-BT-1**

77-BV-1 Blastocyst 4aa before vitrification
77-AW-1 Full expansion after warming
77-BT-1 No contraction after warming, thin cell bridges from inner cell mass to trophectoderm visible

Vitrified/warmed cycle: November 2013

Stimulation	Natural cycle
Endometrium	7.7 mm
Quality before vitrification	Blastocyst 4bc, blastocyst 2cb
Warming day	5
Survival	Yes/Yes
Assisted hatching	No/Yes
Transfer day	5
Quality	Blastocyst 4bb, blastocyst 3bb
Duration of cryostorage	5 months
Time between warming and transfer	3 hours

Outcome: Early pregnancy loss gestation week 8 after one positive heart activity

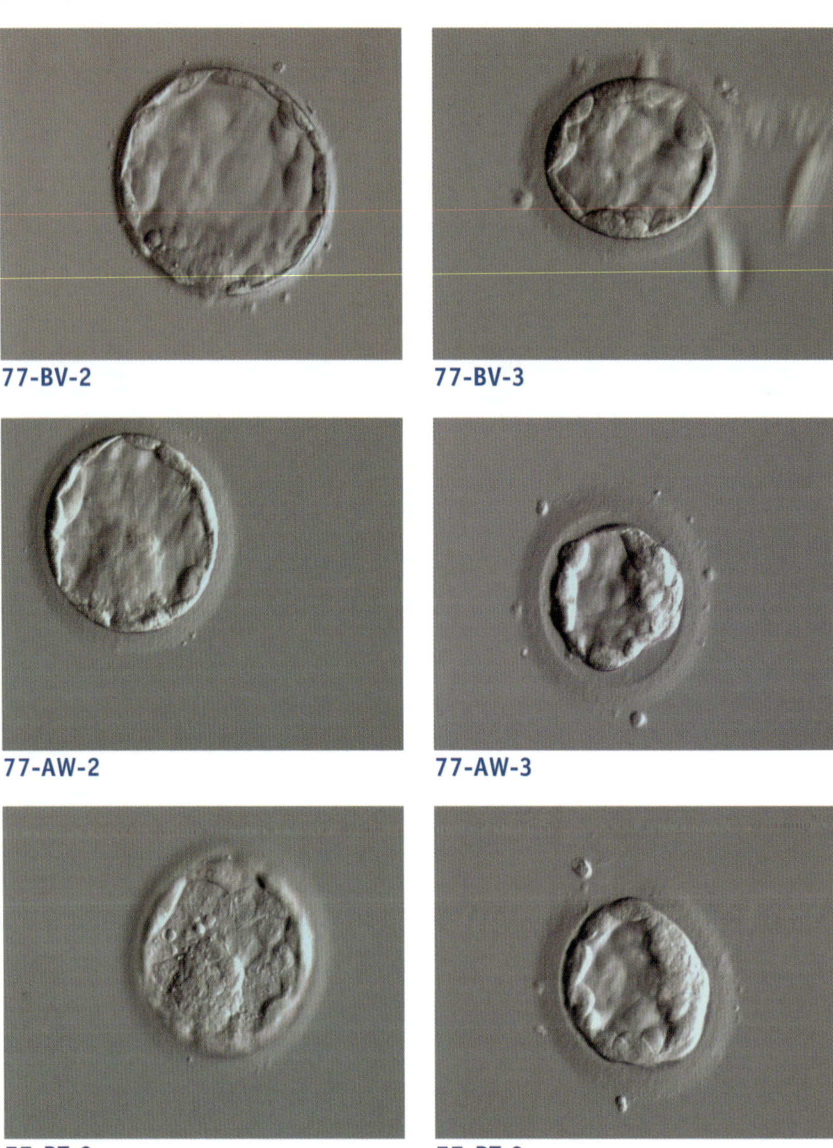

77-BV-2

77-BV-3

77-AW-2

77-AW-3

77-BT-2

77-BT-3

77-BV-2	Blastocyst 4bc before vitrification, loose trophectoderm
77-BV-3	Blastocyst 2cb before vitrification, large trophectoderm cells
77-AW-2	Almost full re-expansion directly after warming, thin cytoplasmic strings from inner cell mass to trophectoderm visible (2 o'clock)
77-AW-3	Blastocyst slightly contracted
77-BT-2	Fully re-expanded blastocyst, inner cell mass clump now visible, some loose fragments
77-BT-3	Re-expanded blastocyst, not hatching yet (opening of the zona at 12 o'clock)

Female partner

Age 37, housewife
Tubal status: patent
MH: 28
BMI: 24.6
Abortion/Deliveries:
Spontaneous conception and
   birth of a healthy girl in 2009
Spontaneous abortion in 2011

Non-smoker, no alcohol consumption
Basal FSH: 6.2 IU/L
Basal LH: 4.9 IU/L
Basal estradiol: 20 pg/mL
Prolactin: 17.4 ng/mL

Male partner

Age 46, technical consultant
History/examination: NAD
BMI: 25.7
Midluteal progesterone: 4.1 ng/mL
Non-smoker, no alcohol consumption
Oligozoospermia

Previous treatments

2013   Intrauterine inseminations ×3 (external)   Not pregnant

Fresh cycle: 2013 IMSI
Semen assessment: oligozoospermia

Volume	1.5 mL
Abstinence	2 days
Concentration	11×10^6/mL
Total sperm number	16.5×10^6/mL
Progressive motility	55%
Non-progressive motility	18%
Immotile	27%
Normal forms	4%
IMSI-Classification	4%/37%/59%
Class I/II/III	

Stimulation protocol and outcome

Stimulation protocol	Long protocol
Days of stimulation	11
Total dose	2325 IU
Number of follicles ≥ 12 mm	25
Total number of COCs	18
Metaphase II	14
Fertilization rate	71%
Cleavage rate	100%
Blastocyst rate	90%

Fresh transfer

Quality of embryo(s)	No fresh transfer because of OHSS
Outcome	
Vitrification	9 blastocysts (day 5)

Vitrified/warmed cycle: 2013

Stimulation	Hormonal substitution protocol
Endometrium	9.0 mm
Quality before vitrification	Blastocyst 5ab, blastocyst 4bb; artificial shrinkage
Warming day	5
Survival	Yes/Yes
Assisted hatching	No/Yes
Transfer day	5
Quality	Blastocyst 5ab, blastocyst 4bb
Duration of cryostorage	1 month
Time between warming and transfer	3.5 hours

Outcome: Live birth, healthy boy

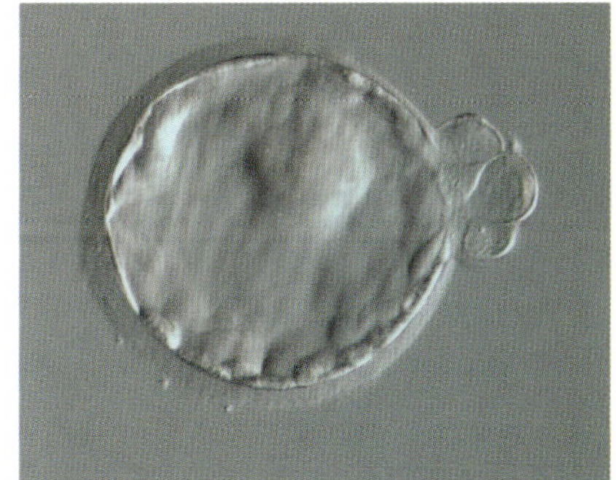

78-BV-1

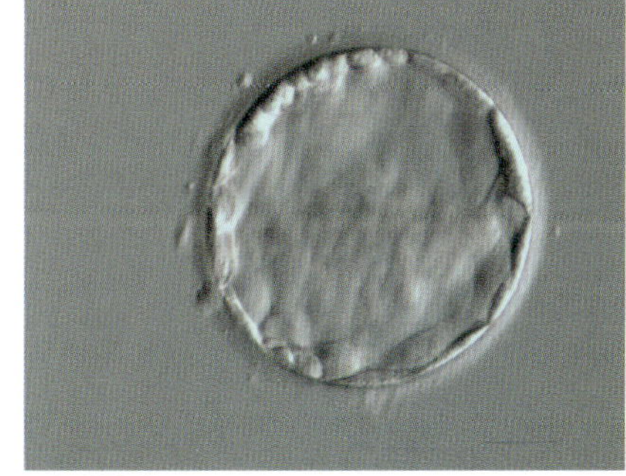

78-BV-2a

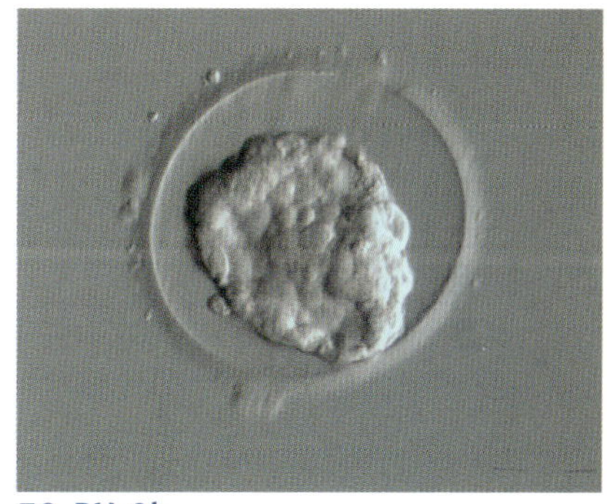

78-BV-2b

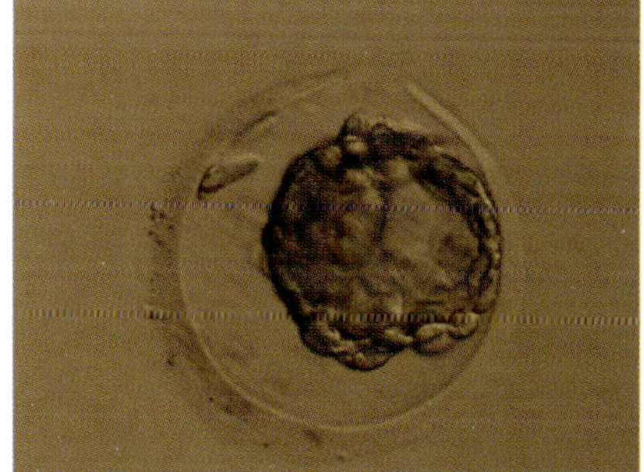

78-AW-1

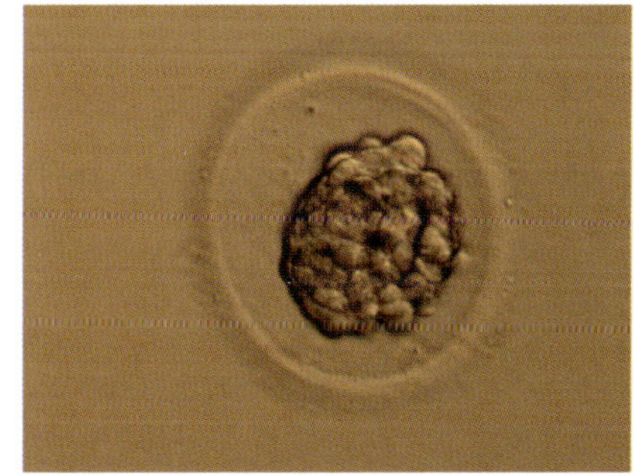

78-AW-2

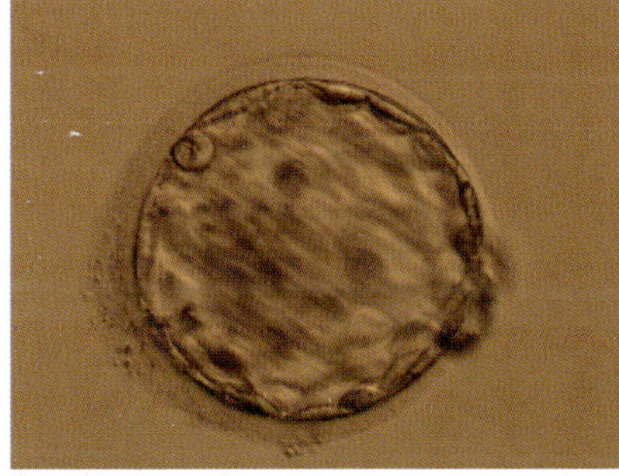

78-BT-1

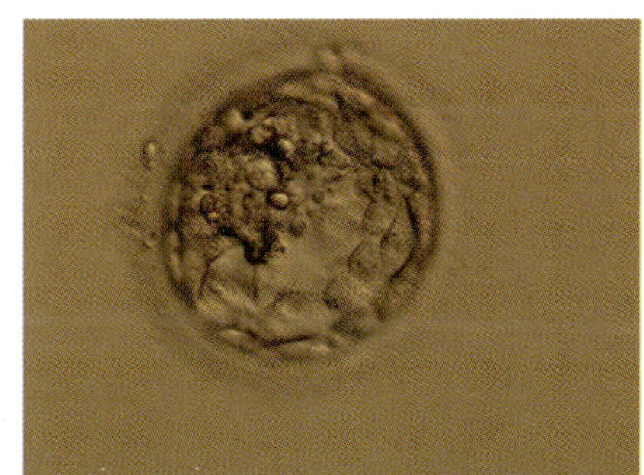

78-BT-2

78-BV-1   Blastocyst 5ab before vitrification, compact inner cell mass in the background at 12 o'clock, hatching at 3 o'clock
78-BV-2a Blastocyst 4bb before artificial shrinkage
78-BV-2b Blastocyst 4bb after artificial shrinkage before vitrification
78-AW-1   Blastocyst half contracted, opening of the zona pellucida at 12 o'clock
78-AW-2   Tightly contracted blastocyst after warming
78-BT-1   Fully re-expanded hatching blastocyst
78-BT-2   Re-expanded blastocyst with some loose fragmentation attached to inner cell mass

Female partner

Age 40, lawyer
Tubal status: patent
MH: 28
BMI: 23.1
Previous surgeries: polyp curettage 2011
Non-smoker, no alcohol consumption

Basal FSH: 6.2 IU/L
Basal LH: 5.7 IU/L
Basal estradiol: 52 pg/mL
AMH: 0.4 µg/L
Midluteal progesterone: 0.4 ng/mL
Prolactin: 18.9 ng/mL

Male partner

Age 38, employee/consultant
History/examination: NAD
BMI: 22.2
Normozoospermia
Non-smoker, no alcohol consumption
Karyogram without pathologic findings for both partners

Previous treatments

2010–2012   Intrauterine inseminations ×4 (external)   Not pregnant ×3 Biochemical pregnancy 2012

Fresh cycle: 2013 IMSI
Semen assessment: normozoospermia

Volume	2 mL
Abstinence	1 day
Concentration	28×10^6/mL
Total sperm number	56×10^6/mL
Progressive motility	36%
Non-progressive motility	11%
Immotile	53%
Normal forms	14%
IMSI-Classification Class I/II/III	14%/48%/38%

Stimulation protocol and outcome

Stimulation protocol	Long protocol
Days of stimulation	11
Total dose	3300 IU
Number of follicles ≥ 12 mm	10
Total number of COCs	9
Metaphase II	6
Fertilization rate	83%
Cleavage rate	100%
Blastocyst rate	60%

Fresh transfer

Quality of embryo(s)	Blastocyst 4ba
Outcome	Not pregnant
Vitrification	2 blastocysts (day 5)

Vitrified/warmed cycle: 2013

Stimulation	Hormonal substitution protocol
Endometrium	7.0 mm
Quality before vitrification	Blastocyst 2cb, early blastocyst
Warming day	5
Survival	Yes / Yes
Assisted hatching	Yes
Transfer day	5
Quality	Blastocyst 2cb, blastocyst 2bb hatching
Duration of cryostorage	4 months
Time between warming and transfer	3.5 hours

Outcome: Biochemical pregnancy

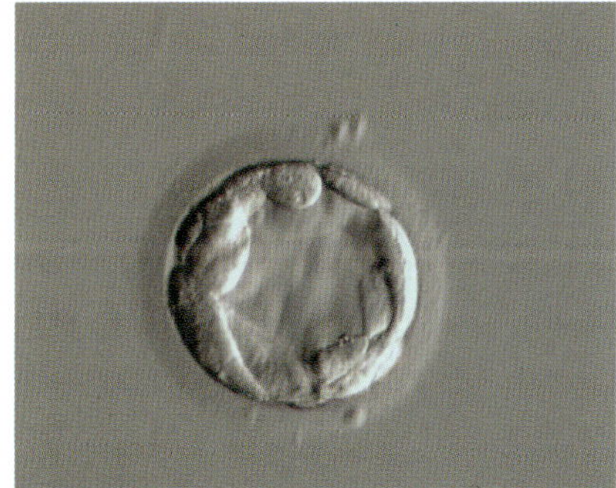

79-BV-1

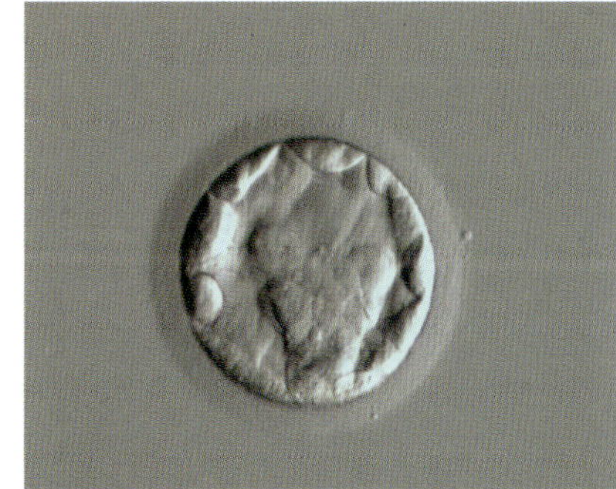

79-BV-2

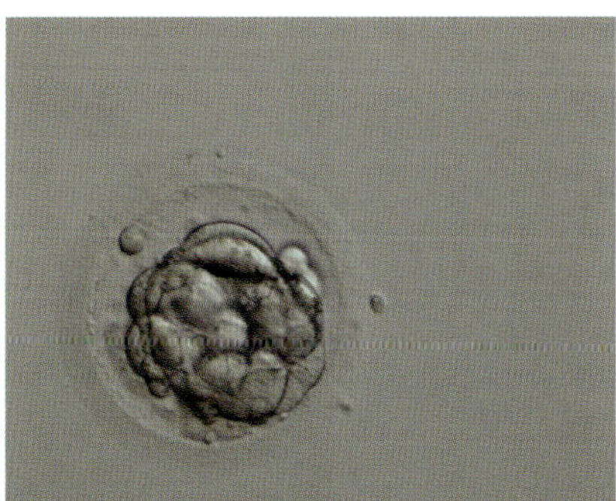
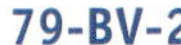

79-AW-1

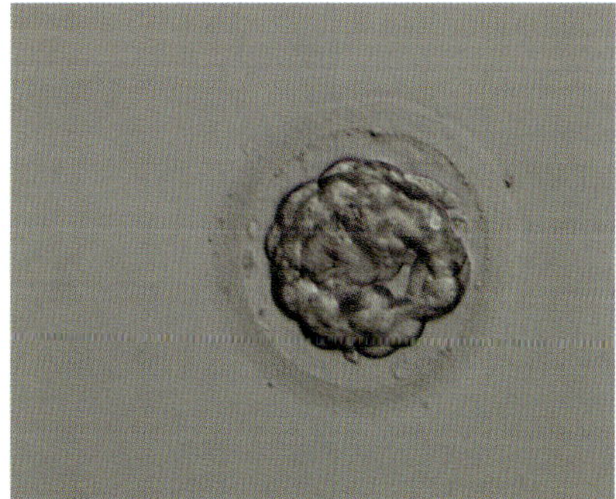

79-AW-2

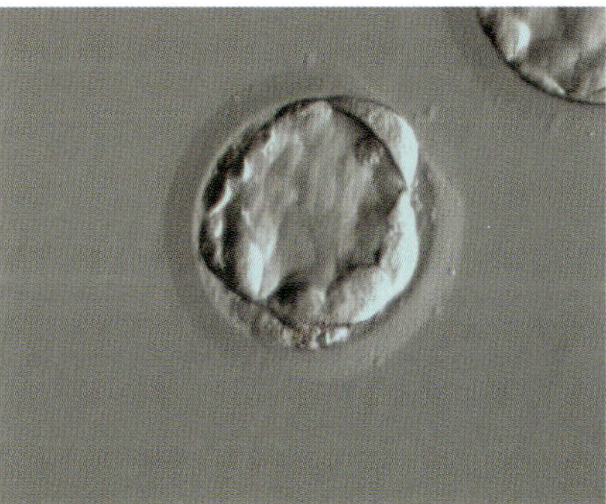

79-BT-1

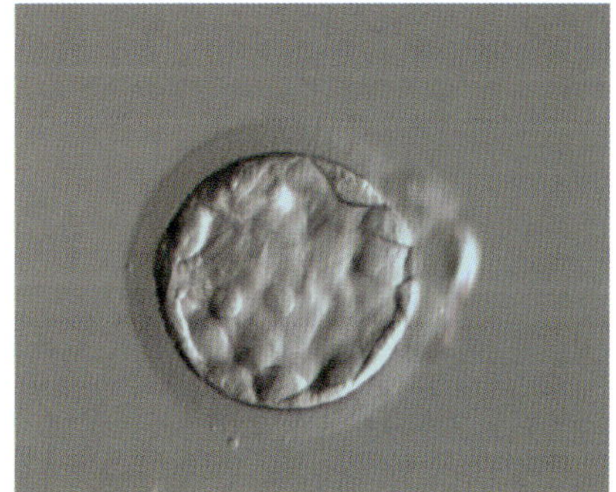

79-BT-2

79-BV-1   Blastocyst 2bc before vitrification, loose trophectoderm, no cohesive cells
79-BV-2   Early blastocyst with thick ZP
79-AW-1   Blastocyst 2bc half contracted after warming, several cells are not included in blastocyst formation
79-AW-2   Early blastocyst with 50% contraction directly after warming
79-BT-1   Blastocyst 2bc starting to hatch through opening, excluded fragments in perivitelline space visible
79-BT-2   Blastocyst 2bb fully expanded and hatching at 3 o'clock position, some loose cells in blastocoelic cavity

Case 80

12 years 2° infertility   Diagnosis: Azoospermia after seminoma and chemotherapy

Female partner

Age 35, teacher
Tubal status: patent
MH: 28

Abortion/Deliveries:
Spontaneous conception and birth of a healthy boy
    in 2001
Non-smoker, no alcohol abuse
BMI: 20.1
Basal FSH: 12 IU/L
Basal LH: 9 IU/L
Basal estradiol: 67 pg/mL
Midluteal progesterone: 1.6 ng/mL

Male partner

Age 52, employee
BMI: 24.3
History/examination: seminoma, extirpation of the
    left testis and TESE on the right testis followed by
    chemotherapy in 2004
Non-smoker, no alcohol abuse

Non-obstructive azoospermia

Previous treatments

None

Fresh cycle: 2013 ICSI with TESE sperm and oocyte activation with ionophore
Semen assessment: frozen TESE material

TESE report: After warming and extraction of TESE material very few motile spermatozoa
                with poor morphology available for injection, artificial oocyte activation after ICSI

Stimulation protocol and outcome

Stimulation protocol	Long protocol
Days of stimulation	11
Total dose	2325 IU
Number of follicles ≥ 12 mm	23
Total number of COCs	21
Metaphase II	11
Fertilization rate	73%
Cleavage rate	100%
Blastocyst rate	50%

Fresh transfer

Quality of embryo(s)	Blastocyst 3bc, blastocyst 3bb
Outcome	Pregnancy with 2 heartbeats, abortion week 9 of gestation
Vitrification	2 blastocysts day 6

Vitrified/warmed cycle: 2013

Stimulation	Hormonal substitution protocol
Endometrium	12.0 mm
Quality before vitrification	Blastocyst 3ba, blastocyst 5cb
Warming day	6
Survival	Yes/Yes
Assisted hatching	No/No
Transfer day	5
Quality	Blastocyst 3bb, blastocyst 5bb
Duration of cryostorage	4.5 months
Time between warming and transfer	4 hours

Outcome: Live birth, healthy boy

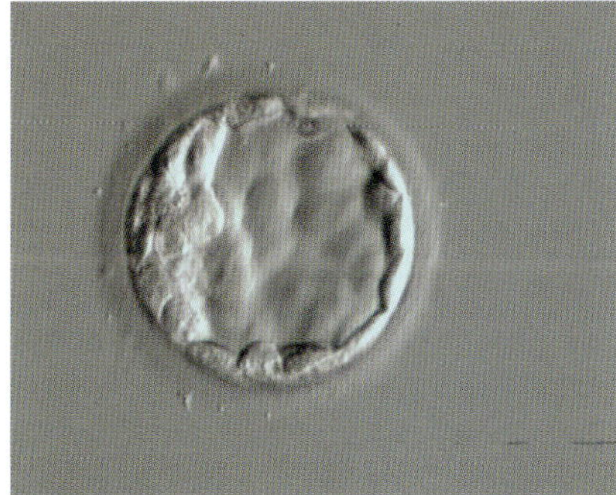

80-BV-1

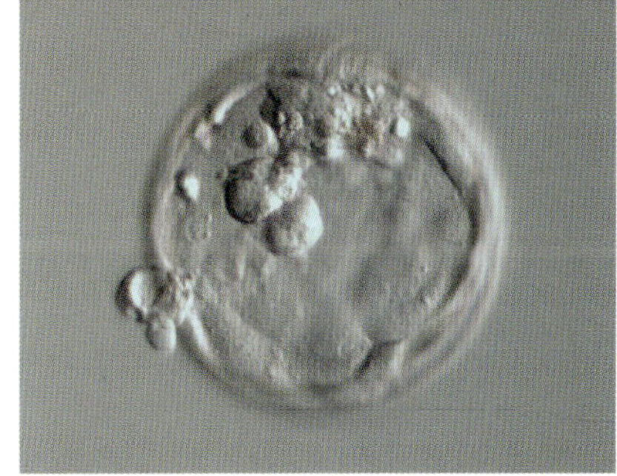

80-BV-2

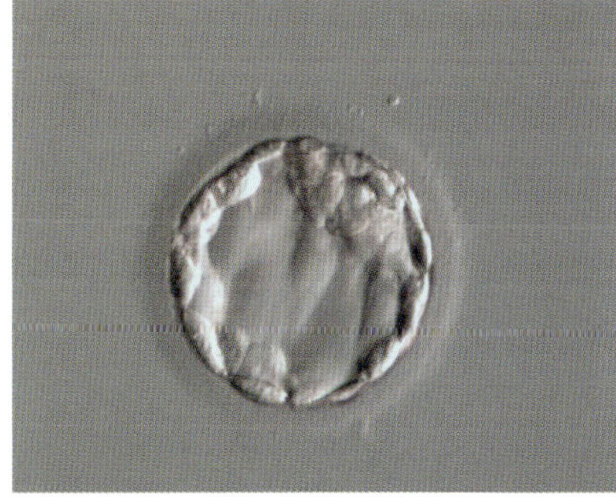

80-AW-1

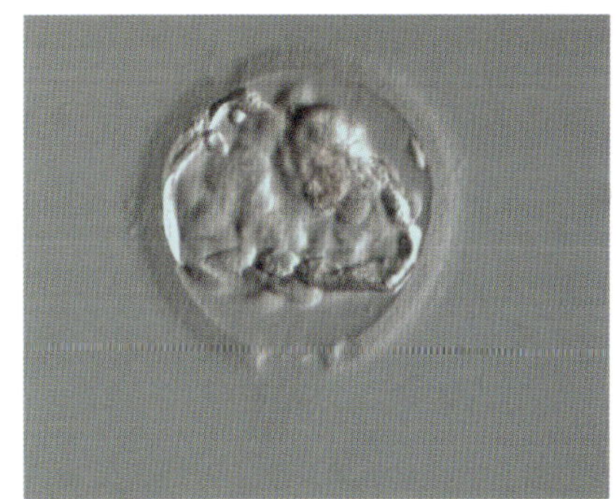

80-AW-2

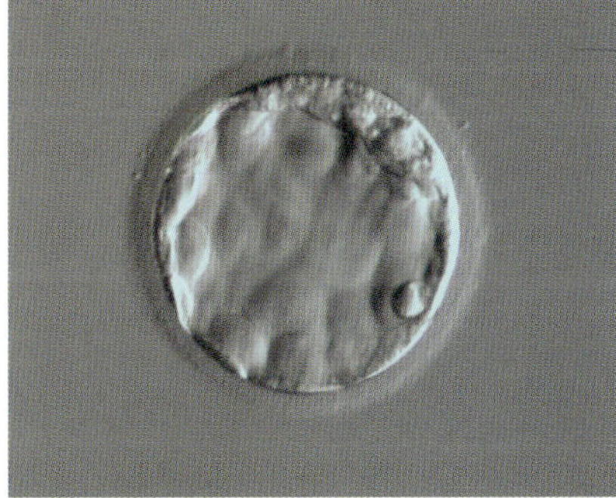

80-BT-1

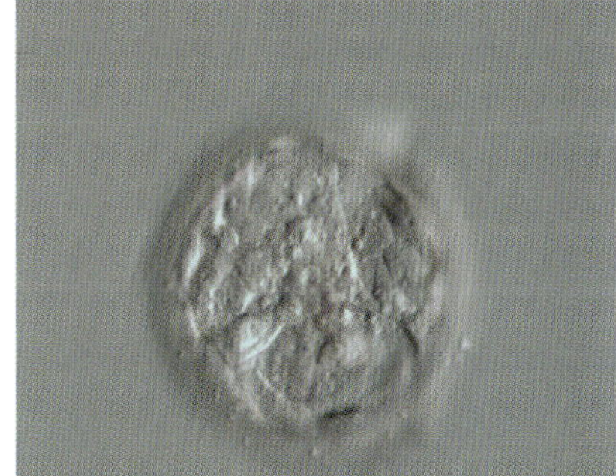

80-BT-2

80-BV-1	Blastocyst 3ba before vitrification, flat inner cell mass, cohesive trophectoderm
80-BV-2	Blastocyst 5cb before vitrification, loose fragments close to inner cell mass and some necrotic cells, hatching at 4 o'clock
80-AW-1	Full re-expansion directly after warming
80-AW-2	Strong contraction after sucrose solutions, trophectoderm attached to zona pellucida at 10 and 4 o'clock
80-BT-1	Intact embryo further expanding before embryo transfer
80-BT-2	Blastocyst 5cb re-expanded with flat, not well defined inner cell mass

Case 81

2 years 2° infertility   Diagnosis: Tubal factor

Female partner

Age 42, teacher

Tubal status: adhesions, not fully patent

MH: 5/28

BMI: 21.9

Mild thrombophilia

Previous surgeries: laparoscopic chromo-perturbation

Abortion/Deliveries:

spontaneous conception and abortion in 2007

Non-smoker, no alcohol consumption

Basal FSH: 6.9 IU/L

Basal LH: 4.7 IU/L

Basal estradiol: 107 pg/mL

Basal AMH: 0.16 ng/mL

Midluteal progesterone: 0.21 ng/mL

Prolactin: 10.4 ng/mL

Male partner

Age 40, engineer

History/examination: NAD

BMI: 24.4

Normozoospermia

Non-smoker, no alcohol consumption

Previous treatments

2009	IVF / ICSI ×3 (external)	Not pregnant
2009	Cryo-ET ×1 (external)	Not pregnant
2010	IVF / ICSI ×2	Not pregnant
2011	IVF / ICSI ×1	Live birth, healthy girl

Fresh cycle: 2013 IMSI

Semen assessment: normozoospermia

Volume	2.6 mL
Abstinence	2 days
Concentration	60×10^6/mL
Total sperm number	156×10^6/mL
Progressive motility	44%
Non-progressive motility	27%
Immotile	29%
Normal forms	14%
IMSI-Classification	14%/39%/47%
Class I/II/III	

Stimulation protocol and outcome

Stimulation protocol	Long protocol
Days of stimulation	12
Total dose	4125 IU
Number of follicles ≥ 12 mm	5
Total number of COCs	5
Metaphase II	4
Fertilization rate	100%
Cleavage rate	100%
Blastocyst rate	75%

Fresh transfer

Quality of embryo(s)	Blastocyst 4ba, blastocyst 4ca
Outcome	Not pregnant
Vitrification	1 expanded blastocyst (day 5)

Vitrified/warmed cycle: 2013

Stimulation	Hormonal substitution protocol
Endometrium	7.2 mm
Quality before vitrification	Expanded blastocyst 4bb
Warming day	5
Survival	Yes
Assisted hatching	No
Transfer day	5
Quality	Blastocyst 4bb
Duration of cryostorage	3 months
Time between warming and transfer	5.5 hours

Outcome: Not pregnant

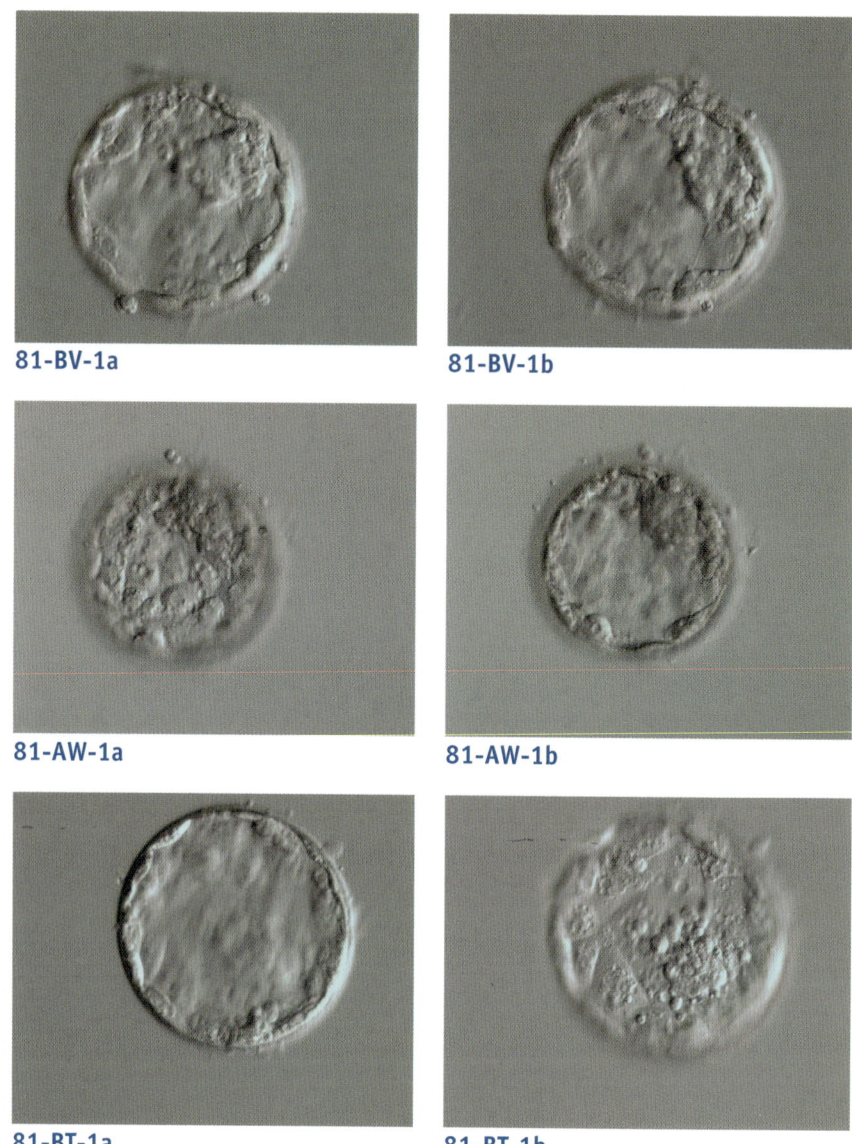

81-BV-1a

81-BV-1b

81-AW-1a

81-AW-1b

81-BT-1a

81-BT-1b

81-BV-1a Blastocyst 4bb before vitrification, a cytoplasmic string extends from the inner cell mass to the trophectoderm (3 o'clock), some TE cells with vacuoles (at 12 o'clock position)

81-BV-1b Large, compact inner cell mass at 1 o'clock position

81-AW-1a After warming in sucrose solution no contraction of blastocyst visible, micro-vacuoles in trophectoderm cells in the background

81-AW-1b Some fragments loosely attached to inner cell mass

81-BT-1a Fully expanded blastocyst before embryo transfer, trophectoderm cells vary in size and appear slightly granular

81-BT-1b Compact inner cell mass with cytoplasmic string extending to trophectoderm

Female partner

Age 29, employee
Tubal status: patent
MH: 28
BMI: 24.2
Psoriasis capitis
Hypothyroidism
Adrenal hyperandrogenemia

Non-smoker, no alcohol
  consumption
Basal FSH: 6.0 IU/L
Basal LH: 5.0 IU/L
Basal estradiol: 324 pg/mL
Midluteal progesterone: 1.8 ng/mL
Prolactin: 10 ng/mL

Male partner

Age 31, business economist
History/examination: orchidopexia
  due to undescended testis age 10
BMI: 22.6
Oligoasthenoteratozoospermia
Non-smoker, no alcohol
  consumption

Previous treatments

2012   Intrauterine inseminations ×3 (external)   Not pregnant ×3

Fresh cycle: 2013 IMSI
Semen assessment: oligoasthenoteratozoospermia

Volume	1.9 mL
Abstinence	2 days
Concentration	4×10^6/mL
Total sperm number	7.6×10^6/mL
Progressive motility	12%
Non-progressive motility	51%
Immotile	37%
Normal forms	3%
IMSI-Classification	3%/56%/41%
Class I/II/III	

Stimulation protocol and outcome

Stimulation protocol	Long protocol
Days of stimulation	14
Total dose	2550 IU
Number of follicles ≥ 12 mm	24
Total number of COCs	17
Metaphase II	13
Fertilization rate	85%
Cleavage rate	100%
Blastocyst rate	91%

Fresh transfer

Quality of embryo(s)	No fresh transfer because of OHSS
Outcome	
Vitrification	10 blastocysts (day 5)

Vitrified/warmed cycle: 2013

Stimulation	Hormonal substitution protocol
Endometrium	9.5 mm
Quality before vitrification	Blastocyst 4aa
Warming day	5
Survival	Yes
Assisted hatching	Yes
Transfer day	5
Quality	Blastocyst 4bb
Duration of cryostorage	4 months
Time between warming and transfer	3 hours

Outcome: Live birth, healthy boy

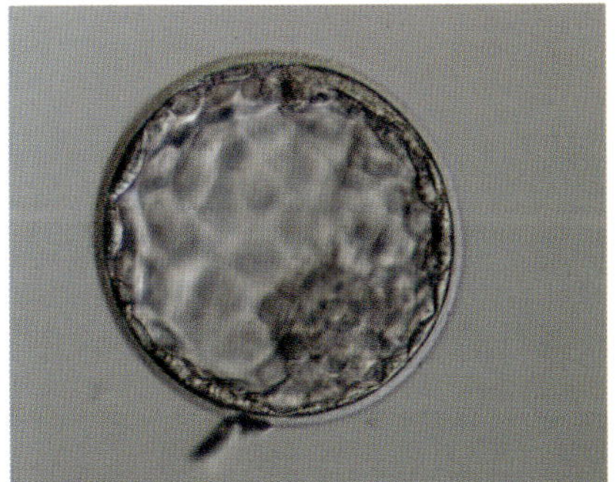

82-BV-1a

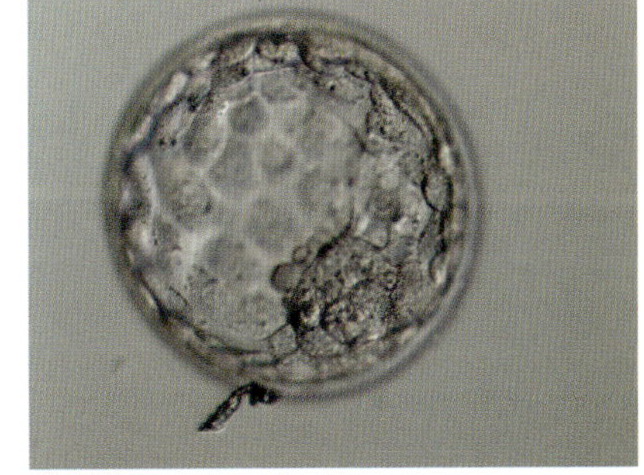

82-BV-1b

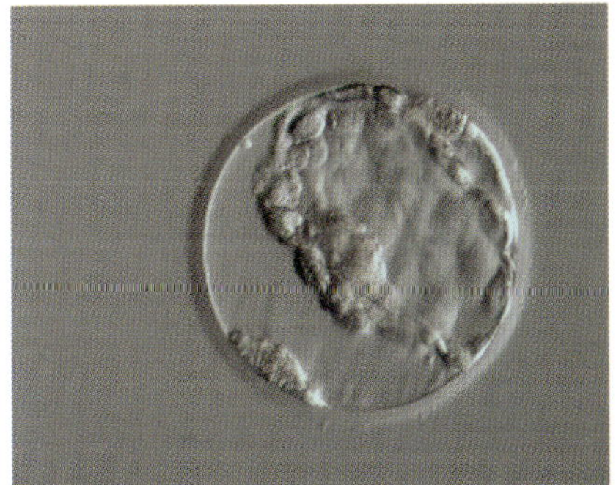

82-AW-1a

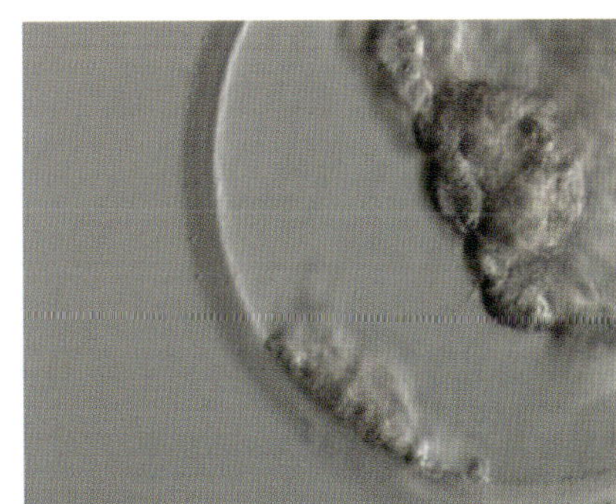

82-AW-1b

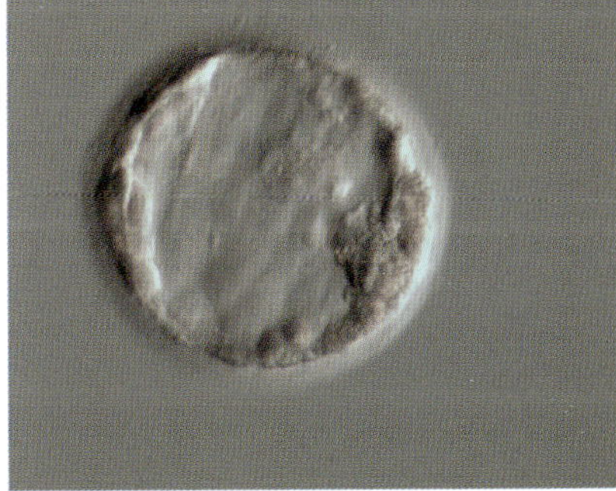

82-BT-1a

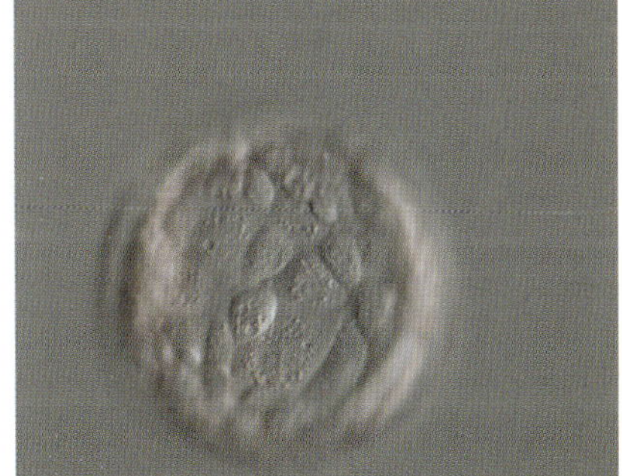

82-BT-1b

82-BV-1a	Before vitrification expanded blastocyst, trophectoderm in focus
82-BV-1b	Nice compact inner cell mass with cytoplasmic string to trophectoderm cells at 3 o'clock
82-AW-1a	Half contracted blastocyst after warming, one excluded fragment attached to ZP at 5 o'clock
82-AW-1b	Compact inner cell mass after warming
82-BT-1a	Before transfer fully re-expanded blastocyst, flat inner cell mass at 3 o'clock
82-BT-1b	Trophectoderm cells viable, no necrotic cells before embryo transfer

Female partner

Age 35, plasterer

Tubal status: patent

MH: 32–45

BMI: 33.2

Previous surgeries: laparoscopic chromoperturbation due to endometriosis in 2012

Non-smoker, no alcohol consumption

Basal FSH: 4.7 IU/L

Basal LH: 5.1 IU/L

Basal estradiol: 71 pg/mL

Midluteal progesterone: 5.3 ng/mL

Prolactin: 14.1 ng/mL

Male partner

Age 30, plasterer

History/examination: NAD

BMI: 26.7

Normozoospermia

Smoker, alcohol consumption occasionally

Previous treatments

2012   IVF cycle ×1 (external)   Not pregnant

Fresh cycle: 2013 IMSI

Semen assessment: normozoospermia

Volume	2 mL
Abstinence	1 day
Concentration	54×10^6/mL
Total sperm number	108×10^6/mL
Progressive motility	43%
Non-progressive motility	33%
Immotile	24%
Normal forms	12%
IMSI-Classification	12%/42%/46%
Class I/II/III	

Stimulation protocol and outcome

Stimulation protocol	Long protocol
Days of stimulation	11
Total dose	2475 IU
Number of follicles ≥ 12 mm	24
Total number of COCs	19
Metaphase II	17
Fertilization rate	88%
Cleavage rate	100%
Blastocyst rate	67%

Fresh transfer

Quality of embryo(s)	Blastocyst 4aa
Outcome	Not pregnant
Vitrification	9 blastocysts (day 5)

Vitrified/warmed cycle: 2013

Stimulation	Hormonal substitution protocol
Endometrium	9.5 mm
Quality before vitrification	Blastocyst 3bc, blastocyst 2bc
Warming day	5
Survival	Yes/Yes
Assisted hatching	No/Yes
Transfer day	5
Quality	Blastocyst 3bc, blastocyst 2bc
Duration of cryostorage	3 months
Time between warming and transfer	3 hours

Outcome: Live birth, healthy girl

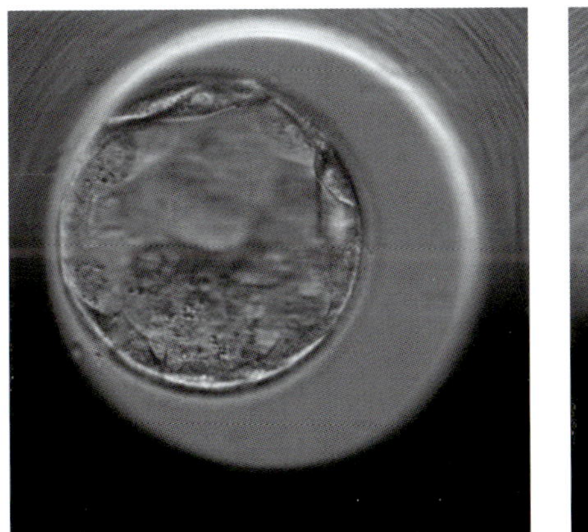

83-BV-1

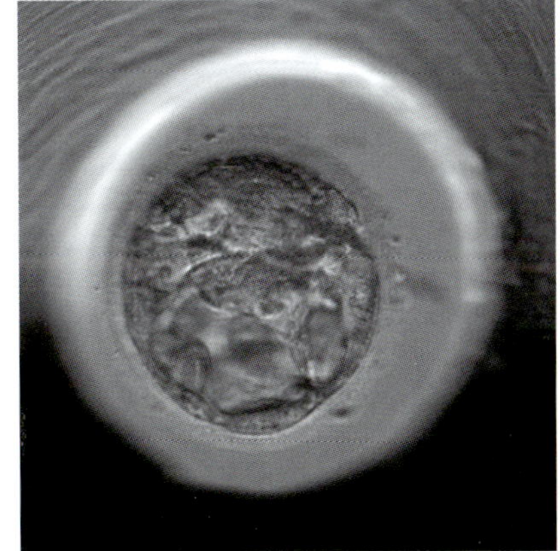

83-BV-2

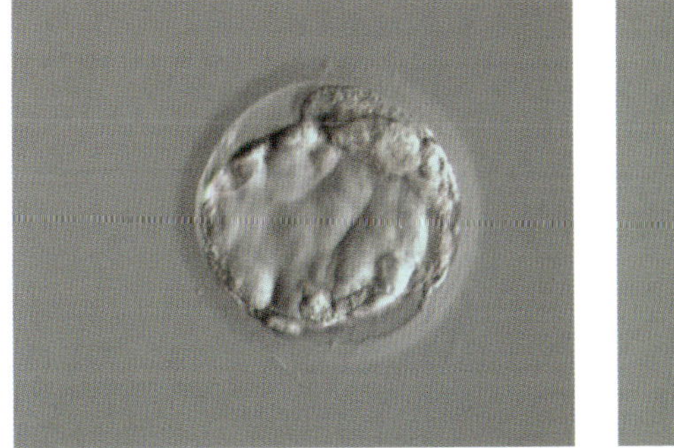

83-AW-1

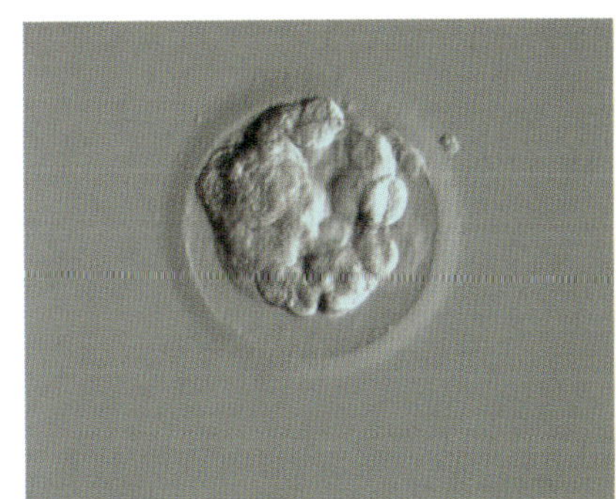

83-AW-2

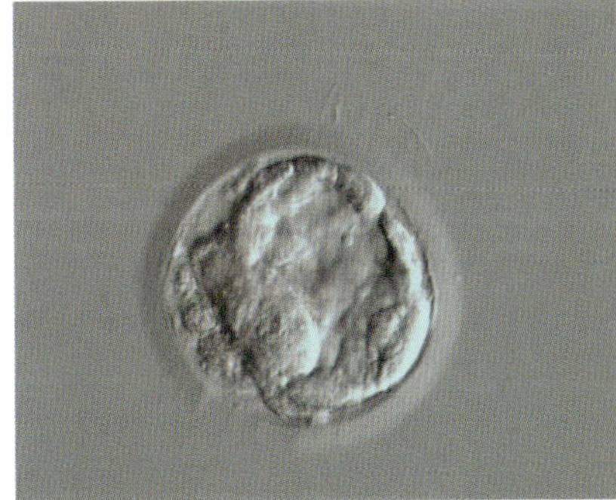

83-BT-1

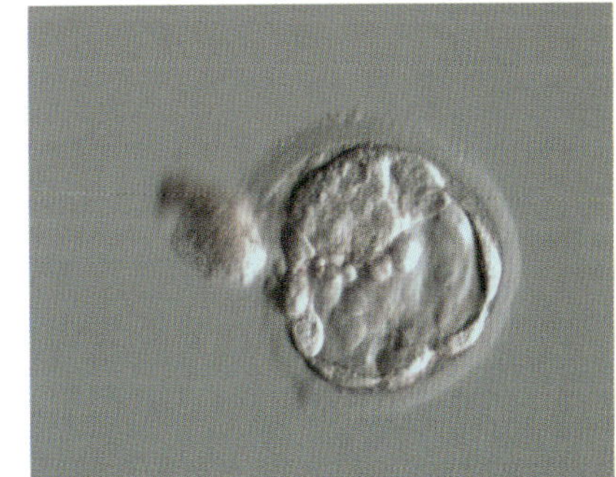

83-BT-2

83-BV-1	Big inner cell mass with loose trophectoderm before vitrification
83-BV-2	Blastocyst 2bc before vitrification
83-AW-1	Almost full re-expansion directly after warming
83-AW-2	Blastocyst half contracted
83-BT-1	Before embryo transfer no full re-expansion, excluded necrotic fragments at 8 o'clock
83-BT-2	Almost full re-expansion before embryo transfer, loose trophectoderm cells, granularity in TE and inner cell mass

Female partner

Age 24, employee
Tubal status: patent
MH: 26
BMI: 28.7
Non-smoker, no alcohol consumption
Basal FSH: 4.5 IU/L
Basal LH: 5.0 IU/L
Basal estradiol: 361 pg/mL
Midluteal progesterone: 1.3 ng/mL
Prolactin: 15 ng/mL

Male partner

Age 41, employee
History/examination: vasectomy in 2002
Failed vasovasostomy in 2012
BMI: 25.6
Obstructive azoospermia after vasectomy
Non-smoker, no alcohol consumption

Previous treatments

None

Fresh cycle: 2013 ICSI with TESE sperm
Semen assessment: fresh TESE material

TESE report: After warming and extraction of TESE material many major
progressive motile spermatozoa

Stimulation protocol and outcome

Stimulation protocol	Long protocol
Days of stimulation	10
Total dose	1500 IU
Number of follicles ≥ 12 mm	17
Total number of COCs	16
Metaphase II	14
Fertilization rate	93%
Cleavage rate	100%
Blastocyst rate	85%

Fresh transfer

Quality of embryo(s)	Blastocyst 4ba
Outcome	Not pregnant
Vitrification	10 blastocysts (day 5)

Vitrified/warmed cycle: 2013

Stimulation	Natural cycle
Endometrium	7.8 mm
Quality before vitrification	Blastocyst 4bb
Warming day	5
Survival	Yes
Assisted hatching	No
Transfer day	5
Quality	Blastocyst 4bb
Duration of cryostorage	5 months
Time between warming and transfer	4 hours

Outcome: Not pregnant

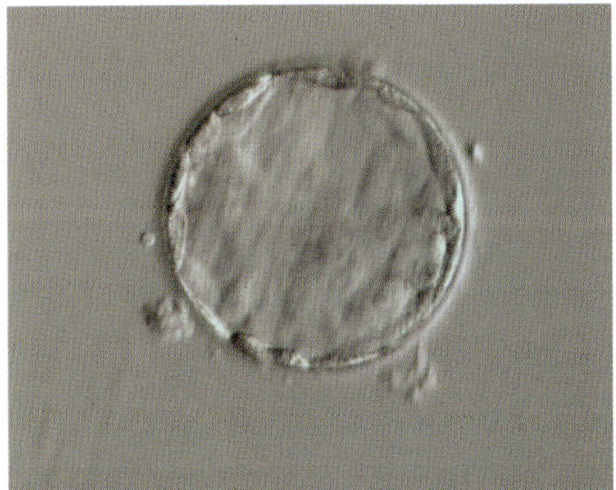
84-BV-1a

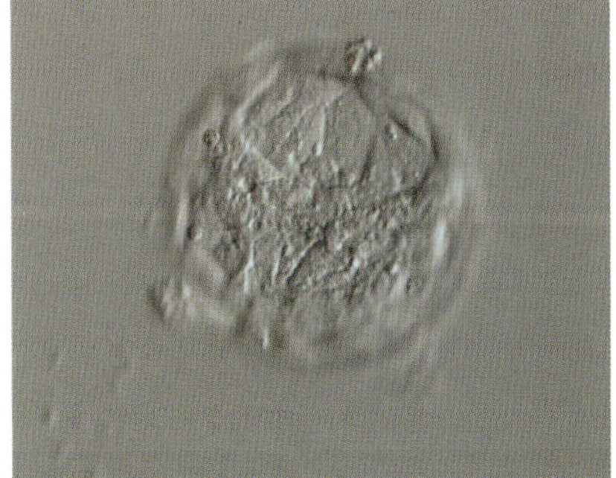
84-BV-1b

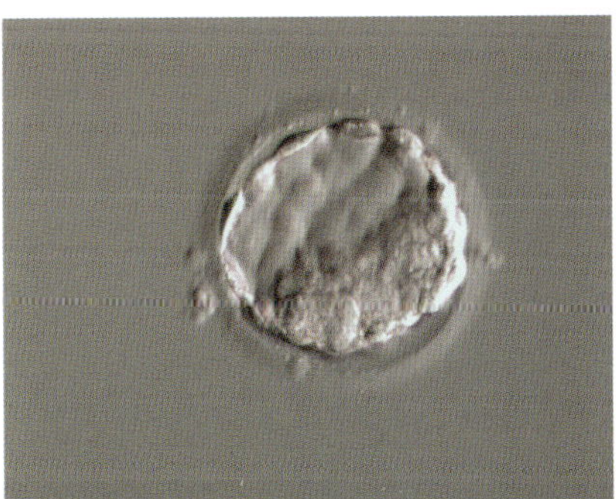
84-AW-1

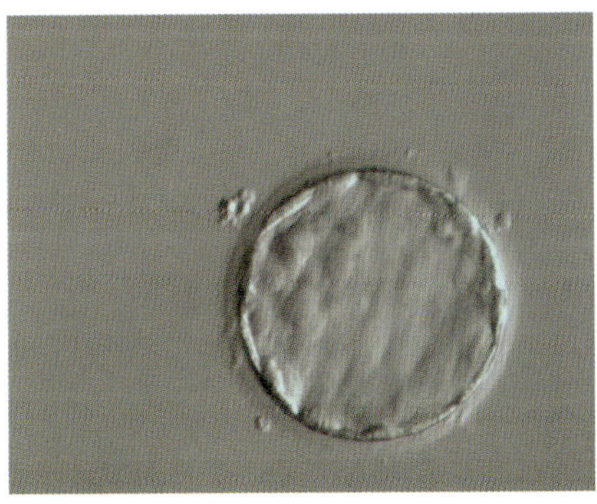
84-BT-1a

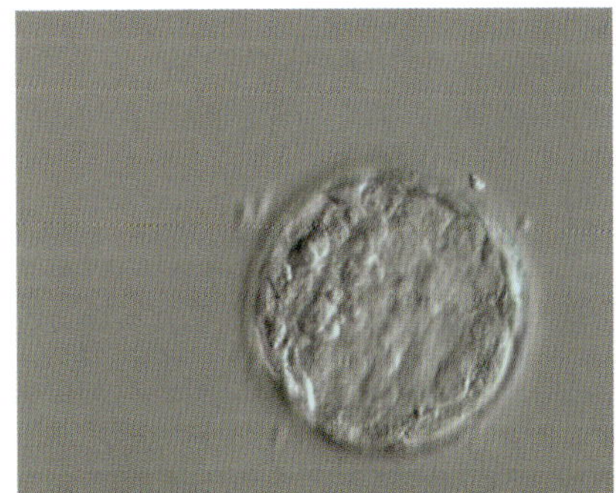
84-BT-1b

84-BV-1a   Trophectoderm with granular cells before vitrification
84-BV-1b   Large and flat inner cell mass
84-AW-1   Slight contraction after warming, no necrotic cells
84-BT-1a   Full re-expansion, trophectoderm with loose, ellipsoid but viable cells
84-BT-1b   Flat inner cell mass with clear viable cells

Female partner

Age 31, no occupation
Tubal status: patent
MH: 30
BMI 16.0

Non-smoker, no alcohol consumption
Basal FSH: 6.7 IU/L
Basal LH: 6.7 IU/L
Basal estradiol: 67 pg/mL
Prolactin: 72.3 ng/mL

Male partner

Age 33, manager
History/examination: NAD
BMI: 25.1
Normozoospermia
Smoker, alcohol consumption
    occasionally

Previous treatments

2008–2009	Intrauterine insemination cycles ×5 (external)	Not pregnant
2009	IVF cycle ×1 (external)	Not pregnant
2010	ICSI cycle	Live birth, healthy girl
2013	Vitrified/warmed cycle	Not pregnant

Fresh cycle: 2010 IMSI

Semen assessment: normozoospermia

Volume	1.2 mL
Abstinence	1 day
Concentration	21×10^6/mL
Total sperm number	25.2×10^6/mL
Progressive motility	66%
Non-progressive motility	14%
Immotile	20%
Normal forms	8%
IMSI-Classification Class I/II/III	8%/42%/50%

Stimulation protocol and outcome

Stimulation protocol	Long protocol
Days of stimulation	10
Total dose	1200 IU
Number of follicles ≥ 12 mm	22
Total number of COCs	19
Metaphase II	17
Fertilization rate	82%
Cleavage rate	100%
Blastocyst rate	64%

Fresh transfer

Quality of embryo(s)	Blastocyst 3bb, blastocyst 3bb
Outcome	Singleton pregnancy, birth of a healthy girl
Vitrification	3 blastocysts (day 5)

Vitrified/warmed cycle: 2013

Stimulation	Natural cycle
Endometrium	7.7 mm
Quality before vitrification	Blastocyst 4bb after warming and re-vitrification in 2013
Warming day	6
Survival	Yes
Assisted hatching	No
Transfer day	5
Quality	Blastocyst 4BC
Duration of cryostorage	3 years
Time between warming and transfer	4 hours

Outcome: Live birth, healthy girl

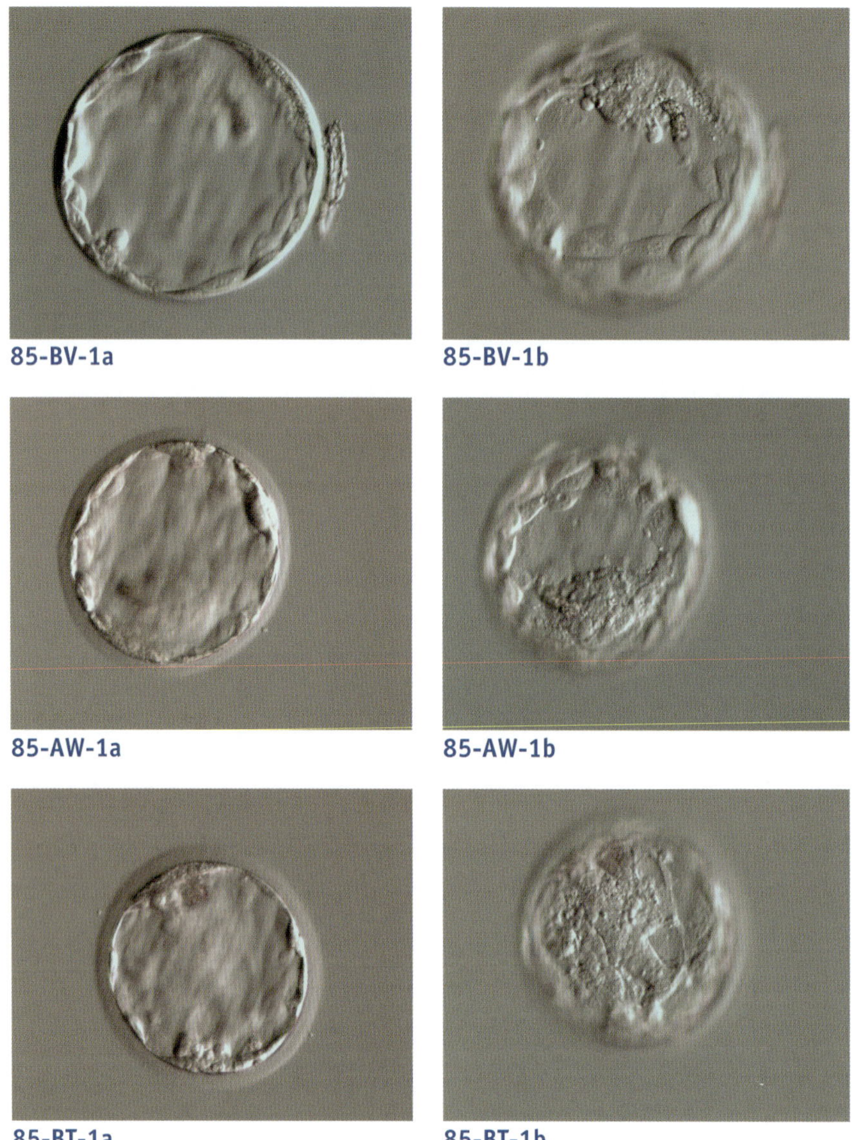

85-BV-1a

85-BV-1b

85-AW-1a

85-AW-1b

85-BT-1a

85-BT-1b

85-BV-1a Cohesive trophectoderm of fully expanded blastocyst before re-vitrification
85-BV-1b Inner cell mass with presence of some loose and necrotic cells before re-vitrification
85-AW-1a Focus on trophectoderm, no signs of contraction
85-AW-1b Inner cell mass directly after warming, with few necrotic cells close to ICM
85-BT-1a Before embryo transfer loose granular trophectoderm structure, one dark TE cell at 12 o'clock
85-BT-1b Inner cell mass appears larger and more flat as compared with before

Female partner

Age 34, social worker
Tubal status: not patent
MH: >=30
BMI: 22.5
Previous surgeries: laparoscopy with chromotuberation and ovarian drilling 2011
Abortion/deliveries:
Spontaneous conception and birth of a healthy boy in 2009

Non-smoker, no alcohol consumption
Basal FSH: 7.1 IU/L
Basal LH: 6.7 IU/L
Basal estradiol: 38 pg/mL
Midluteal progesterone: 0.4 ng/mL
Prolactin: 8.3 ng/mL

Male partner

Age 36, constructional engineer
History/examination: NAD
BMI: 25.0
Normozoospermia
Smoker, alcohol consumption occasionally

Previous treatments

None

Fresh cycle: 2013 IVF
Semen assessment: normozoospermia

Volume	3 mL
Abstinence	1 day
Concentration	29×10^6/mL
Total sperm number	87×10^6/mL
Progressive motility	62%
Non-progressive motility	10%
Immotile	20%
Normal forms	28%

Stimulation protocol and outcome

Stimulation protocol	Long protocol
Days of stimulation	13
Total dose	2325 IU
Number of follicles ≥ 12 mm	14
Total number of COCs	14
Metaphase II	14
Fertilization rate	79%
Cleavage rate	100%
Blastocyst rate	91%

Fresh transfer

Quality of embryo(s)	Blastocyst 5ab
Outcome	Clinical pregnancy without heart activity, spontaneous abortion gestation week 7
Vitrification	9 blastocysts (day 5)

Vitrified/warmed cycle: 2013

Stimulation	Hormonal substitution protocol
Endometrium	10.0 mm
Quality before vitrification	Blastocyst 4ab, blastocyst 4bb
Warming day	5
Survival	Yes/Yes
Assisted hatching	No/No
Transfer day	5
Quality	Blastocyst 4bb, blastocyst 4bb
Duration of cryostorage	4 months
Time between warming and transfer	3 hours

Outcome: After detection of 2 embryos with positive heart activity live birth of one healthy girl

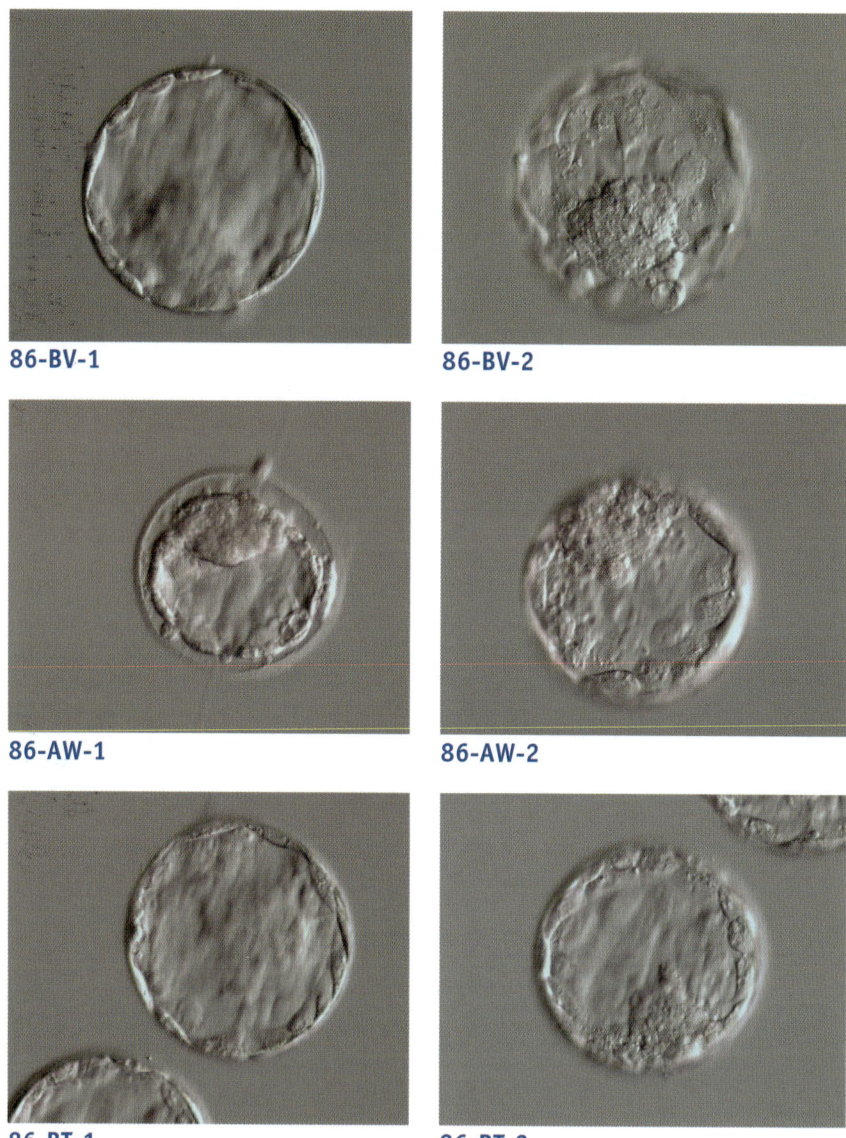

86-BV-1

86-BV-2

86-AW-1

86-AW-2

86-BT-1

86-BT-2

86-BV-1 Blastocyst 4ab before vitrification, clump inner cell mass slightly visible at 6 o'clock, trophectoderm with loose cells which are slightly granular

86-BV-2 Blastocyst 4bb before vitrification with focus on inner cell mass, on cytoplasmic string to the trophectoderm visible in the center, one TE cell with a vacuole at 6 o'clock

86-AW-1 Slightly collapsed blastocyst after warming, well compacted inner cell mass, granular vacuolated trophectoderm cells

86-AW-2 Second blastocyst stays fully expanded, light cells, presence of vacuoles in the majority of trophectoderm cells (notice the different behaviour during vitrification procedure in terms of contraction and expansion: embryo 1 contracted, embryo 2 no signs of collapsing)

86-BT-1 Full re-expansion of the blastocyst, nice compact inner cell mass slightly visible in the background

86-BT-2 Inner cell mass as well as trophectoderm cells with granulation and vacuoles

Female partner

Age 36, receptionist
Tubal status: not patent
MH: 31
BMI: 21.3
Previous surgeries: laparo-
  scopic chromopertubation
  due to tubal adhesions 2012
Abortions/deliveries:
Spontaneous conception and
  birth of a healthy girl in 2007

Non-smoker, no alcohol
  consumption
Basal FSH: 3.7 IU/L
Basal LH: 4.2 IU/L
Basal estradiol: 64.5 pg/mL
Midluteal progesterone: 3.4 ng/mL
Prolactin: 13.2 ng/mL

Male partner

Age 36, carpenter
History/examination: NAD
BMI: 23.1
Normozoospermia
Non-smoker, no alcohol
  consumption

Previous treatments

None

Fresh cycle: 2013 ICSI
Semen assessment: normozoospermia

Volume	1.2 mL
Abstinence	1 day
Concentration	51×10^6/mL
Total sperm number	61.2×10^6/mL
Progressive motility	76%
Non-progressive motility	6%
Immotile	18%
Normal forms	12%

Stimulation protocol and outcome

Stimulation protocol	Long protocol
Days of stimulation	11
Total dose	1950 IU
Number of follicles ≥ 12 mm	37
Total number of COCs	18
Metaphase II	16
Fertilization rate	86%
Cleavage rate	100%
Blastocyst rate	79%

Fresh transfer

Quality of embryo(s)	No fresh transfer because of OHSS
Outcome	
Vitrification	11 blastocysts (day 5)

Vitrified/warmed cycle: 2013

Stimulation	Hormonal substitution protocol
Endometrium	7.0 mm
Quality before vitrification	Blastocyst 4ba
Warming day	5
Survival	Yes
Assisted hatching	No
Transfer day	5
Quality	Blastocyst 4ba
Duration of cryostorage	1 month
Time between warming and transfer	2.5 hours

Outcome: Biochemical pregnancy

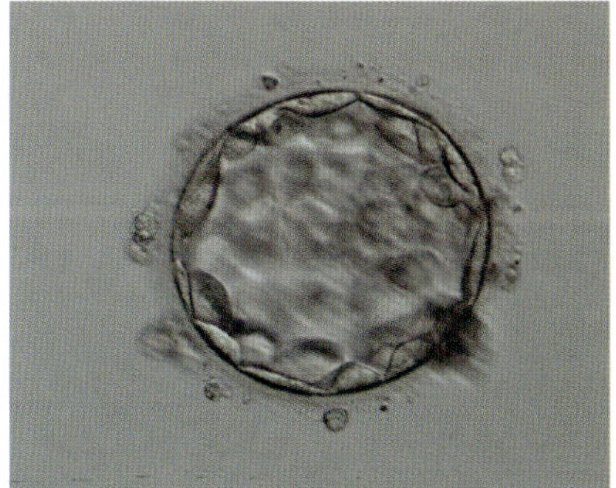

87-BV-1a

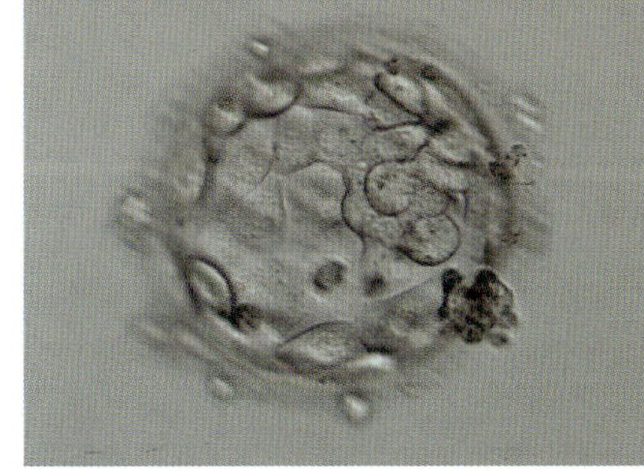

87-BV-1b

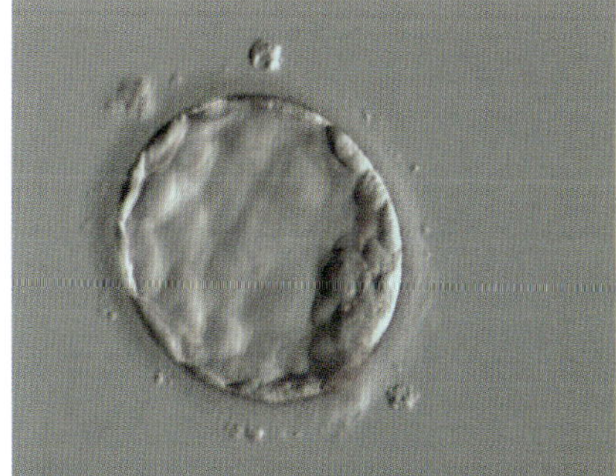

87-AW-1a

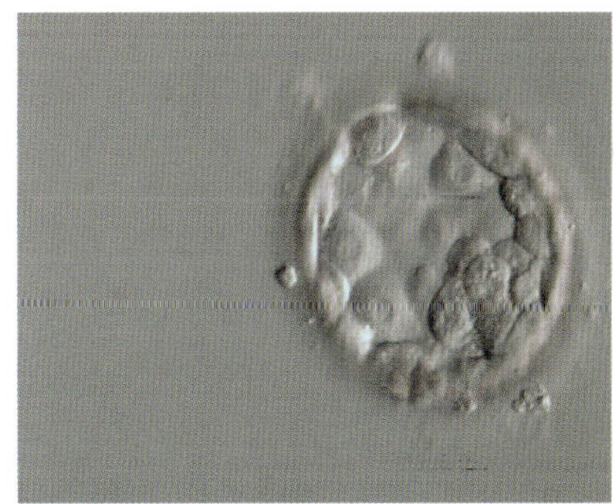

87-AW-1b

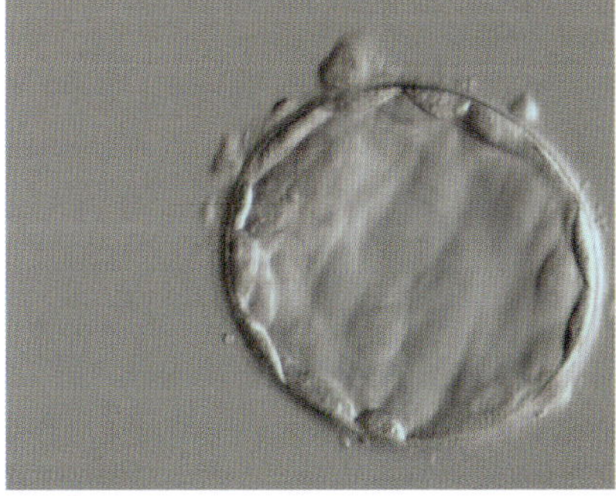

87-BT-1a

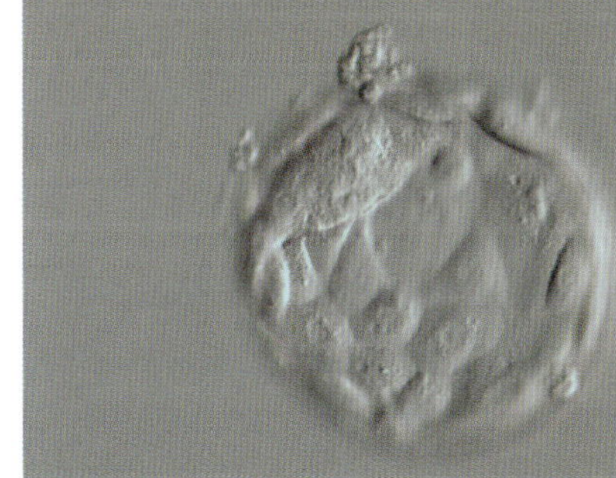

87-BT-1b

87-BV-1a	Before vitrification well-defined cohesive trophectoderm cells
87-BV-1b	Inner cell mass compact but consisting of few cells
87-AW-1a	No sign of contraction after warming
87-AW-1b	Clear inner cell mass cells, well-defined trophectoderm cells with nucleus visible
87-BT-1a	Before embryo transfer further expansion and thinning of the ZP
87-BT-1b	Cells forming the inner cell mass in one cluster

Female partner

Age 35, employee
Tubal status: patent
MH: >30
BMI: 25.3
Celiac disease
Non-smoker, no alcohol
  consumption

Basal FSH: 9 IU/L
Basal LH: 9.1 IU/L
Basal estradiol: 30.9 pg/mL
Midluteal progesterone: 0.5 ng/mL
Prolactin: 211 ng/mL

Male partner

Age 35, electrician
History/examination: Surgery due to
  undescended testicles at age 5
BMI: 34.9
Oligozoospermia
Smoker, alcohol consumption
  occasionally
Spontaneous conception with
  previous partner

Previous treatments

2011–2012   Intrauterine insemination cycles ×6 (external)   Not pregnant

Fresh cycle: 2013 IMSI
Semen assessment: oligozoospermia

Volume	1.8 mL
Abstinence	1 day
Concentration	7×10^6/mL
Total sperm number	12.6×10^6/mL
Progressive motility	80%
Non-progressive motility	5%
Immotile	15%
Normal forms	9%
IMSI-Classification	9%/47%/44%
Class I/II/III	

Stimulation protocol and outcome

Stimulation protocol	Long protocol
Days of stimulation	11
Total dose	1650 IU
Number of follicles ≥ 12 mm	18
Total number of COCs	20
Metaphase II	15
Fertilization rate	80%
Cleavage rate	100%
Blastocyst rate	75%

Fresh transfer

Quality of embryo(s)	No fresh transfer because of OHSS
Outcome	
Vitrification	9 blastocysts (day 5)

Vitrified/warmed cycle: 2013

Stimulation	Hormonal substitute protocol
Endometrium	6.5 mm
Quality before vitrification	Blastocyst 3aa
Warming day	5
Survival	Yes
Assisted hatching	Yes
Transfer day	5
Quality	Blastocyst 3ab
Duration of cryostorage	1 month
Time between warming and transfer	4 hours

Outcome: Live birth, healthy boy

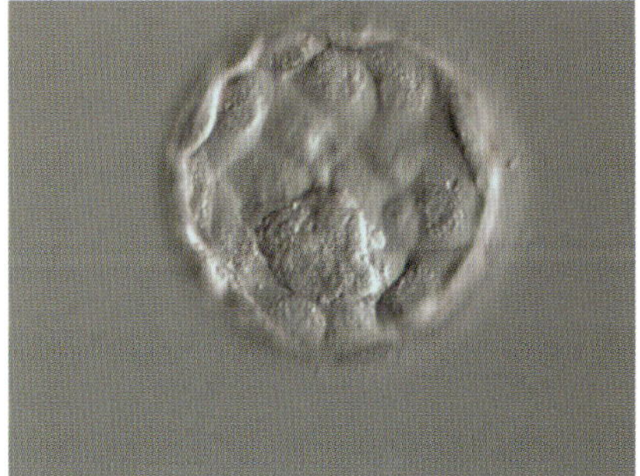

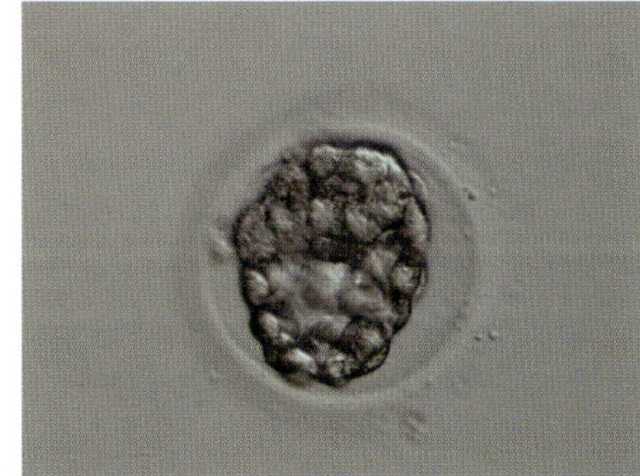

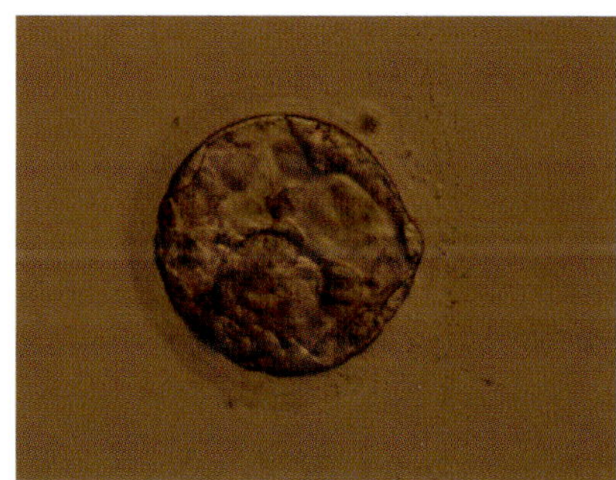

88-BV-1   **88-AW-1**   **88-BT-1**

88-BV-1 Compact inner cell mass before vitrification
88-AW-1 Half collapsed blastocyst after warming
88-BT-1 Before embryo transfer full re-expansion, trophectoderm appears less cohesive than before vitrification, no hatching yet

Female partner

Age 29, no occupation

Tubal status: not fully patent after chlamydia infection

MH: 28

BMI: 18.7

Hashimoto's thyroiditis

Non-smoker, no alcohol consumption

TSH: 1.63 µU/mL

Basal FSH: 7.9 IU/L

Basal LH: 4.6 IU/L

Basal estradiol: 45.8 pg/mL

AMH: 1.6 µg/L

Midluteal progesterone: 0.2 ng/mL

Prolactin: 9.9 ng/mL

Male partner

Age 34, footballer

History/examination: surgery due to varicocele in 2012

BMI: 26.0

Normozoospermia

Previous treatments

2012   Intrauterine insemination ×1 (external)   Not pregnant

Fresh cycle: 2010 IMSI

Semen assessment: normozoospermia

Volume	1.5 mL
Abstinence	5 days
Concentration	58×10^6/mL
Total sperm number	87×10^6/mL
Progressive motility	44%
Non-progressive motility	23%
Immotile	33%
Normal forms	7%
IMSI-Classification	7%/49%/44%
Class I/II/III	

Stimulation protocol and outcome

Stimulation protocol	Long protocol
Days of stimulation	11
Total dose	1725 IU
Number of follicles ≥ 12 mm	12
Total number of COCs	13
Metaphase II	12
Fertilization rate	100%
Cleavage rate	100%
Blastocyst rate	50%

Fresh transfer

Quality of embryo(s)	No fresh transfer because of uterine polyp
Outcome	
Vitrification	6 blastocysts (day 5)

Vitrified/warmed cycle: 2013

Stimulation	Hormonal substitution protocol
Endometrium	14.0 mm
Quality before vitrification	Blastocyst 5ac
Warming day	5
Survival	Yes
Assisted hatching	No
Transfer day	5
Quality	Blastocyst 5ac hatching
Duration of cryostorage	4.5 months
Time between warming and transfer	2.5 hours

Outcome: Live birth, healthy girl

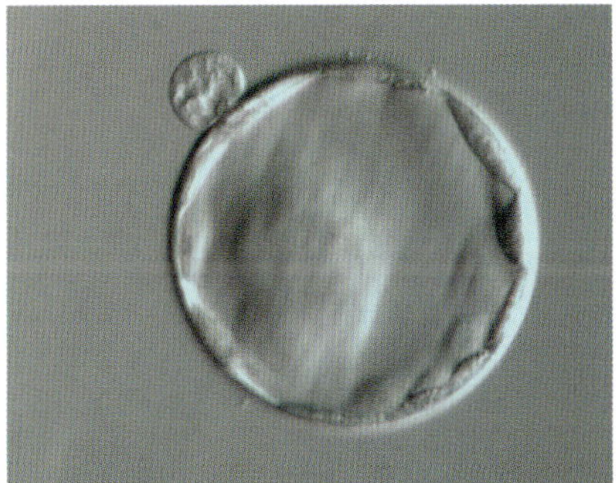

89-BV-1a

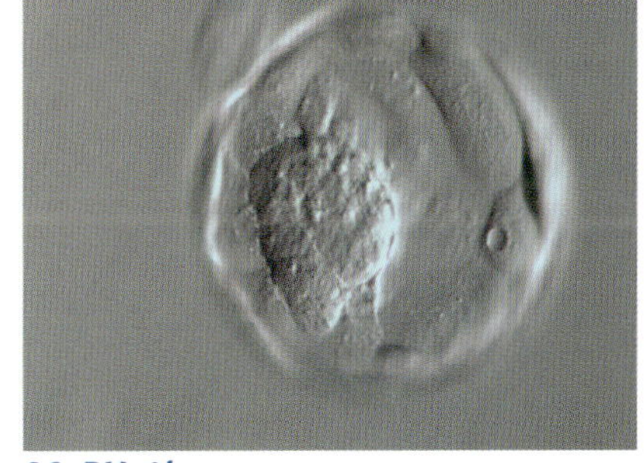

89-BV-1b

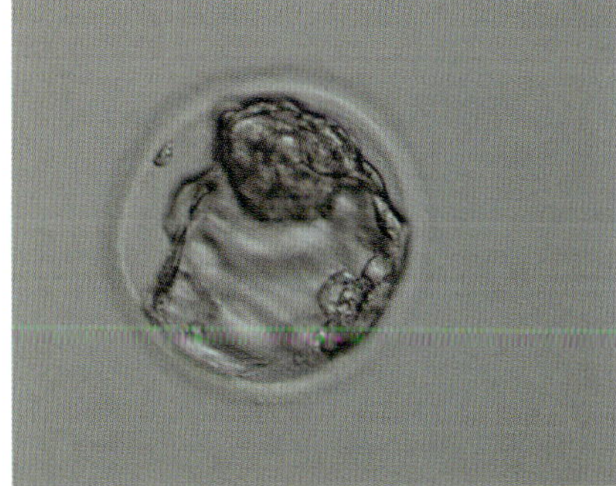

89-AW-1a

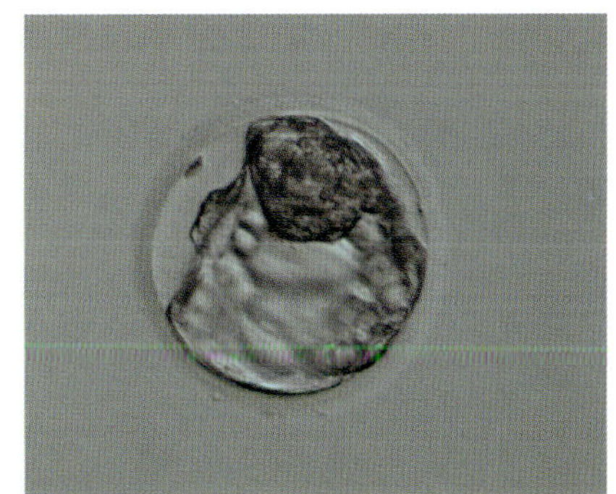

89-AW-1b

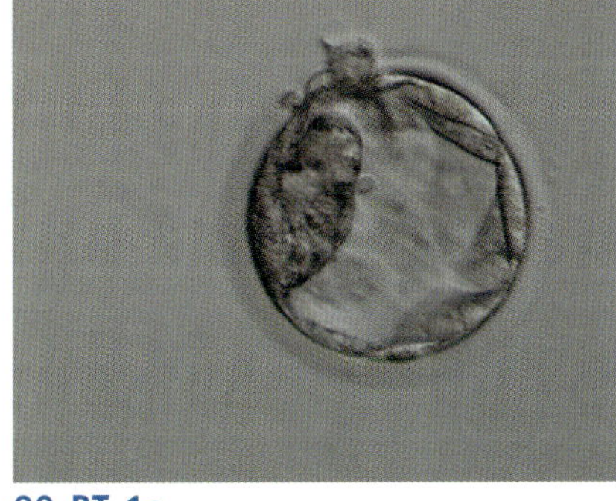

89-BT-1a

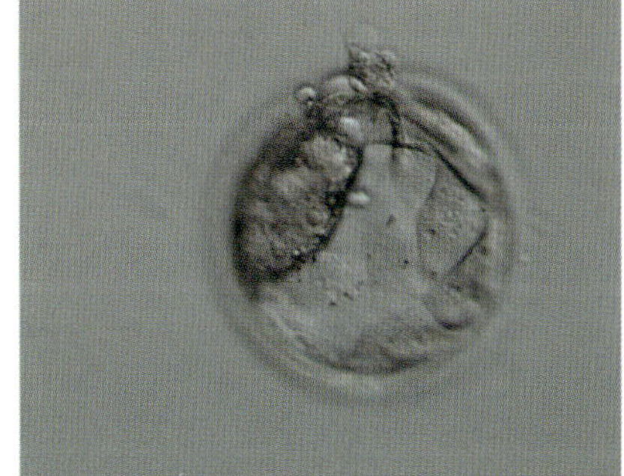

89-BT-1b

89-BV-1a	Few elypsoid trophectoderm cells
89-BV-1b	Large compact inner cell mass
89-AW-1a	After warming contraction of the blastocysts whereas the majority of the trophectoderm cells stay attached to the ZP (zona anchorage)
89-AW-1b	Inner cell mass clearly visible after warming
89-BT-1a	Full re-expansion before embryo transfer, clear cells
89-BT-1b	Blastocyst starts to hatch at the 12 o'clock position

1 year 2° infertility   Diagnosis: Amenorrhea, tubal factor

Female partner

Age 39, teacher

Tubal status: not fully patent after chlamydia infection

MH: amenorrhea

BMI: 18.4

Previous surgeries: conization in 2009, laparoscopic hysteroscopy in 2011

Before 2012 oligomenorrhea with menstrual cycles between 31 and 52 days, after curettage in 2012 amenorrhea

Non-smoker, no alcohol consumption

TSH: 1.4 µU/mL

Basal FSH: 6.7 IU/L

Basal LH: 6.4 IU/L

Basal estradiol: 31 pg/mL

Prolactin: 8.4 ng/mL

Male partner

Age 44, lawyer

History/examination: NAD

BMI: 24.6

Normozoospermia

Non-smoker, no alcohol consumption

Previous treatments

2011	ICSI cycle ×1 (external)	Biochemical pregnancy
2012	ICSI cycle ×1 (external)	Abortion in gestation week 8

Fresh cycle: 2013 IMSI

Semen assessment: normozoospermia

Volume	2 mL
Abstinence	2 days
Concentration	54×10^6/mL
Total sperm number	108×10^6/mL
Progressive motility	26%
Non-progressive motility	20%
Immotile	54%
Normal forms	6%
IMSI-Classification Class I/II/III	6%/30%/64%

Stimulation protocol and outcome

Stimulation protocol	Long protocol
Days of stimulation	12
Total dose	1950 IU
Number of follicles ≥ 12 mm	18
Total number of COCs	14
Metaphase II	12
Fertilization rate	100%
Cleavage rate	100%
Blastocyst rate	75%

Fresh transfer

Quality of embryo(s)	Blastocyst 4aa
Outcome	Not pregnant
Vitrification	7 blastocysts (day 5)

Vitrified/warmed cycle: 2013

Stimulation	Hormonal substitution protocol
Endometrium	7.0 mm
Quality before vitrification	Blastocyst 4bb, blastocyst 2bb
Warming day	5
Survival	Yes/Yes
Assisted hatching	Yes/Yes
Transfer day	5
Quality	Blastocyst 4bc hatching, blastocyst 2bb hatching
Duration of cryostorage	4 months
Time between warming and transfer	3 hours

Outcome: Not pregnant

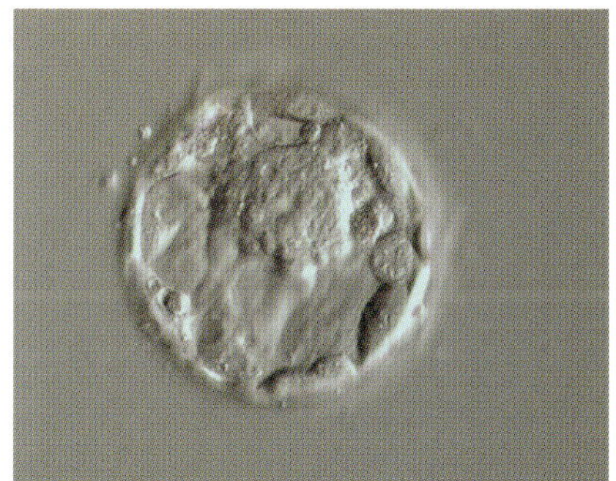

90-BV-1

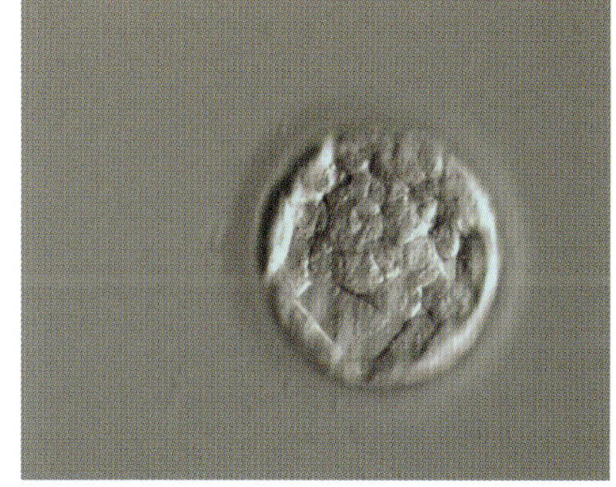

90-BV-2

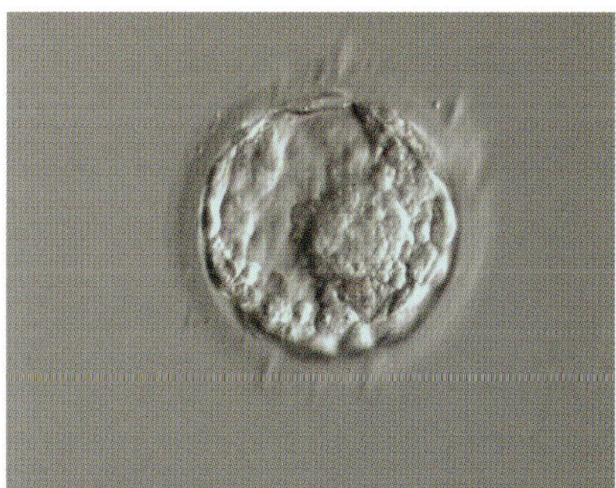

90-AW-1

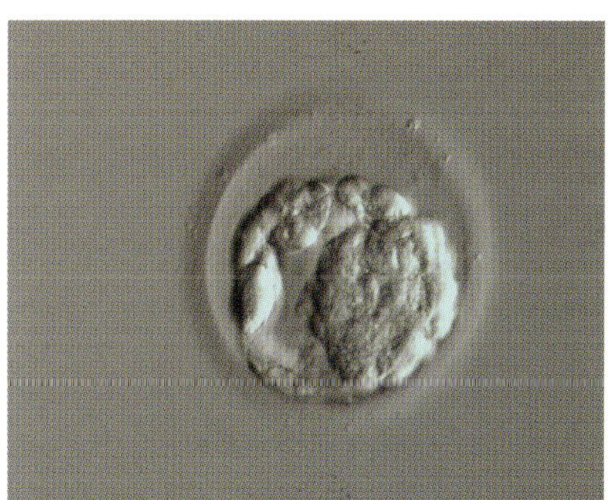

90-AW-2

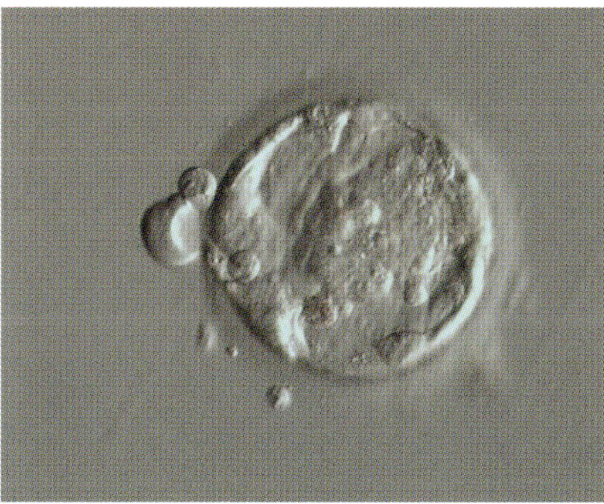

90-BT-1

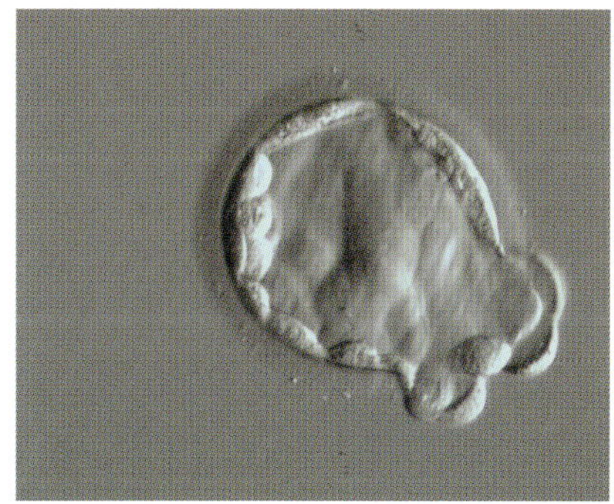

90-BT-2

90-BV-1 Blastocyst 4bb before vitrification, one necrotic cell at 2 o'clock, granular trophectoderm cells

90-BV-2 Before vitrification blastocyst 2bb with large cells visible in inner cell mass

90-AW-1 No contraction after warming

90-AW-2 Half contracted after warming

90-BT-1 Blastocyst re-expanded with granular trophectoderm cells, flat inner cell mas, blastocyst starting to hatch, one necrotic cell (already present before vitrification) at 7 o'clock

90-BT-2 Fully re-expanded blastocyst nicely hatching

Female partner

Age 36, illustrator
Tubal status: patent
MH: 28
BMI: 27.2
Previous surgeries: ovarectomy right in 1983 during appendicitis, plastic surgery of artificial cervix in 1993 due to cervical aplasia
Non-smoker, no alcohol consumption
TSH: 1.9 μU/mL

Basal FSH: 8.6 IU/L
Basal LH: 9.7 IU/L
Basal estradiol: 40 pg/mL
Midluteal progesterone: 1 ng/mL
Prolactin: 9.9 ng/mL

Male partner

Age 37, customer relationship manager
History/examination: NAD
BMI: 25.0
Normozoospermia
Non-smoker, no alcohol consumption

Previous treatments

2011	Intrauterine inseminations ×3 (external)	Not pregnant
2011	ICSI cycle ×1 (external)	Not pregnant
2011	Frozen/thawed cycle ×2 (external)	Not pregnant
2012	ICSI cycle ×1 (external)	Not pregnant
2012	Frozen/thawed cycle ×2 (external)	Not pregnant

Fresh cycle: 2013 IMSI

Semen assessment: normozoospermia

Volume	2.4 mL
Abstinence	2 days
Concentration	14×10^6/mL
Total sperm number	33.6×10^6/mL
Progressive motility	41%
Non-progressive motility	38%
Immotile	54%
Normal forms	9%
IMSI-Classification Class I/II/III	9%/47%/44%

Stimulation protocol and outcome

Stimulation protocol	Short protocol
Days of stimulation	9
Total dose	2700 IU
Number of follicles ≥ 12 mm	14
Total number of COCs	14
Metaphase II	9
Fertilization rate	67%
Cleavage rate	83%
Blastocyst rate	83%

Fresh transfer

Quality of embryo(s)	Blastocyst 5aa
Outcome	Not pregnant
Vitrification	3 blastocysts (day 5)

Vitrified/warmed cycle: 2013

Stimulation	Natural cycle
Endometrium	7.0 mm
Quality before vitrification	Blastocyst 2bb
Warming day	5
Survival	Yes
Assisted hatching	Thinning
Transfer day	5
Quality	Blastocyst 2bb
Duration of cryostorage	4 months
Time between warming and transfer	3 hours

Outcome: Live birth, healthy boy

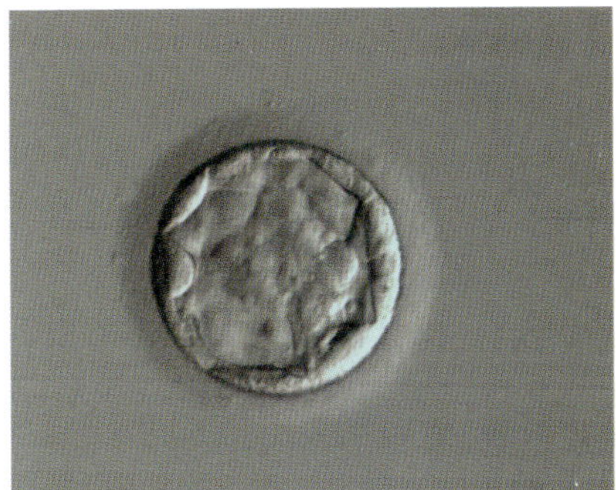

91-BV-1

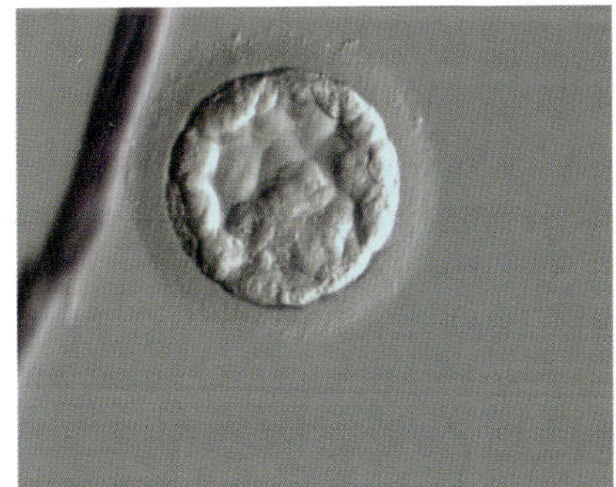

91-AW-1

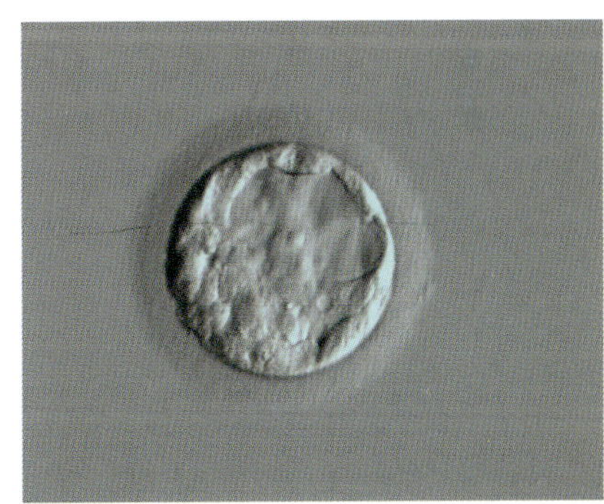

91-BT-1

91-BV-1 Before vitrification, notable a relatively thick ZP
91-AW-1 No contraction after warming, cells appear clear and viable
91-BT-1 Before embryo transfer full re-expansion, trophectoderm cells partly granular, some with vacuoles

Case 92

1 year 2° infertility   **Diagnosis: Endometriosis, male factor infertility**

Female partner

Age 38, restorer
Tubal status: patent
MH: 28
BMI: 24.2
Previous surgeries: cervical coni-
  zation in 1998, hysteroscopy
  because of endometriosis in
  2008
Non-smoker, no alcohol
  consumption
TSH: 0.9 µU/mL
Basal FSH: 8.1 IU/L

Basal LH: 2.2 IU/L
Basal estradiol: 42.5 pg/mL
AMH: 1.6 µg/L
Midluteal progesterone: 0.5 ng/mL
Prolactin: 156 ng/mL

Male partner

Age 44, librarian
History/examination: NAD
BMI: 25.2
Asthenoteratozoospermia
Smoker, no alcohol consumption
Karyogram without pathological
  findings for both partners

Previous treatments

2009	External ICSI/IMSI ×3	Not pregnant
2009	External frozen/thawed cycle	Not pregnant
2010	External ICSI/IMSI	Not pregnant
2010	External ICSI/IMSI	Gemini pregnancy with abortion in gestation week 17
2010	External frozen/thawed cycle	Not pregnant
2011	External ICSI/IMSI	Not pregnant
2011	External frozen/thawed cycle ×2	Not pregnant
2012	External ICSI/IMSI	Clinical pregnancy and curettage in gestation week 8

Fresh cycle: 2013 IMSI

Semen assessment: asthenoteratozoospermia

Volume	1.8 mL
Abstinence	1 day
Concentration	16×10^6/mL
Total sperm number	28.8×10^6/mL
Progressive motility	13%
Non-progressive motility	12%
Immotile	75%
Normal forms	1%
IMSI-Classification Class I/II/III	1%/40%/59%

Stimulation protocol and outcome

Stimulation protocol	Long protocol
Days of stimulation	12
Total dose	2850 IU
Number of follicles ≥ 12 mm	8
Total number of COCs	6

Metaphase II	3
Fertilization rate	100%
Cleavage rate	100%
Blastocyst rate	100%

Fresh transfer

Quality of embryo(s)	Blastocyst 4ab
Outcome	Biochemical pregnancy
Vitrification	2 blastocysts (day 5)

Vitrified/warmed cycle: 2013

Stimulation	Hormonal substitution protocol
Endometrium	14.0 mm
Quality before vitrification	Blastocyst 2bc
Warming day	5
Survival	Yes
Assisted hatching	Yes
Transfer day	5
Quality	Blastocyst 2bc
Duration of cryostorage	4 months
Time between warming and transfer	4 hours

Outcome: Live birth, healthy girl

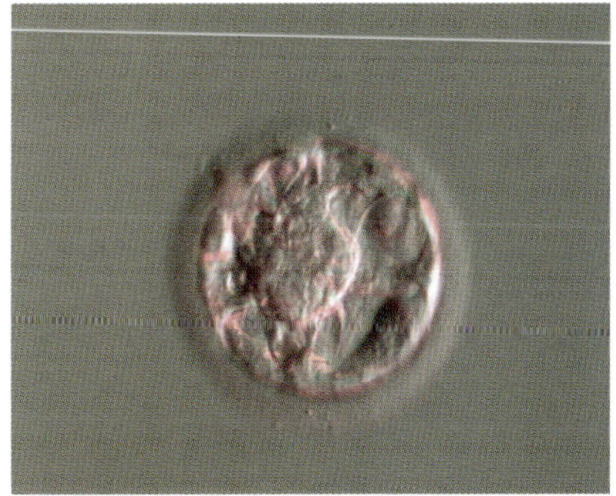
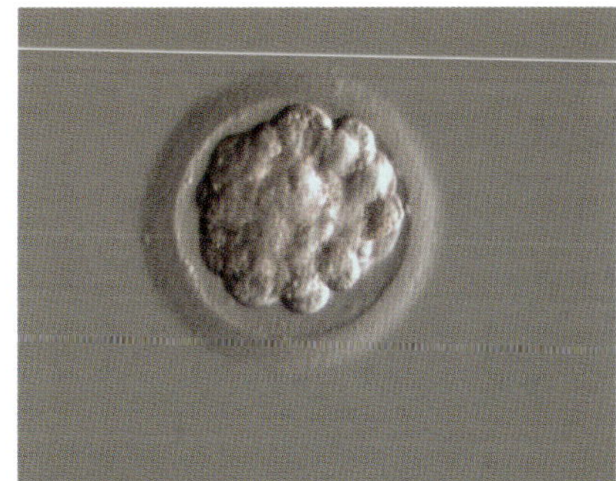
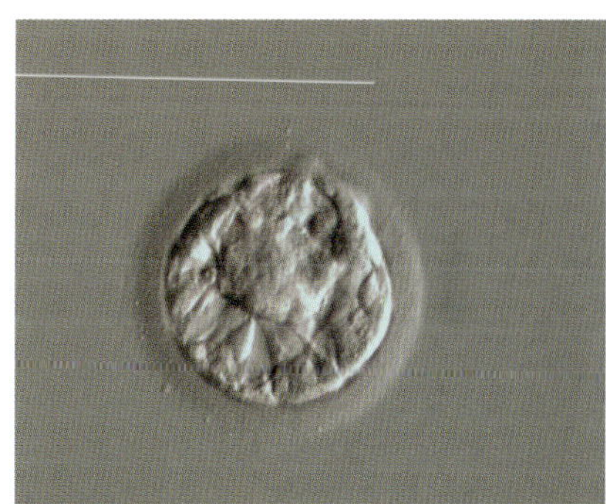

92-BV-1 **92-AW-1** **92-BT-1**

92-BV-1 Blastocyst with big, compact inner cell mass, several cytoplasmic strings between ICM and trophectoderm
92-AW-1 Contracted blastocyst, some trophectoderm cells appear granular with some small vacuoles
92-BT-1 Blastocyst resuming its initial appearance, no hatching yet

Female partner

Age 35, employee
Tubal status: patent
MH: oligomenorrhea
BMI: 23.2
Non-smoker, no alcohol
  consumption
TSH: 1.21 μU/mL

Basal FSH: 4.2 IU/L
Basal LH: 1.5 IU/L
Basal estradiol: 125 pg/mL
AMH: 0.9 μg/L
Midluteal progesterone: 1.1 ng/mL
Prolactin: 89 ng/mL

Male partner

Age 39, car mechanic
History/examination: NAD
BMI: 23.3
Teratozoospermia
Non-smoker, no alcohol consumption

Previous treatments

2010	Intrauterine inseminations ×3 (external)	Not pregnant
2011	ICSI cycle (external)	Not pregnant
2011	Frozen/thawed cycle ×2 (external)	Not pregnant
2012	ICSI cycle (external)	Twin pregnancy, early onset preeclampsia and cesarean section in gestation week 25, both children died postpartum
2013	Frozen/thawed cycle ×1 (external)	Not pregnant

Fresh cycle: 2013 IMSI
Semen assessment: teratozoospermia

Volume	1.4 mL
Abstinence	2 days
Concentration	22×10^6/mL
Total sperm number	30.8×10^6/mL
Progressive motility	27%
Non-progressive motility	46%
Immotile	27%
Normal forms	0%
IMSI-Classification	0%/42%/58%
Class I/II/III	

Stimulation protocol and outcome

Stimulation protocol	Antagonist
Days of stimulation	13
Total dose	2550 IU
Number of follicles ≥ 12 mm	27
Total number of COCs	23
Metaphase II	20
Fertilization rate	50%
Cleavage rate	100%
Blastocyst rate	40%

Fresh transfer

Quality of embryo(s)	Blastocyst 4aa
Outcome	Not pregnant
Vitrification	3 blastocysts (day 5)

Vitrified/warmed cycle: 2013

Stimulation	Hormonal substitution protocol
Endometrium	7.1 mm
Quality before vitrification	Blastocyst 4bb
Warming day	5
Survival	Yes
Assisted hatching	No
Transfer day	5
Quality	Blastocyst 4bb
Duration of cryostorage	10 months
Time between warming and transfer	2.5 hours

Outcome: Live birth, healthy girl

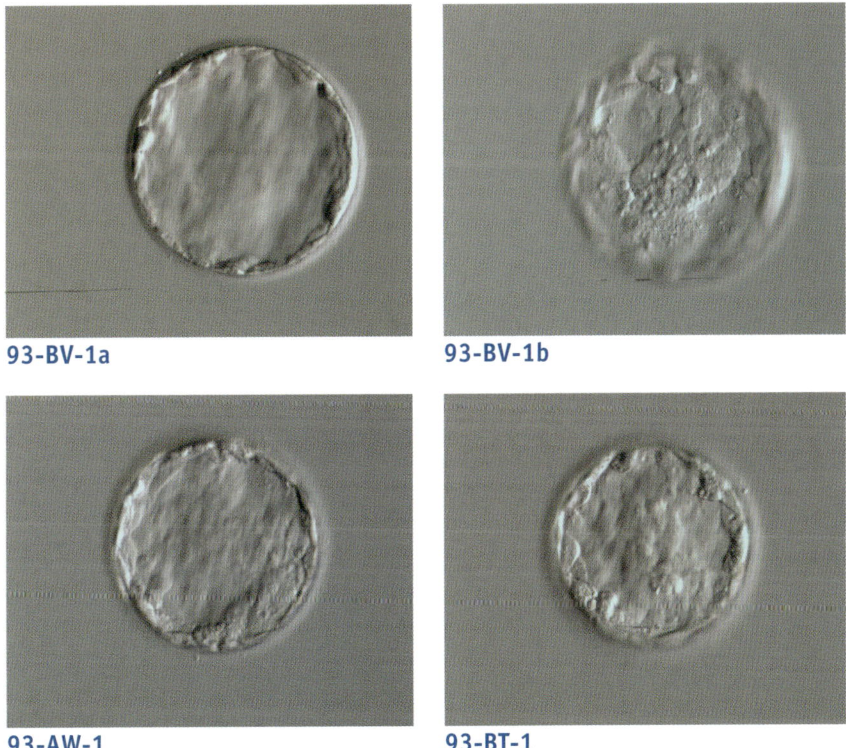

93-BV-1a

93-BV-1b

93-AW-1

93-BT-1

93-BV-1a   Expanded blastocyst with cohesive but slightly granular trophectoderm cells
93-BV-1b   The inner cell mass appears very flat
93-AW-1   Full re-expansion directly after warming
93-BT-1   Viable but granular trophectoderm and inner cell mass cells, blastocyst fully expanded

Female partner

Age 28, accountant
Tubal status: patent
MH: 27–35
BMI: 36.1
Previous surgeries: conization in 1998, hysteroscopy because of endometriosis in 2008
After OPU in 2013 three morphological abnormal oocytes with polyfragmentation and vacuolization
Non-smoker, no alcohol consumption

TSH: 1.1 µU/mL
Basal FSH: 4.5 IU/L
Basal LH: 0.7 IU/L
Basal estradiol: 15 pg/mL
Midluteal progesterone: 0.1 ng/mL
Prolactin: 12.4 ng/mL

Male partner

Age 30, controller
History/examination: NAD
BMI: 25.5
Oligoasthenoteratozoospermia
Non-smoker, no alcohol consumption

Previous treatments

2013   Vitrified/warmed cycle ×1   Not pregnant

Fresh cycle: 2013 IMSI
Semen assessment: oligoasthenoteratozoospermia

Volume	3 mL
Abstinence	1 day
Concentration	4.4×10^6/mL
Total sperm number	13.2×10^6/mL
Progressive motility	4%
Non-progressive motility	15%
Immotile	81%
Normal forms	0%
IMSI-Classification	0%/29%/71%
Class I/II/III	

Stimulation protocol and outcome

Stimulation protocol	Long protocol
Days of stimulation	12
Total dose	2475 IU
Number of follicles ≥ 12 mm	48
Total number of COCs	30
Metaphase II	17
Fertilization rate	82%
Cleavage rate	100%
Blastocyst rate	93%

Fresh transfer

Quality of embryo(s)	No fresh transfer because of OHSS
Vitrification	13 blastocysts (day 5)

Vitrified/warmed cycle: 2013

Stimulation	Hormonal substitution protocol
Endometrium	11.1 mm
Quality before vitrification	Blastocyst 4ab, blastocyst 4bb
Warming day	5
Survival	Yes/Yes
Assisted hatching	Yes/Yes
Transfer day	5
Quality	Blastocyst 4ab hatching, blastocyst 4bb hatching
Duration of cryostorage	6 months
Time between warming and transfer	3 hours

Outcome: After detection of 2 embryos with positive heart activity live birth of one healthy boy

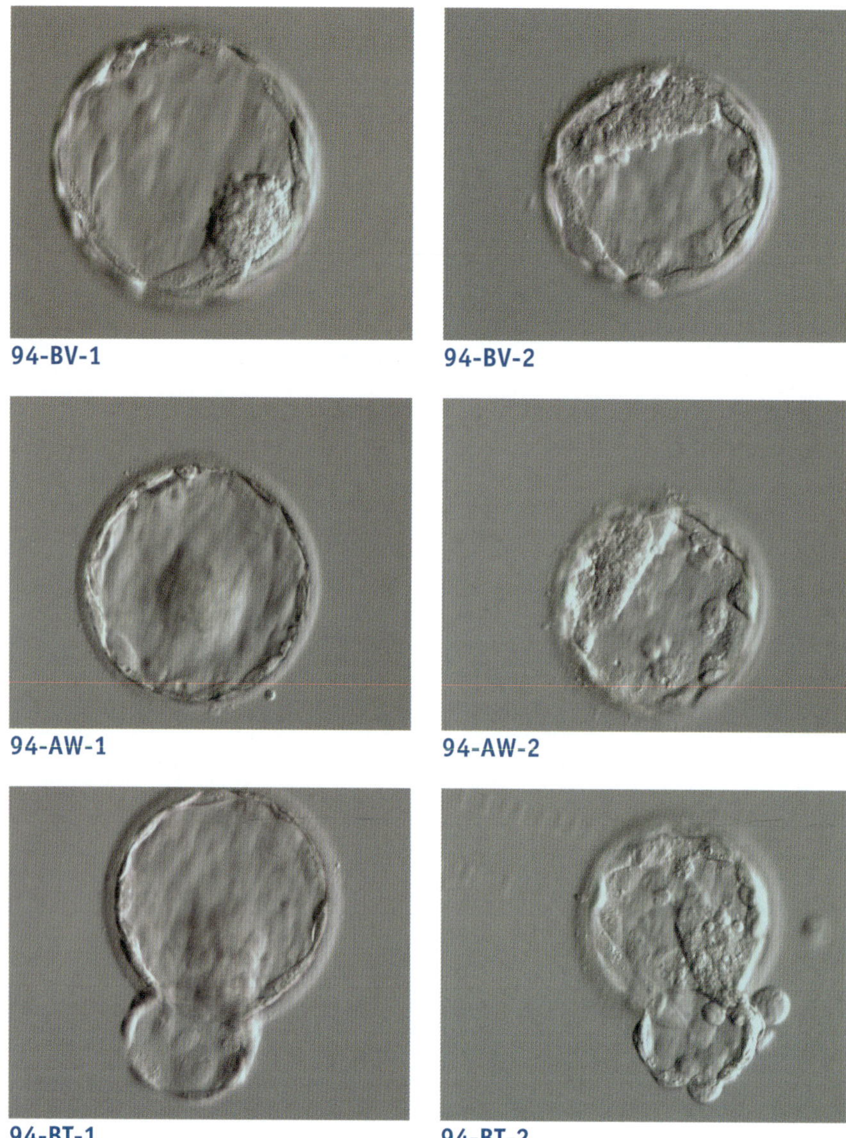

94-BV-1   94-BV-2

94-AW-1   94-AW-2

94-BT-1   94-BT-2

94-BV-1 Blastocyst 4ab before vitrification with nice clumped inner cell mass, slightly granular trophectoderm cells

94-BV-2 Blastocyst 4bb with elongated, flat inner cell mass, ICM and trophectoderm cells with granulation

94-AW-1 No contraction directly after warming, no degenerated cells (15 min later blastocyst contracted)

94-AW-2 No contraction directly after warming, no degenerated cells (15 min later blastocyst contracted)

94-BT-1 Blastocyst 4ab fully re-expanded and hatching

94-BT-2 Blastocyst 4bb fully re-expanded and starting to hatch with some loose fragments not integrated in blastocyst formation at 3 o'clock

2 years 2° infertility **Diagnosis: Tubal factor, endometriosis**

Female partner

Age 31, housewife
Tubal status: not patent
MH: 28
BMI: 19.4
Previous surgeries: laparoscopic hysteroscopy in 2008 and 2011 due to endometriosis
Non-smoker, no alcohol consumption
TSH: 0.9 µU/mL
Basal FSH: 5 IU/L
Basal LH: 2.3 IU/L
Basal estradiol: 100 pg/mL
Midluteal progesterone: 0.64 ng/mL

Male partner

Age 34, engineer
History/examination: NAD
BMI: 24.8
Normozoospermia
Non-smoker, no alcohol consumption

Previous treatments

2011   ICSI cycle ×1   Term birth of a healthy girl

Fresh cycle: 2013 IMSI
Semen assessment: normozoospermia (parvisemia)

Volume	1.2 mL
Abstinence	1 day
Concentration	23×10^6/mL
Total sperm number	27.6×10^6/mL
Progressive motility	69%
Non-progressive motility	13%
Immotile	18%
Normal forms	5%
IMSI-Classification	5%/52%/43%
Class I/II/III	

Stimulation protocol and outcome

Stimulation protocol	Long protocol
Days of stimulation	12
Total dose	1140 IU
Number of follicles ≥ 12 mm	21
Total number of COCs	15
Metaphase II	5
Fertilization rate	100%
Cleavage rate	100%
Blastocyst rate	60%

Fresh transfer

Quality of embryo(s)	Blastocyst 4aa
Outcome	Not pregnant
Vitrification	2 blastocysts (day 5)

Vitrified/warmed cycle: 2013

Stimulation	Hormonal substitution protocol
Endometrium	9.2 mm
Quality before vitrification	Blastocyst 2cb, blastocyst 3bb contracted
Warming day	5
Survival	Yes/Yes
Assisted hatching	Yes/Yes
Transfer day	5
Quality	Blastocyst 2cb hatching, blastocyst 3bc hatching
Duration of cryostorage	3 months
Time between warming and transfer	3.3 hours

Outcome: Live birth of a healthy twin pair (one girl and one boy)

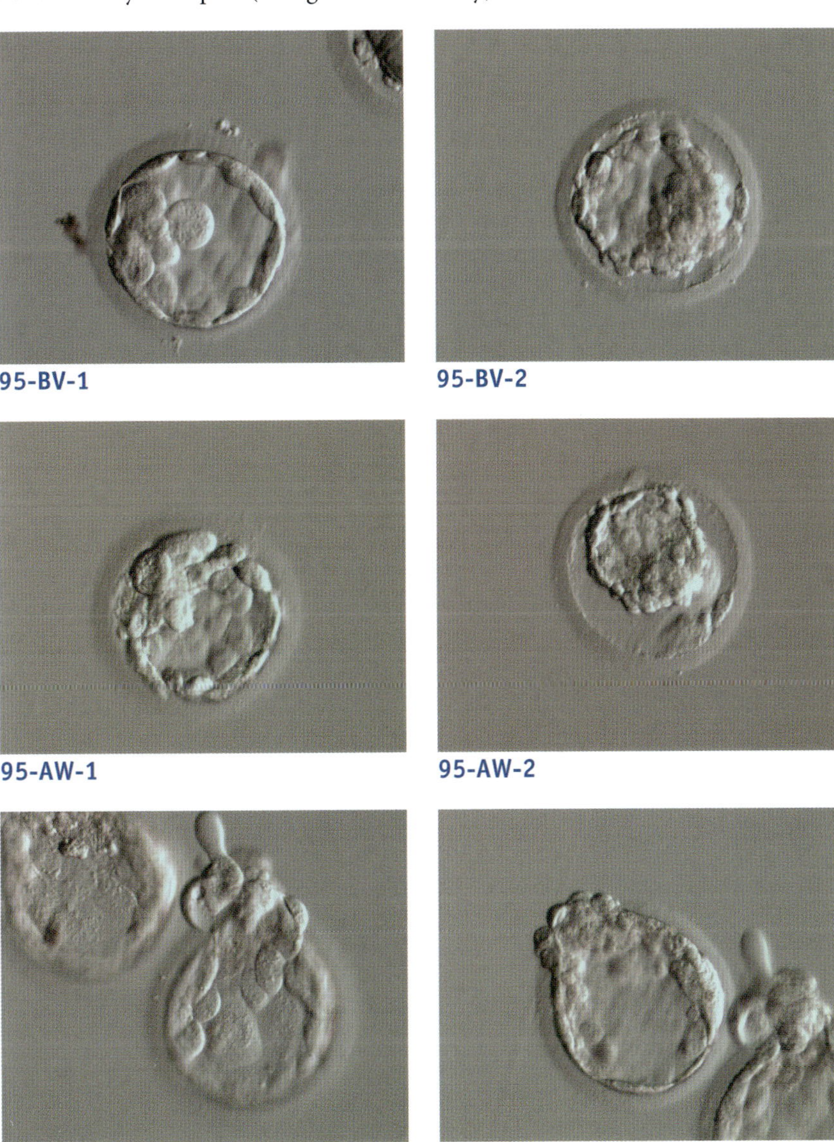

95-BV-1

95-BV-2

95-AW-1

95-AW-2

95-BT-1

95-BT-2

95-BV-1   Blastocyst 2cb before vitrification, no defined inner cell mass visible, instead large blastomeres in blastocoel with apparent granulation in trophectoderm

95-BV-2   Contracted blastocyst before vitrification, cells appear dark granular

95-AW-1   After warming poor contraction of the blastocyst, excluded fragments in perivitelline space between 9 and 12 o'clock

95-AW-2   Blastocyst contracted 50% directly after sucrose solutions

95-BT-1   After 3 hours fully expanded and hatching blastocyst

95-BT-2   Full re-expansion of blastocyst before embryo transfer, trophectoderm and inner cell mass cells with strong, dark granulation

Case 96

2 years 1° infertility   Diagnosis: PCOS

Female partner

Age 34, medical doctor
Tubal status: patent
MH: severe oligomenorrhea
BMI: 18.3
PCOS
Reduced fertilization rate after IVF (external cycles)
Non-smoker, no alcohol abuse
Basal FSH: 6.1 IU/L
Basal LH: 13.7 IU/L
Basal estradiol: 82 pg/mL
Prolactin: 22.7 ng/mL
Midluteal progesterone: 1.2 ng/mL

Male partner

Age 40, medical doctor
History/examination: NAD
BMI: 27.6
Normozoospermia
Smoker, no alcohol abuse

Previous treatments

2012	Timed intercourse ×3 (external)	Not pregnant (×3)
2013	IVF-cycle ×2 (external) fertilization rate 30%	Not pregnant (×2)

Fresh cycle: 2013 IMSI, AOA
Semen assessment: normozoospermia

Volume	1.8 mL
Abstinence	2 days
Concentration	82×10^6/mL
Total sperm number	147.6×10^6/mL
Progressive motility	40%
Non-progressive motility	40%
Immotile	20%
Normal forms	15%
IMSI-Classification Class I/II/III	15%/41%/55%

Stimulation protocol and outcome

Stimulation protocol	Long protocol
Days of stimulation	10
Total dose	1500 IU
Number of follicles ≥ 12 mm	25
Total number of COCs	25
Metaphase II	21
Fertilization rate	86%
Cleavage rate	100%
Blastocyst rate	100%

Fresh transfer

Quality of embryo(s)	No fresh transfer because of OHSS
Vitrification	11 blastocysts day 5
	7 blastocysts day 6

Vitrified/warmed cycle: 2013

Stimulation	Hormonal substitution protocol
Endometrium	5.8 mm
Quality before vitrification	Blastocyst 4bb
Warming day	5
Survival	Yes
Assisted hatching	No
Transfer day	5
Quality	Blastocyst 4bb
Duration of cryostorage	1 month
Time between warming and transfer	2.5 hours

Outcome: Live birth, healthy girl

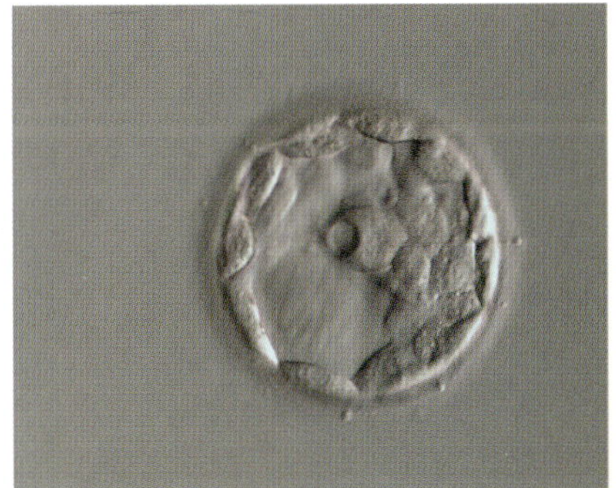

96-BV-1

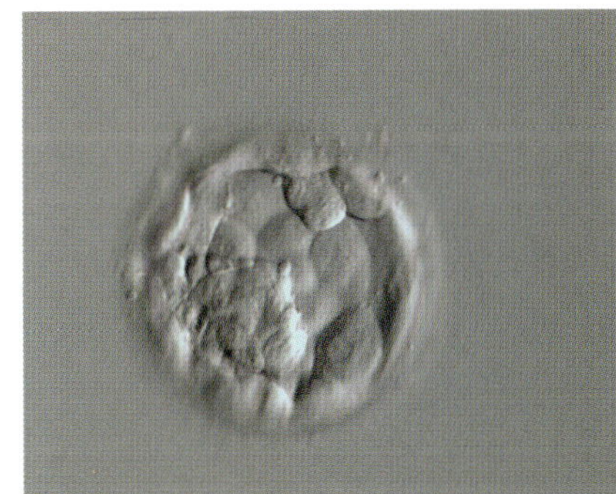

96-AW-1

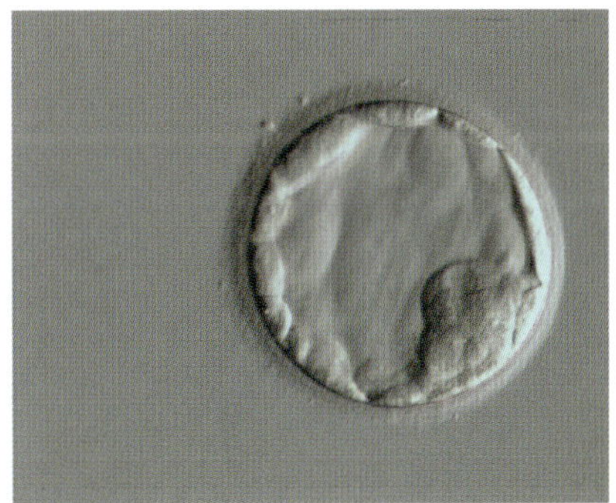

96-BT-1

96-BV-1 Expanded blastocyst with high inner cell mass, peak cell with a vacuole
96-AW-1 Full re-expansion after exposure to sucrose solution
96-BT-1 Cells clear and viable before transfer

Female partner

Age 31, vendor
Tubal status: patent
MH: 28–33
BMI: 27.2
Previous surgeries: cervical conization in 1998,
    hysteroscopy because of endometriosis in 2008
Abortion/Deliveries:
Spontaneous conceptions and birth of two healthy girls in
    2004 and 2009
Spontaneous abortion in 2007
All in previous relationship
Non-smoker, no alcohol consumption
TSH: 1.1 µU/mL
Basal FSH: 7.1 IU/L
Basal LH: 4.0 IU/L
Basal estradiol: 45 pg/mL
Midluteal progesterone: 0.5 ng/mL
Prolactin: 7.2 ng/mL

Male partner

Age 49, employee
History/examination: vasectomy in 2001
BMI: 26.6
Obstructive azoospermia after vasectomy
Smoker, no alcohol consumption
One son from previous relationship born 1993

Previous treatments

None

Fresh cycle: 2013 ICSI with TESE sperm
Semen assessment: fresh TESE tissue

TESE report: After dilation of tubuli several motile spermatozoa detected, after preparation
               of tissue selection of sperm with moderate morphology for injection

Stimulation protocol and outcome

Stimulation protocol	Long protocol
Days of stimulation	11
Total dose	2475 IU
Number of follicles ≥ 12 mm	31
Total number of COCs	15
Metaphase II	14
Fertilization rate	64%
Cleavage rate	100%
Blastocyst rate	67%

Fresh transfer

Quality of embryo(s)	No fresh transfer because of OHSS
Vitrification	6 blastocysts (day 5)

Vitrified/warmed cycle: 2013

Stimulation	Hormonal substitution protocol
Endometrium	10.0 mm
Quality before vitrification	Blastocyst 4bb
Warming day	5
Survival	Yes
Assisted hatching	Yes
Transfer day	5
Quality	Blastocyst 4bb hatching
Duration of cryostorage	4 months
Time between warming and transfer	4 hours

Outcome: Live birth, healthy girl

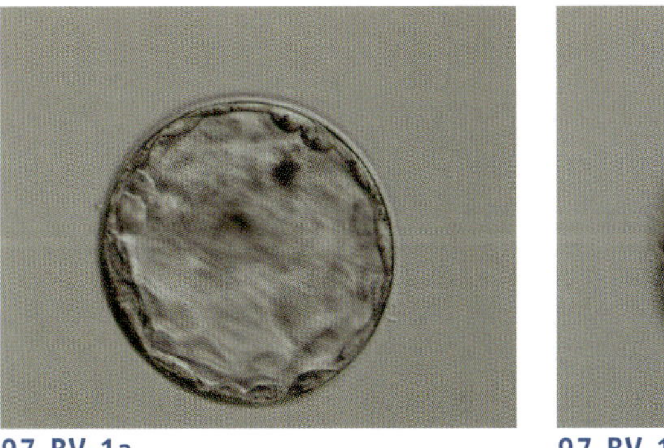

97-BV-1a

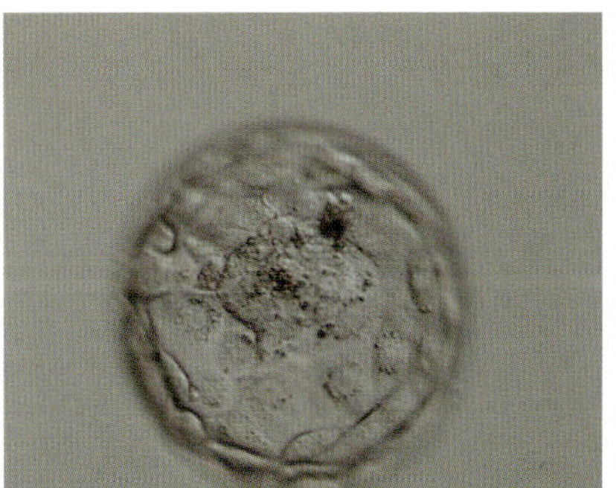

97-BV-1b

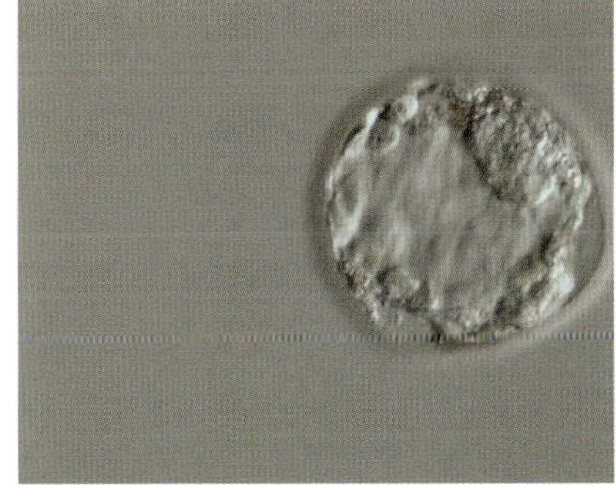

97-AW-1a

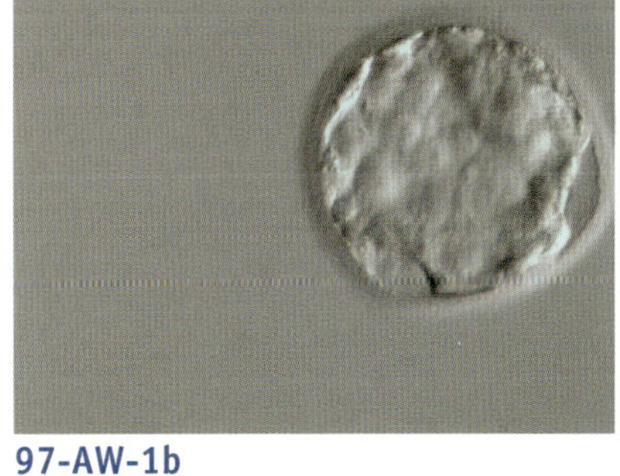

97-AW-1b

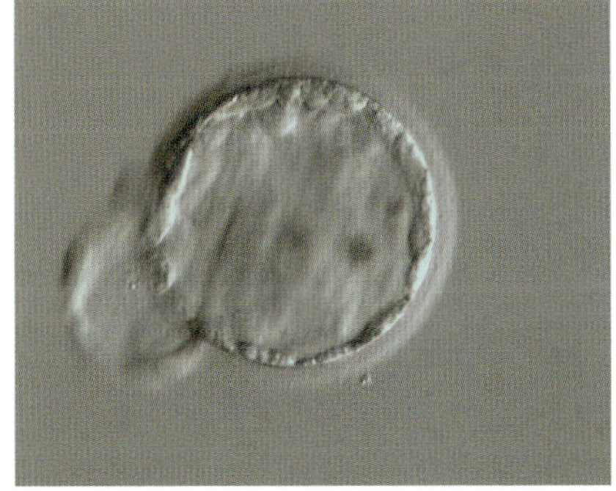

97-BT-1a

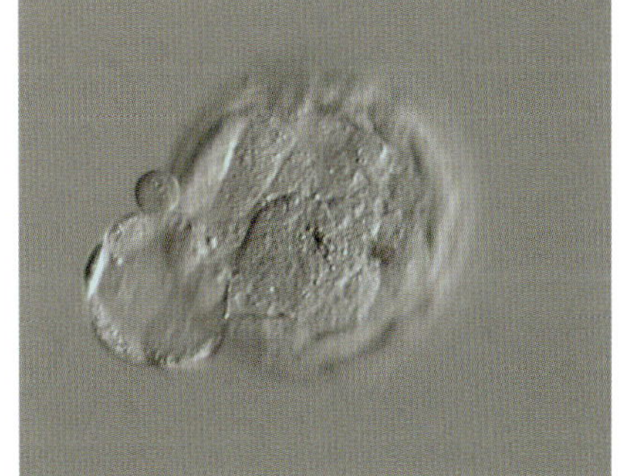

97-BT-1b

97-BV-1a	Coherent trophectoderm
97-BV-1b	Inner cell mass compact and well defined, some dark granulation on the surface
97-AW-1a	Poor contraction after warming, granular appearance of cells
97-AW-1b	Depressions in ZP
97-BT-1a	Full re-expansion, trophectoderm coherent and starting to hatch
97-BT-1b	Inner cell mass compact and clear

Female partner

Age 38, employee

Tubal status: patent

MH: 28

BMI: 23.4

Previous surgeries: laparoscopic hysteroscopy due to uterine polyps and endometriosis in 2010 and 2011

Non-smoker, no alcohol consumption

TSH: 1.32 μU/mL

Basal FSH: 6.6 IU/L

Basal LH: 3.1 IU/L

Basal estradiol: 146 pg/mL

AMH: 0.9 μg/L

Prolactin: 137 ng/mL

Male partner

Age 41, teacher

History/examination: orchidopexy age 5

BMI: 26.1

Teratozoospermia

Non-smoker, occasional alcohol consumption

Previous treatments

2011–2012	Intrauterine insemination ×6 (external)	Not pregnant
2012	ICSI cycle ×1 (external)	Not pregnant
2012	Frozen/thawed cycle ×1 (external)	Not pregnant
2013	ICSI cycle ×1 (external)	Not pregnant
2013	Frozen/thawed cycle ×2 (external)	Not pregnant

Fresh cycle: 2013 IMSI

Semen assessment: teratozoospermia

Volume	1.8 mL
Abstinence	1 day
Concentration	22×10^6/mL
Total sperm number	39.6×10^6/mL
Progressive motility	50%
Non-progressive motility	14%
Immotile	36%
Normal forms	3%
IMSI-Classification	3%/34%/63%
Class I/II/III	

Stimulation protocol and outcome

Stimulation protocol	Long protocol
Days of stimulation	1
Total dose	2700 IU
Number of follicles ≥ 12 mm	9
Total number of COCs	9
Metaphase II	7
Fertilization rate	71%
Cleavage rate	100%
Blastocyst rate	40%

Fresh transfer

Quality of embryo(s)	No fresh ET due to hypertrophic and already transformed endometrial lining
Vitrification	2 blastocysts (day 5)

Vitrified/warmed cycle: 2013

Stimulation	Hormonal substitution protocol
Endometrium	11.0 mm
Quality before vitrification	Blastocyst 2bb, early blastocyst (b)
Warming day	5
Survival	Yes/Yes
Assisted hatching	No/Yes
Transfer day	5
Quality	Blastocyst 3bb, early blastocyst grade (d)
Duration of cryostorage	3 months
Time between warming and transfer	3 hours

Outcome: Live birth, healthy twin pair (one girl and one boy)

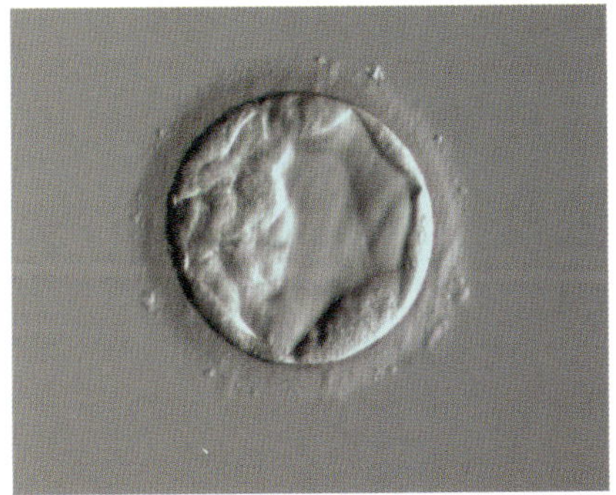

98-BV-1

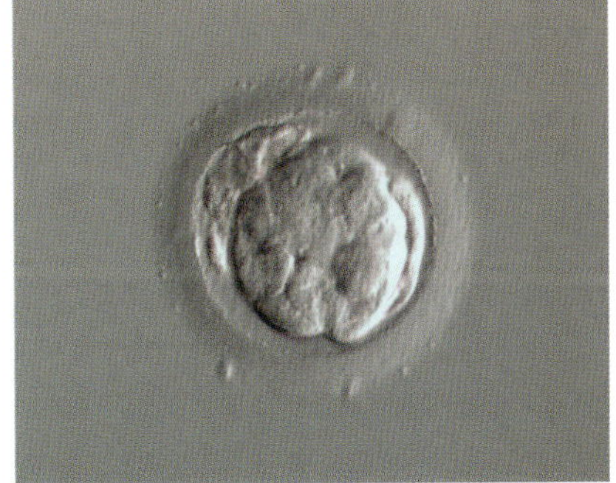

98-BV-2

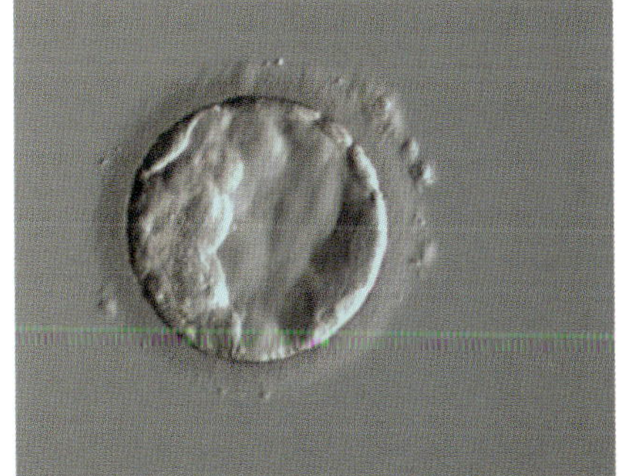

98-AW-1

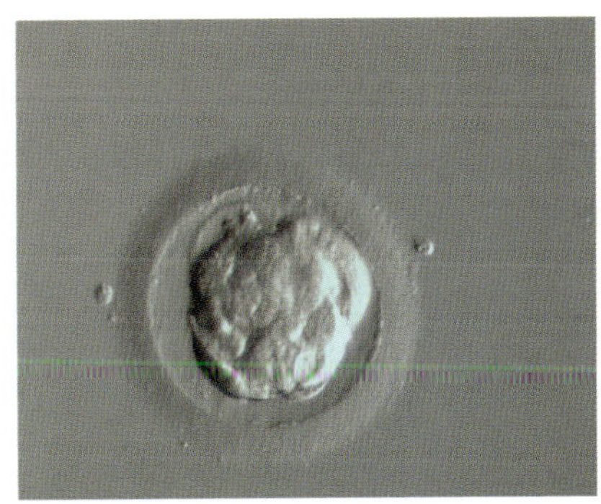

98-AW-2

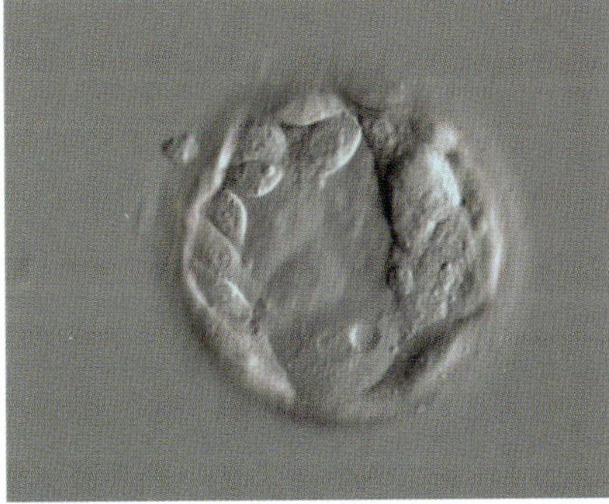

98-BT-1

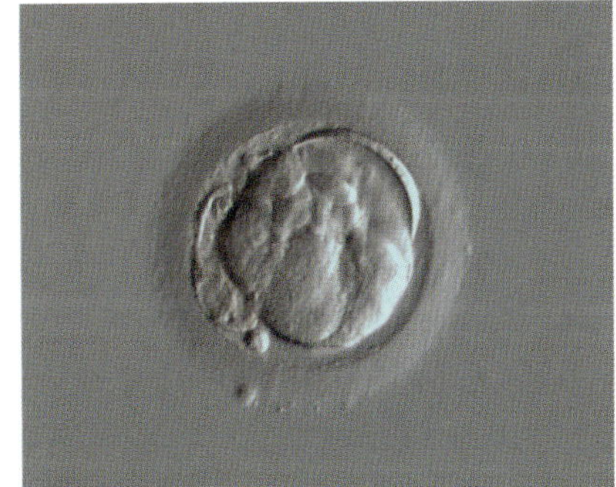

98-BT-2

98-BV-1	Blastocyst 2bb with defined inner cell mass and long, ellipsoid cells in trophectoderm
98-BV-2	Early blastocyst slightly contracted with degenerated excluded fragments between 9 and 12 o'clock position and thick zona pellucida
98-AW-1	Fully expanded blastocyst after warming
98-AW-2	Early blastocyst 40% contracted after warming
98-BT-1	Blastocyst further expanding with clear viable cells in inner cell mass and trophectoderm
98-BT-2	Early blastocyst in re-expansion, one trophectoderm cell starting to blow up

Case 99

1 year 2° infertility

Diagnosis: Tubal factor, uterus anomaly, male factor infertility

Female partner

Age 35, business economist
Tubal status: not patent
MH: 28–30
BMI: 22.4
Previous surgeries:
  salpingectomy after
  ectopic pregancy in 2012
Uterus arcuatus and
  myomatosus
Hashimoto's thyroiditis

Non-smoker, no alcohol
  consumption
TSH: 0.9 μU/mL
Basal FSH: 4.2 IU/L
Basal LH: 4.9 IU/L
Basal estradiol: 72 pg/mL
Midluteal progesterone: 5.4 ng/mL
Prolactin: 19.1 ng/mL

Male partner

Age 44, plumber
History/examination: NAD
BMI: 26.9
Teratozoospermia
Smoker, no alcohol consumption

Previous treatments

2012	ICSI cycle ×1 (external)	Not pregnant
2012	ICSI cycle ×1 (external)	Ectopic pregnancy with salpingectomy
2012	Frozen/thawed cycle ×2 (external)	Not pregnant

Fresh cycle: 2013 IMSI

Semen assessment: teratozoospermia

Volume	2.0 mL
Abstinence	1 day
Concentration	24×10^6/mL
Total sperm number	48×10^6/mL
Progressive motility	66%
Non-progressive motility	5%
Immotile	29%
Normal forms	1%
IMSI-Classification	1%/35%/64%
Class I/II/III	

Stimulation protocol and outcome

Stimulation protocol	Long protocol
Days of stimulation	11
Total dose	1800 IU
Number of follicles ≥ 12 mm	7
Total number of COCs	20
Metaphase II	19
Fertilization rate	68%
Cleavage rate	100%
Blastocyst rate	77%

Fresh transfer

Quality of embryo(s)	No fresh transfer because of OHSS
Vitrification	10 blastocysts (day 5)

Vitrified/warmed cycle: 2013

Stimulation	Hormonal substitution protocol
Endometrium	6.3 mm
Quality before vitrification	Blastocyst 4bc, blastocyst 2bc
Warming day	5
Survival	Yes/Yes
Assisted hatching	Yes/Yes
Transfer day	5
Quality	Blastocyst 3cc, blastocyst 2bc
Duration of cryostorage	2 months
Time between warming and transfer	3 hours

Outcome: Triplet pregnancy, loss of one embryo after positive heart activity, birth of monozygotic twins gestation week 36 (healthy girls)

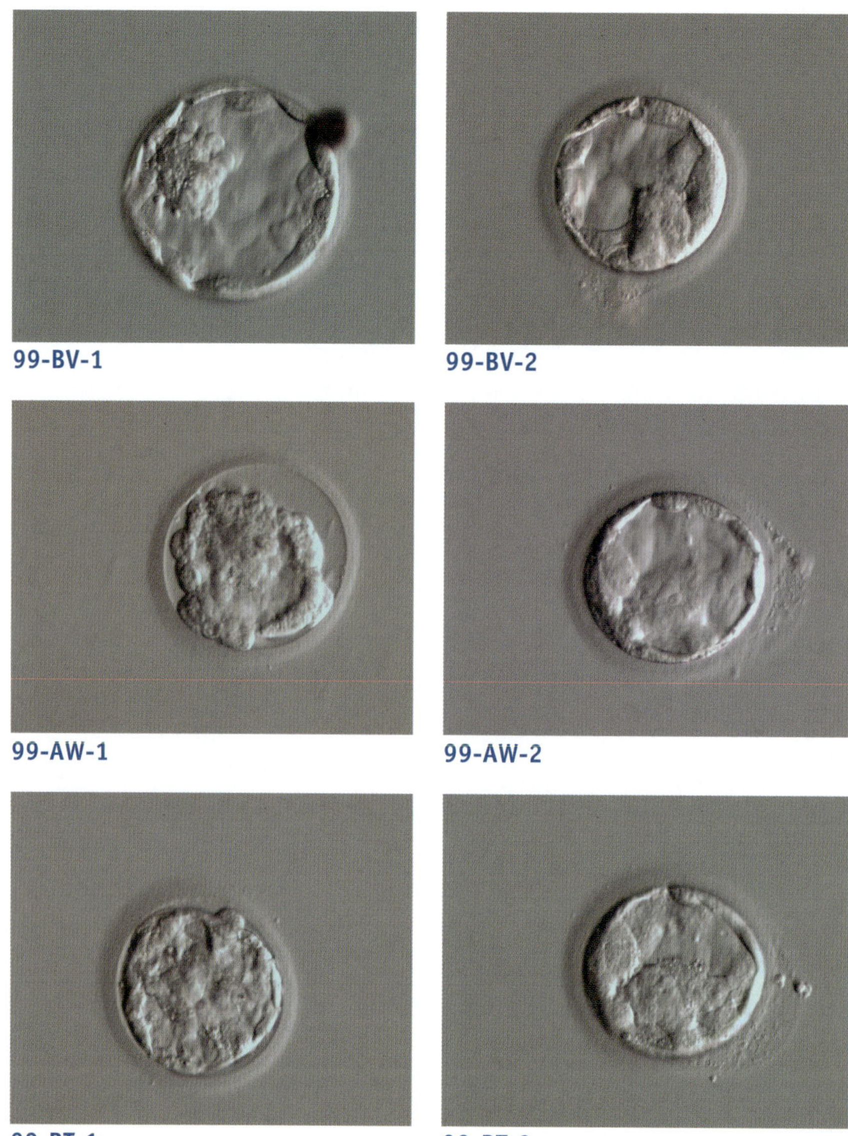

99-BV-1 99-BV-2

99-AW-1 99-AW-2

99-BT-1 99-BT-2

199-BV-1 Blastocyst 4bc, inner cell mass compact but with loose fragments on surface, trophectoderm with few ellipsoid cells (dark black spot on 2o'clock is artefact)

99-BV-2 Blastocyst 2bc with flat inner cell mass and few trophectoderm cells, abnormal shape of zona pellucida at 7 o'clock position

99-AW-1 After sucrose solutions 30% contracted blastocyst with dark, strongly granulated cells

99-AW-2 Blastocyst 2bc with no apparent contraction directly after warming

99-BT-1 Blastocyst appears severely stressed, re-expanded but not fully yet, one excluded fragment at 1 o'clock visible in peri-vitelline space, all cells with strong granulation and some with vacuoles (e.g. 6 o'clock), inner cell mass not visible

99-BT-2 Blastocyst still fully expanded, cells in inner cell mass and trophectoderm clear and viable

Case 100

3 years 2° infertility   **Diagnosis: Male factor infertility, recurrent pregnancy loss**

Female partner

Age 35, economist

Tubal status: patent

MH: 28

BMI: 25.5

Previous surgeries: curettage after missed abortion in 2013

Abortions/deliveries:

2011 spontaneous pregnancy and abortion in gestation week 9

2012 spontaneous pregnancy and abortion in gestation week 13, Turner syndrome with hydrops fetalis

Non-smoker, no alcohol consumption

TSH: 0.81 µU/mL

Basal FSH: 8.8 IU/L

Basal LH: 3.6 IU/L

Midluteal progesterone: 19.7 ng/mL

Prolactin: 13 ng/mL

Male partner

Age 36, engineer

History/examination: NAD

BMI: 22.3

Oligozoospermia

Non-smoker, no alcohol consumption

Karyogram without pathological findings for both partners

Previous treatments

None

Fresh cycle: 2013 IMSI

Semen assessment: oligozoospermia, parvisemia

Volume	0.8 mL
Abstinence	0 day
Concentration	12×10^6/mL
Total sperm number	9.6×10^6/mL
Progressive motility	43%
Non-progressive motility	7%
Immotile	50%
Normal forms	6%
IMSI-Classification	6%/37%/57%
Class I/II/III	

Stimulation protocol and outcome

Stimulation protocol	Long protocol
Days of stimulation	10
Total dose	2400 IU
Number of follicles $\geq$ 12 mm	11
Total number of COCs	8
Metaphase II	5
Fertilization rate	80%
Cleavage rate	100%
Blastocyst rate	75%

Fresh transfer

Quality of embryo(s)	Blastocyst 4aa
Outcome	Not pregnant
Vitrification	2 blastocysts (day 5)

Vitrified/warmed cycle: 2013

Stimulation	Hormonal substitution protocol
Endometrium	14.0 mm
Quality before vitrification	Blastocyst 5bb, blastocyst 4bb
Warming day	5
Survival	Yes/Yes
Assisted hatching	No/Yes
Transfer day	5
Quality	Blastocyst 5bb, blastocyst 4bb
Duration of cryostorage	5 months
Time between warming and transfer	3 hours

Outcome: Live birth, healthy girl

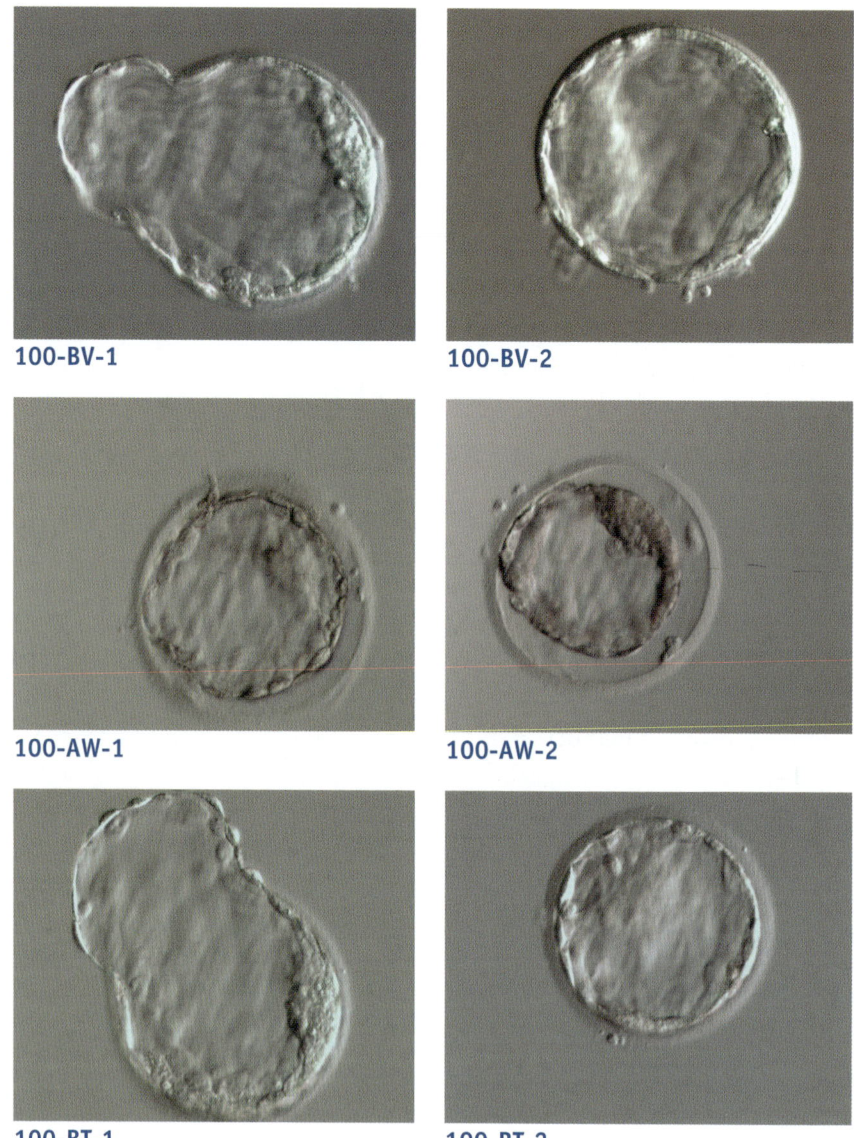

100-BV-1

100-BV-2

100-AW-1

100-AW-2

100-BT-1

100-BT-2

100-BV-1 Hatching blastocyst with flat inner cell mass at 2 o'clock and some loose fragments around ICM

100-BV-2 Fully expanded blastocyst with large, compact but flat inner cell mass at the left side

100-AW-1 After warming blastocyst pulled back in contraction its ZP

100-AW-2 40% contraction directly after exposure to sucrose solutions

100-BT-1 Full re-expansion and hatching blastocyst, cells clear and viable

100-BT-2 Re-expansion but not yet thinning of ZP before embryo transfer, cells appear granular

INDEX